The Unofficial Guide to ECGs

The Unofficial Guide to ECGs

Series Editor

Zeshan Qureshi, BM, BSc (Hons), MSc, MRCPCH, FAcadMEd, MRCPS(Glasg)
Paediatric Registrar
London Deanery
United Kingdom

Edited by

Ali B.A.K. Al-Hadithi, MB BChir, MA(Cantab), MRCP(UK), AFHEA, PGCert (Med Ed)
Academic Clinical Fellow (Cardiology and Internal Medicine)
University of Cambridge;
Cambridge University Hospitals NHS Trust
United Kingdom

Associate Editors

Alex R Hobson, MBBS, BSc (Hons), MD (Res), FRCP
Department of Cardiology
Portsmouth University Hospitals NHS Trust;
British Cardiovascular Intervention Society
United Kingdom

Senthil Kirubakaran, MD, FRCP, FHRS
Portsmouth University Hospitals NHS Trust
United Kingdom

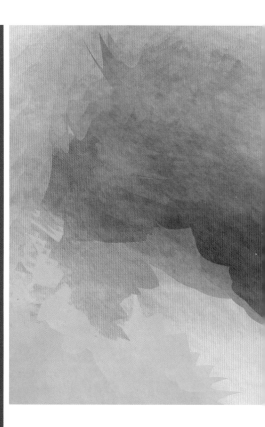

ELSEVIER

Notices

Practitioners and researchers must always rely on their own experience and knowledge in evaluating and using any information, methods, compounds or experiments described herein. Because of rapid advances in the medical sciences, in particular, independent verification of diagnoses and drug dosages should be made. To the fullest extent of the law, no responsibility is assumed by Elsevier, authors, editors or contributors for any injury and/or damage to persons or property as a matter of products liability, negligence or otherwise, or from any use or operation of any methods, products, instructions, or ideas contained in the material herein.

ISBN: 978-0-323-93189-2

Content Strategist: Jeremy Bowes
Content Project Manager: Shubham Dixit
Design: Miles Hitchen
Illustration Manager: Akshaya Mohan
Marketing Manager: Deborah Watkins

Printed in India by Replika Press Pvt. Ltd.

Last digit is the print number: 9   8   7   6   5   4   3   2   1

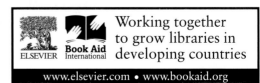

This book is dedicated to Bara, Suhair, Ahmed and Miriam for their continuous support.

Series Editor Foreword

The Unofficial Guide to Medicine is not just about helping students study, it is also about allowing those that learn to take back control of their own education. Since its inception, it has been driven by the voices of students, and through this, democratised the process of medical education, blurring the line between learners and teachers.

Medical education is an evolving process, and the latest iteration of our titles has been rewritten to bring them up to date with modern curriculums, after extensive deliberation and consultation. We have kept the series up to date, incorporating new guidelines and perspectives from a wide range of students, junior doctors, and senior clinicians. There is greater consistency across the titles, more illustrations, and through these and other changes, I hope the books will now be even better study aids.

These books though are a process of continual improvement. By reading this book, I hope that you not only get through your exams but also consider contributing to a future edition. You may be a student now, but you are also the future of medical education.

I wish you all the best with your future career and any upcoming exams.

Zeshan Qureshi
November 2022

Introduction

Despite its widespread use in clinical practice, ECG interpretation presents a challenge at all stages of training. Indeed, the median accuracy of interpretation across all training levels is less than 60% and even cardiologists have an accuracy of approximately 75%.

The Unofficial Guide to ECGs aims to address these difficulties by providing a foundation on what is needed to interpret ECGs, including their underlying electrophysiology, anatomy, pathophysiology and diagnostic reasoning. While these are the pillars that support the analytic skills required for ECG interpretation, these alone would not be sufficient for becoming skilled in the subject – an application of this knowledge to real-life scenarios is essential to mastering this crucial skill. Therefore, the latter half of the book is designed to allow the reader to apply what they learnt to real-life ECG cases, each with their own annotations and full explanations of the diagnosis and further management plans.

The book starts by building a solid framework on the essential basics of interpretation. The introductory chapter is dedicated to the foundations of ECGs – their purpose, practicalities of recording, electrophysiology of the heart and how this relates to the tracings recorded. The first half of the book is structured according to the individual components of ECG tracings and their interpretation, including their definitions, electrophysiology and variations. These are then elaborated upon with the relevant pathologies to look for in each part of the ECG tracing, including their clinical significance. Every chapter ends with a 'Key Points' box that summarises and provides reminders of the pertinent ECG features to look for at each stage.

Chapter 11 shifts focus towards applying the learnt information to clinical cases. 40 clinical scenarios with real ECGs are provided alongside 120 multiple-choice questions. ECGs range in difficulty from plain normal ECGs up to rarely seen pathologies, such as digoxin toxicity, that allow readers from all abilities to test their learning. In the answers section, every ECG is annotated and described with an ideal interpretation answer that explains each ECG feature. Every MCQ option, be it correct or incorrect, has an explanation as to the rationale for the answer.

Written by recently qualified junior doctors with review by senior clinicians, we have ensured that the book is accessible to complete newcomers to ECGs as well as offering a key revision tool for those that are more familiar with the subject. Through reading this book, we hope you will become more confident and competent in interpreting ECGs, both in exams and in clinical practice.

We are grateful to all those who have helped us throughout the process of producing this book, including our families, friends, colleagues and students, without whom this would not have been possible.

Ali B.A.K. Al-Hadithi
November 2022

Contributors

Alistair Roddick, MBBS, BSc
Oxford University Hospitals NHS
Foundation Trust
United Kingdom

Chung Shen Chean, MBChB, PGCe (Med Ed)
University Hospitals of Leicester NHS Trust
United Kingdom

Hugh Johnson, BA (Hons), BMBCh
Queen Charlotte's and Chelsea Hospital
United Kingdom

Wayne Swann, BSc (Hons), DipHE, ALNP
Broomwell Healthwatch, Manchester
School of Medicine & Dentistry
University of Central Lancashire
United Kingdom

Contents

1 ECG Basics, 1

What are ECGS?, 1
The Utility of ECGS, 1
Normal Pacemakers and Heart Conduction, 1
  Cardiac Anatomy, 1
  Electrical Conduction, 1
ECG Paper Basics, 2
ECG of a Single Heart Beat, 2
Electrode Placement, 3
Leads and the 12-Lead ECG, 3
  Leads and their anatomical correlation, 4
Types of ECG Recordings, 4
  12-Lead ECG, 4
  Three-Lead ECG, 5
  Holter or Ambulatory ECG Monitoring, 5
  Implantable Loop Recorder, 5
  Exercise ECG, 8
  Smartphone Apps, 11
Presenting an ECG, 11

2 Rate and Rhythm, 13

Overview, 13
  Definition, 13
Normal Variants, 15
  Sinus Arrhythmia, 15
Regular Narrow-Complex Tachycardia, 15
  Sinus Tachycardia, 17
  Atrial Tachycardia, 17
  Atrial Flutter, 19
  Atrioventricular Nodal Re-Entrant Tachycardia, 19
  Atrioventricular Re-Entrant Tachycardia, 20
Irregular Narrow-Complex Tachycardia, 21
  Atrial Fibrillation, 21
Regular Broad-Complex Tachycardia, 22
  Ventricular Tachycardia, 23
Irregular Broad-Complex Tachycardia, 25
  Ventricular Fibrillation, 25
  Torsades De Pointes Ventricular Tachycardia, 26
Bradycardias, 26
  Sinus Bradycardia, 27
  Sinus Node Disease, 29
  Escape Rhythms, 30
Ectopic Beats, 31

3 The Cardiac Axis, 34

Overview, 34
  Definition, 34
  Electrophysiology, 34
  Interpretation, 34

Axis Deviation, 38
  Left-Axis Deviation, 38
  Right-Axis Deviation, 38
  Extreme Axis Deviation, 39

4 P Wave, 41

Overview, 41
  Definition, 41
  Electrophysiology, 41
  Interpretation, 41

5 PR Segment, 46

Overview, 46
  Definition, 46
  Electrophysiology, 46
  Interpretation, 46
Atrioventricular Block, 46
  Definition, 46
  Classification, 47
First-Degree Heart Block, 47
  ECG Findings, 47
  Clinical Features, 47
  Management, 47
Second-Degree Heart Block, 47
  ECG Findings, 47
  Clinical Features, 49
  Management, 50
Third-Degree Heart Block, 50
  ECG Findings, 50
  Clinical Features, 50
  Management, 50

6 QRS Complex, 53

Overview, 53
  Definition, 53
  Electrophysiology, 53
  Interpretation, 54
Left Ventricular Hypertrophy, 57
  Definition, 57
  ECG Findings, 58
  Clinical Features, 59
  Management, 60
Right Ventricular Hypertrophy, 60
  Definition, 60
  ECG Findings, 60
  Clinical Features, 61
  Management, 61
Pericardial Effusion, 61
  Definition, 61
  ECG Findings, 61

Clinical Features, 61
Management, 61
Bundle Branch Block, 61
Definition, 61
Classification, 62
Right Bundle Branch Block, 62
ECG Findings, 63
Clinical Features, 64
Management, 64
Left Bundle Branch Block, 64
ECG Findings, 64
Clinical Features, 64
Management, 65
Left Anterior Fascicular Block, 65
ECG Findings, 65
Clinical Features, 65
Management, 65
Left Posterior Fascicular Block, 65
ECG Features, 65
Clinical Features, 68
Management, 68
Bifascicular Block, 68
ECG Findings, 68
Clinical Features, 68
Management, 68
Trifascicular Block, 68
ECG Findings, 68
Clinical Features, 69
Management, 69
Pulmonary Embolism, 69
ECG Findings, 69
Clinical Features, 69
Management, 70

7 QT Interval, 71

Overview, 71
Definition, 71
Electrophysiology, 71
Interpretation, 71
Hypercalcaemia, 72
Definition, 72
ECG findings, 72
Clinical Features, 72
Management, 72
Hypocalcaemia, 72
Definition, 72
ECG findings, 72
Clinical Features, 74
Management, 74

8 ST Segment, 75

Overview, 75
Definition, 75
Electrophysiology, 75
Interpretation, 75
Acute Coronary Syndrome, 75
Definition, 75
Classification, 75

STEMI, 75
ECG Findings, 76
Clinical Features, 77
Management, 77
Myocardial Ischaemia and NSTEMI, 79
ECG Findings, 79
Clinical Features, 82
Management, 82
Pericarditis, 83
Definition, 83
ECG findings, 83
Clinical Features, 84
Management, 84
Brugada Syndrome, 84
Definition, 84
ECG findings, 84
Clinical Features, 84
Management, 85
Digoxin, 85
Definition, 85
ECG Findings, 85
Clinical Features, 85
Management, 85

9 T Wave, 87

Overview, 87
Definition, 87
Electrophysiology, 87
Interpretation, 87
Hyperkalaemia, 88
Definition, 88
ECG Findings, 88
Clinical Features, 89
Management, 89

10 Abnormal Extra Waves, 90

U Wave, 90
Definition, 90
ECG Findings, 90
Hypokalaemia, 90
Clinical Features, 91
Management, 91
Delta Waves and Pre-Excitation, 91
Definition, 91
ECG Findings, 91
Clinical Findings, 93
Management, 93
Osborn Wave, 94
Definition, 94
ECG Findings, 94
Clinical Features, 94
Management, 94
Pacemakers, 94
Definition, 94
ECG Findings, 96
Clinical Features, 96
Management, 96
Normal ECG Variants, 96

ECGs in Athletes, 96
Pregnancy, 99
Paediatric Cases, 99

11 Cases 101

Case 1– Questions, 101
Questions for Candidate, 102
Case 2 – Questions, 102
Questions for Candidate, 103
Case 3 – Questions, 103
Questions for Candidate, 104
Case 4 – Questions, 104
Questions for Candidate, 105
Case 5 – Questions, 105
Questions for Candidate, 106
Case 6 – Questions, 106
Questions for Candidate, 107
Case 7 – Questions, 107
Questions for Candidate, 108
Case 8 – Questions, 108
Questions for Candidate, 109
Case 9 – Questions, 109
Questions for Candidate, 110
Case 10 – Questions, 110
Questions for Candidate, 111
Case 11 – Questions, 111
Questions for Candidate, 112
Case 12 – Questions, 112
Questions for Candidate, 113
Case 13 – Questions, 113
Questions for Candidate, 114
Case 14 – Questions, 114
Questions for Candidate, 115
Case 15 – Questions, 115
Questions for Candidate, 116
Case 16 – Questions, 116
Questions for Candidate, 117
Case 17 – Questions, 117
Questions for Candidate, 118
Case 18 – Questions, 118
Questions for Candidate, 119
Case 19 – Questions, 119
Questions for Candidate, 120
Case 20 – Questions, 120
Questions for Candidate, 121
Case 21 – Questions, 121
Questions for Candidate, 122
Case 22 – Questions, 122
Questions for Candidate, 123
Case 23 – Questions, 123
Questions for Candidate, 124
Case 24 – Questions, 124
Questions for Candidate, 125
Case 25 – Questions, 125
Questions for Candidate, 126
Case 26 – Questions, 126
Questions for Candidate, 127

Case 27 – Questions, 127
Questions for Candidate, 128
Case 28 – Questions, 128
Questions for Candidate, 129
Case 29 – Questions, 129
Questions for Candidate, 130
Case 30 – Questions, 130
Questions for Candidate, 131
Case 31 – Questions, 131
Questions for Candidate, 132
Case 32 – Questions, 132
Questions for Candidate, 133
Case 33 – Questions, 133
Questions for Candidate, 134
Case 34 – Questions, 134
Questions for Candidate, 135
Case 35 – Questions, 135
Questions for Candidate, 136
Case 36 – Questions, 136
Questions for Candidate, 137
Case 37 – Questions, 137
Questions for Candidate, 138
Case 38 – Questions, 138
Questions for Candidate, 139
Case 39 – Questions, 139
Questions for Candidate, 140
Case 40 – Questions, 140
Questions for Candidate, 141
Case 1 – Answers, 141
Answers for Candidates, 142
Case 2 – Answers, 144
Answers for Candidates, 144
Case 3 – Answers, 146
Answers for Candidates, 146
Case 4 – Answers, 148
Answers for Candidates, 148
Case 5 – Answers, 150
Answers for Candidates, 150
Case 6 – Answers, 152
Answers for Candidates, 152
Case 7 – Answers, 154
Answers for Candidates, 154
Case 8 – Answers, 156
Answers for Candidates, 156
Case 9 – Answers, 158
Answers for Candidates, 158
Case 10 – Answers, 160
Answers for Candidates, 160
Case 11 – Answers, 162
Answers for Candidates, 163
Case 12 – Answers, 164
Answers for Candidates, 165
Case 13 – Answers, 166
Answers for Candidates, 167
Case 14 – Answers, 168
Answers for Candidates, 169
Case 15 – Answers, 170

Answers for Candidates, 171
Case 16 – Answers, 172
Answers for Candidates, 173
Case 17 – Answers, 174
Answers for Candidates, 175
Case 18 – Answers, 176
Answers for Candidates, 177
Case 19 – Answers, 178
Answers for Candidates, 179
Case 20 – Answers, 180
Answers for Candidates, 180
Case 21 – Answers, 181
Answers for Candidates, 182
Case 22 – Answers, 183
Answers for Candidates, 184
Case 23 – Answers, 185
Answers for Candidates, 186
Case 24 – Answers, 187
Answers for Candidates, 188
Case 25 – Answers, 189
Answers for Candidates, 190
Case 26 – Answers, 191
Answers for Candidates, 192
Case 27 – Answers, 193
Answers for Candidates, 194
Case 28 – Answers, 195
Answers for Candidates, 196
Case 29 – Answers, 197
Answers for Candidates, 198
Case 30 – Answers, 199
Answers for Candidates, 200

Case 31 – Answers, 201
Answers for Candidates, 202
Case 32 – Answers, 203
Answers for Candidates, 204
Case 33 – Answers, 205
Answers for Candidates, 206
Case 34 – Answers, 207
Answers for Candidates, 208
Case 35 – Answers, 209
Answers for Candidates, 210
Case 36 – Answers, 211
Answers for Candidates, 212
Case 37 – Answers, 214
Answers for Candidates, 215
Case 38 – Answers, 216
Answers for Candidates, 216
Case 39 – Answers, 218
Answers for Candidates, 218
Case 40 – Answers, 220
Answers for Candidates, 221

12 Quick Reference Guide, 223

ECG Basics (Figs 12.1–12.3), 223
  Normal Values, 223
Interpretation Structure, 224
  Cardiac Axis (Fig. 12.4), 224
  Arrhythmias, 225
  Intervals and Wave Morphology, 225
Important Conditions (Tables 12.1 and 12.2), 226
Case List, 229
Index, 230

ECG Basics

WHAT ARE ECGS?

An electrocardiogram (ECG) is a recording of the heart's electrical activity. It is derived from electrodes placed on the skin which measures small changes in voltage due to depolarisation and repolarisation of cardiac myocytes. Just like all muscle cells, contraction of heart myocytes is caused by depolarisation, so every time the heart beats, there is a wave of electrical charge spreading through the heart.

THE UTILITY OF ECGS

ECGs are an indispensable, non-invasive tool that constitute part of the basic clinical work-up. They provide information on the function of the cardiac electrical system which can be affected by a wide range of cardiac and non-cardiac pathologies (Box 1.1). In terms of cardiac pathology, ECGs can offer evidence of electrical as well as structural pathology. Furthermore, they are key to diagnosing arrhythmias and myocardial infarction.

NORMAL PACEMAKERS AND HEART CONDUCTION

An understanding of cardiac anatomy and electrophysiology is key for effective interpretation of ECGs.

Box 1.1 Pathologies that produce ECG changes

- Electrical conditions
  - Cardiac arrhythmias
  - Conduction block
  - Channelopathies
  - Pacemakers
- Structural pathologies
  - Ventricular hypertrophy
  - Atrial dilatation
- Myocardial ischaemia and infarction
- Electrolyte abnormalities
  - Potassium (hypokalaemia/hyperkalaemia)
  - Calcium (hypocalcaemia/hypercalcaemia)
  - Magnesium (hypomagnesaemia)
- Pulmonary disease, e.g. pulmonary embolism
- Metabolic, e.g. digoxin toxicity
- Hypothermia

CARDIAC ANATOMY

The heart is normally made up of four chambers: the left and right atria and the left and right ventricles (Figs 1.1 and 1.2). The right atrium and ventricle are separated by the tricuspid valve; the left atrium and ventricle are separated by the mitral valve. The left and right sides of the heart are divided by the septum, a wall of muscular and connective tissue. In the ventricular septum, there are vital components of the heart's conduction system: the bundle of His, the left and right bundle branches and the Purkinje fibres. Since the left and right side normally depolarise and repolarise simultaneously, we can often consider both atria as a single unit, and both ventricles as a single unit, for the purpose of ECG interpretation.

ELECTRICAL CONDUCTION

The sinoatrial node (SAN) in the wall of the right atrium initiates depolarisation in the heart due to its inbuilt pacemaker activity. This wave of depolarisation spreads through the atria, causing them to contract. Electricity is unable to pass from the atria to the ventricles except at the atrioventricular node (AVN), which acts to slow down conduction between the atria and the ventricles to make sure the ventricles do not

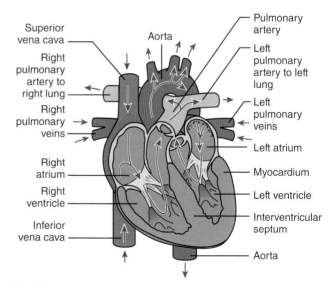

Fig. 1.1 Anatomy of the heart – chambers and valves. Illustration of the four chambers: left and right atria, and left and right ventricles. Their associated blood vessels are also shown (blue for right-sided vessels, red for left-sided vessels). (Source: Aehlert, B. (2009) Anatomy and physiology. In: *ECGs Made Easy*, 4th ed. Maryland Heights, MO: Elsevier.)

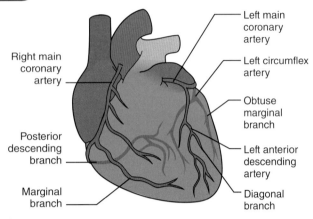

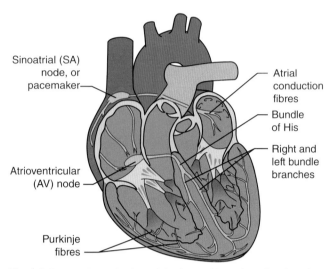

Fig. 1.2 Anatomy of the heart – vessels. The left anterior descending artery supplies the anterior two-thirds of the interventricular septum (septal perforators), anterior and lateral wall of the left ventricle (LV: diagonal branches) and sometimes part of the right ventricle (RV).

Circumflex (Cx) supplies the LV lateral (anterolateral marginal branches) and posterior walls, and occasionally its inferior aspect (posterior LV arteries: 15% of patients) and the posterior septum.

The right coronary artery (RCA) supplies the RV wall, and usually the posterior septum and inferior (diaphragmatic) wall of the LV (posterior LV arteries; 85% of people). The RCA is 'dominant' (as opposed to the Cx) if it gives rise to the posterior descending coronary artery and the posterior left ventricular arteries. (Source: Bersten, A., Handy, J. M. (2018). Acute cardiac syndromes, investigations and interventions. In: *Oh's Intensive Care Manual*, 8th ed. Elsevier.)

Fig. 1.3 Electrical conduction of the heart. Normal cardiac impulses start in the sinoatrial node and then get passed to the atrioventricular node and down the His–Purkinje fibres. (Source: Elsevier collection – Cardiovascular Electrical conduction of the heart.)

contract until the atria have fully contracted, allowing the atrium to push blood into the ventricle.

After a short pause at the AVN, electricity moves down the septum through the bundle of His, into the bundle branches and then the Purkinje fibres all the way to the apex of the heart before moving up the ventricular walls (Fig. 1.3). This causes the ventricles to contract, and then relax as the cells repolarise. After a certain amount of time (depending on what the heart rate is), the SAN will depolarise again, and the whole process will repeat.

ECG PAPER BASICS

ECG paper conventionally shows recordings over a period of 10 s. The horizontal axis represents time moving from left to right. The vertical axis represents the level of electrical activity (voltage) (Fig. 1.4).

The ECG is printed on a grid at a rate of 25 mm/s; each small square is 1 mm in length while larger squares are 5 mm. Therefore, each small square represents 40 ms of time and larger squares represent 200 ms.

The amplitude (voltage) of electrical activity is represented by the vertical axis. Conventionally, 1 mV is represented by 10 mm. A rectangular calibration pulse of 1 mV is produced at the edge of the page to calibrate the amplitude of recordings.

ECG OF A SINGLE HEART BEAT

Several important ECG waves and intervals occur in a single heart beat that directly relate to the cardiac conduction described above (Figs 1.5 and 1.6).

WAVE		DESCRIPTION	SIGNIFICANCE
P wave		First wave (usually upwards deflection) before the QRS complex	Atrial depolarisation. Abnormalities in the P wave can tell us about the size and function of the atria
QRS complex	Q	Downwards deflection preceding the first positive deflection (R wave, as defined below)	The narrow width of the QRS complex depends on speed of depolarisation through the ventricles via the His–Purkinje fibres
	R	First positive deflection	
	S	Downwards deflection immediately following the R wave	
T wave		First wave (usually upwards deflection) after the QRS complex	Ventricular repolarisation
PR interval		Beginning of the P wave to the beginning of the QRS complex	Represents the time from atrial to ventricular depolarisation
PR segment		End of the P wave to the beginning of the QRS complex	Time for depolarisation to conduct from the atria to the ventricles

WAVE	DESCRIPTION	SIGNIFICANCE
ST segment	The end of the QRS complex to the beginning of the T wave	Represents the beginning of ventricular repolarisation. The junction between the end of the QRS complex and the start of the ST segment is termed the J-point. Abnormalities can indicate cardiac ischaemia and/or infarction
QT interval	Start of the QRS complex to the end of the T wave	Represents the time it takes for the ventricles to depolarise and then repolarise

ECG Graph Paper

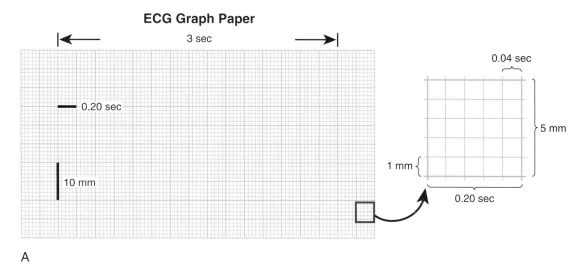

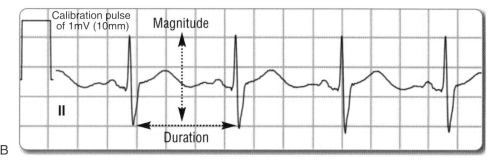

Fig. 1.4 ECG paper axes. The ECG is recorded on graph paper divided into millimetre squares, with darker lines marking 5-mm squares.

(A) Time is presented horizontally and voltage vertically on ECG tracings. With a paper speed of 25 mm/s, a large box represents 200 ms of time and a small box represents 40 ms. Most ECG recordings are done over a total period of 10 s.

(B) A calibration pulse (left side of image) represents 1 mV (10 mm amplitude) of electrical activity. (Source: Goldberger, A., Goldberger, Z., Shvilkin, A. (2017). ECG basics. In: *Goldberger's Clinical Electrocardiography: A Simplified Approach*, 9th ed. Elsevier.)

ELECTRODE PLACEMENT

An ECG trace is recorded by placing several sticky electrodes on various parts of the body. Measuring electrical activity between electrodes allows us to produce 'leads' that are placed at specific anatomical locations (Figs 1.7 and 1.8). In order to obtain a 12 lead ECG, 10 electrodes are placed at specific locations to give a comprehensive spatial picture of the cardiac electrical propagation. It is important to record the ECG accurately as incorrect electrode placement can lead to misdiagnosis.

Studies have shown that precordial ECG electrode placement is often poor, and this can lead to incorrect interpretation. The anterior chest leads are frequently placed too high and the lateral precordial leads too superiorly and posteriorly (Fig. 1.9).

LEADS AND THE 12-LEAD ECG

ECG traces display information using leads. A lead is simply a measure of electrical activity between two electrodes. Depolarisation travelling in the direction of a lead produces a positive deflection, while depolarisation travelling away from a lead produces a negative deflection (Fig. 1.10). This means that leads can look at the heart from different directions and measure the flow of electricity in that particular direction.

The typical 12-lead ECG is made up of two types of leads: six limb leads and six chest leads. While the limb leads measure electricity in the frontal (coronal) plane, the chest leads all look at the heart in the horizontal (transverse) plane. The leads include:

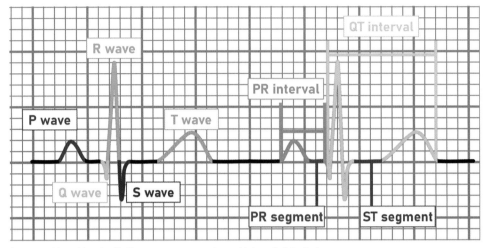

Fig. 1.5 ECG trace of a normal heart beat with the waves, segments and intervals labelled.

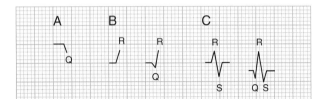

Fig. 1.6 Definitions of the individual waves in a QRS complex. Defining the parts of the QRS complex can be confusing as the nomenclature changes depending on whether the first deflection after the P wave is positive or negative.
(A) If the wave following the P wave is negative, it is a Q wave.
(B) If a positive deflection follows the P wave, it is called an R wave, whether it is preceded by a Q wave or not.
(C) Any following negative deflection is known as an S wave, whether there is a preceding Q wave or not. (Source: Horton-Szar, D. (2015). Cardiac electrophysiology and arrhythmia. In: *Crash Course: Cardiovascular System*, 4th ed. Elsevier.)

SITE	LEADS	CORONARY ARTERY
Septal	$V_1–V_2$	Left anterior descending
Anterior	$V_3–V_4$	Left anterior descending
Lateral	I, aVL, $V_5–V_6$	Left circumflex; left anterior descending
Inferior	II, III, aVF	Right coronary
Posterior	$V_7–V_9$ (with dominant R wave and ST depression in $V_1–V_3$)	Right coronary

- Limb Leads and Augmented Limb Leads: I, II, III and aVL, aVR, aVF
- Chest or precordial Leads: V1, V2, V3, V4, V5, V6.

LEADS AND THEIR ANATOMICAL CORRELATION

The limb leads and augmented limbs lead compare electrical activity in the coronal plane, which corresponds to the inferior (II, aVF, III) and lateral (I and aVL) regions (Fig. 1.11).

The chest leads are recorded using six electrodes placed on the front and left side of the chest, called $V_1–V_6$. Each chest lead compares electrical activity from the centre of the chest to each of these electrodes in the horizontal plane. As you can see from Fig. 1.12, V_1 and V_2 are placed approximately over the right ventricle and so measure electrical activity there. V_3 and V_4 look at the septum and anterior wall of the left ventricle, while V_5 and V_6 look at the anterior and lateral left ventricular walls.

To illustrate how to interpret the direction of depolarisation, let us think about lead I (Fig. 1.13): this lead measures electricity flowing from right to left. If depolarisation in the heart spreads from right to left, there will be a positive (upwards) deflection in lead I, while if depolarisation spreads from left to right, there will be a negative (downwards) deflection.

It is worth taking time to understand and learn the leads and which areas of the heart each ECG lead looks at (Fig. 1.14). This information can be important clinically; for example, if a patient comes in with an ST elevation myocardial infarction (STEMI), it is important to know exactly where in the heart the infarct is. If the ST elevation is greatest in leads V_5 and V_6, you can use your knowledge of the direction ECG leads to say that there is lateral infarction.

Each of the 12 ECG leads looks at the heart in a slightly different direction, so the waves will be predominantly upwards in some leads and negative in some leads depending on whether depolarisation is moving towards or away from that lead; by analysing this, you can calculate the cardiac axis (see Chapter 3).

TYPES OF ECG RECORDINGS

12-LEAD ECG

As described above, the 12-lead ECG is the routine type of ECG done in clinical settings. This is performed using 10 electrodes placed on the limbs and chest. These electrodes generate 12 leads, which measure the electrical activity of the heart in 12 directions (Fig. 1.15).

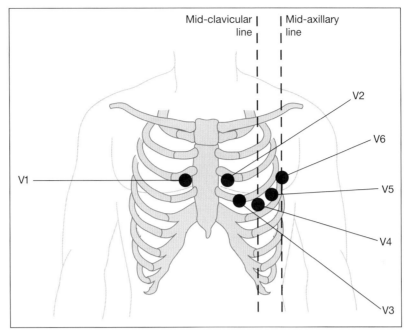

Fig. 1.7 Electrode placement on the chest. V_1, Right fourth intercostal space on sternal border; V_2, left fourth intercostal space on sternal border; V_3, midway between V_2 and V_4; V_4, left fifth intercostal space in mid-clavicular line; V_5, left fifth intercostal space between V_4 and V_6; V_6, left fifth intercostal space in mid-axillary line. (Source: Brown, A., Cadogan, M., Celenza, T. (2016). Cardiac monitoring and the electrocardiograph. In: *Marshall & Ruedy's On Call: Principles & Protocols*, 3rd ed. Elsevier.)

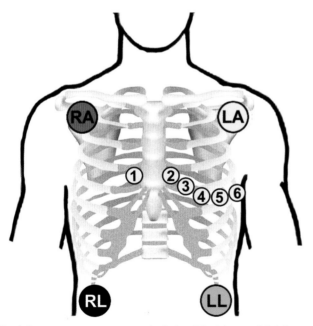

Fig. 1.8 Electrode placement on the limbs. RA, right arm; LA, left arm; RL, right leg; LL, left leg. (Source: Offenstadt, G., Bollaert, P.-E., Mercat, A., Mira, J.-P. (2020). Monitorage ECG: conditions d'interprétation et analyse du signal en reanimation. In: *Réanimation: Les Essentiels en Médecine Intensive*, 4th ed. Elsevier.)

THREE-LEAD ECG

The three-lead ECG is more commonly used for continuous monitoring of cardiac patients or in pre-hospital settings. This uses three electrodes on the limbs to generate three leads (Fig. 1.16). Three-lead ECGs only record the rhythm on leads I, II and III and so are not as informative as a 12-lead ECG. However, they are less restrictive for patients than 12-lead ECGs and so are more useful for continuous monitoring on the ward.

HOLTER OR AMBULATORY ECG MONITORING

Continuous ECG monitoring can be done over a period of 24 h or longer (up to 7 days) using Holter monitors (Fig. 1.17). Electrodes are placed on the chest and limbs and recordings are made on a portable recorder. Patients are advised to keep a diary and make notes on any symptoms they develop. At the end of the monitoring period, the recorder device is returned for analysis.

Continuous monitoring allows intermittent arrhythmias to be detected and we can check if they correspond with symptoms. Holter monitoring can be offered in an outpatient setting while patients go about their daily activities. Indications include palpitations and fainting episodes.

IMPLANTABLE LOOP RECORDER

Similar to a Holter monitor, implantable loop recorders (ILRs) can record ECGs in an outpatient setting over a long period of time, spanning months to years (Fig. 1.18). Therefore, they are useful in cases where Holter monitoring has not detected an abnormality yet there remains a high clinical suspicion of an arrhythmia. ILRs are implanted in the chest under the skin under local anaesthetic. Although ILRs monitor the ECG, they only save recordings whenever the device detects an arrhythmia. Recordings are also saved when patients activate the device when they are symptomatic.

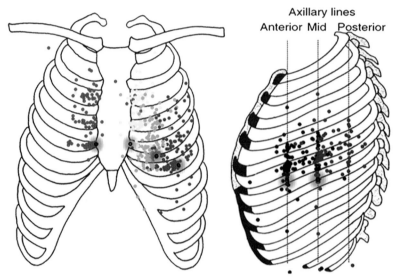

Fig. 1.9 Schematic showing suggested precordial ECG lead placement by 100 health staff who often perform ECGs (V_1 red; V_2 yellow; V_3 green; V_4 brown; V_5 black and V_6 purple). (with permission from Kishto, 0.)

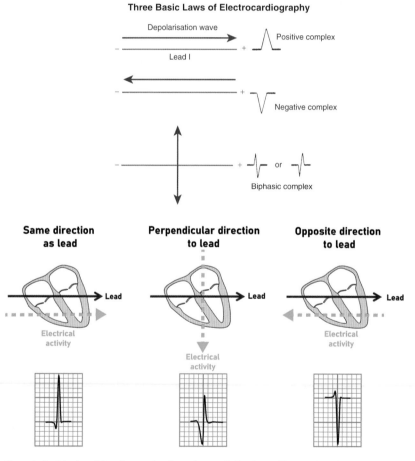

Fig. 1.10 Direction of electrical activity along a lead produces deflections. Electrical activity travelling towards a lead produces a positive deflection, while negative deflections indicate that electrical activity is travelling away from the lead. Electrical activity perpendicular to the direction of the lead produces biphasic deflections. (Source: Goldberger, A., Goldberger, Z., Shvilkin, A. (2017). The normal ECG. In: *Goldberger's Clinical Electrocardiography: A Simplified Approach*, 9th ed. Elsevier.)

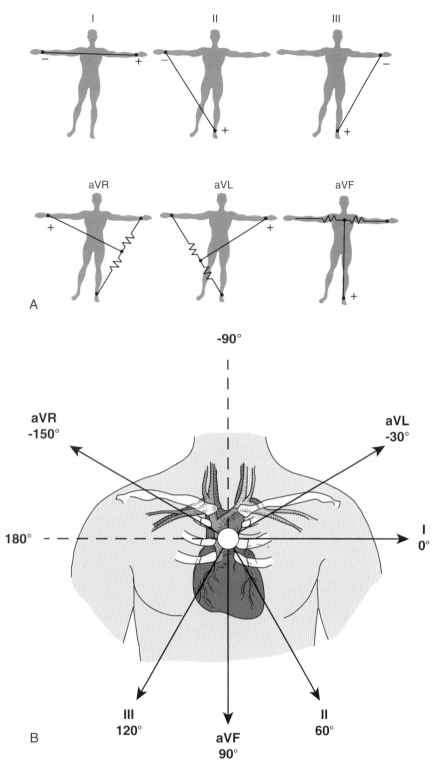

Fig. 1.11 Limb leads measure electrical activity in the coronal plane. (A) The individual directions of the six limb leads. Note that leads aVR, aVL and aVF use an 'augmented' rather than a real electrode for the negative terminal; therefore, these leads can also be referred to as unipolar leads. (B) Directions of the limb leads as shown from the centre of the chest. (Source: (A) Grimnes, S., Martinsen, O. G. (2014). Selected applications. In: *Bioimpedance and Bioelectricity Basics*, 3rd ed. Elsevier. (B) Adapted from Griffin Perry, A., Potter, P. A., Ostendorf, W., Laplante, N. (2021). *Clinical Nursing Skills & Techniques*, 10th ed. Elsevier.)

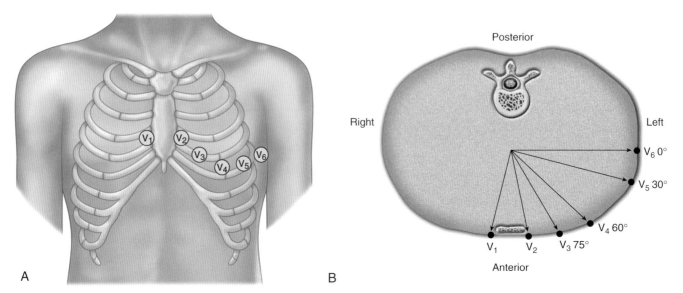

Fig. 1.12 (A, B) Pracordial leads measure electrical activity in the transverse plane. Lead direction is from the centre of the chest to the corresponding electrode. Leads V_1 and V_2 look at the right ventricle, V_3 and V_4 at the interventricular septum and V_5 and V_6 at the left ventricle. The normal QRS complex in each lead is shown. The R wave in the chest (precordial) leads steadily increases in amplitude from lead V_1 to V_6 with a corresponding decrease in S-wave depth, culminating in a predominantly positive complex in V_6.

(A) Source: Griffin Perry, A., Potter, P. A., Ostendorf, W., Laplante, N. (2021). Cardiac care. In: *Clinical Nursing Skills & Techniques*, 10th ed. Elsevier.

(B) Source: Zipes, D. P., Libby, P. (2018). *Braunwald's Heart Disease: A Textbook of Cardiovascular Medicine*, 11th ed. Elsevier.

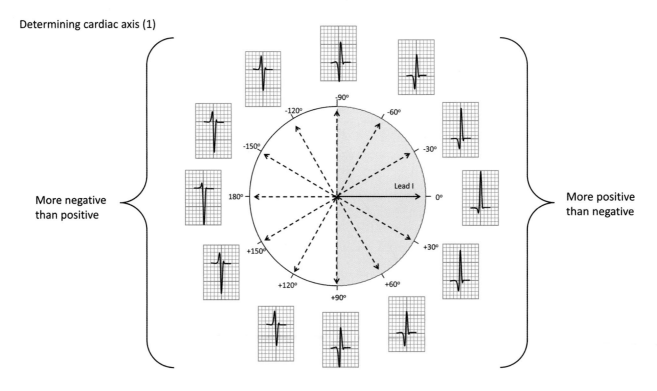

Fig. 1.13 Direction of electrical activity in lead I and its corresponding ECG deflection.

EXERCISE ECG

Exercise tolerance tests (also known as cardiac stress tests) record an ECG under conditions of increasing activity. This is commonly used to assess for coronary heart disease by stressing the heart. Recordings are made while the patient is exercising, such as on a treadmill or exercise bike. The test becomes gradually harder over a period of approximately 15 min. This stresses the heart and checks for cardiac ischaemia, whether symptomatic and/or on the ECG. The pattern

Anterior infarct

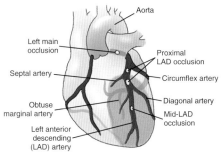

I Lateral	aVR	V₁ Septum	V₄ Anterior
II Inferior	aVL Lateral	V₂ Septum	V₅ Lateral
III Inferior	aVF Inferior	V₃ Anterior	V₆ Lateral

A

Lateral infarct

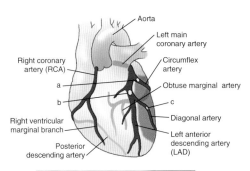

I Lateral	aVR	V₁ Septum	V₄ Anterior
II Inferior	aVL Lateral	V₂ Septum	V₅ Lateral
III Inferior	aVF Inferior	V₃ Anterior	V₆ Lateral

B

Inferior infarct

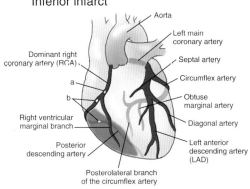

I Lateral	aVR	V₁ Septum	V₄ Anterior
II Inferior	aVL Lateral	V₂ Septum	V₅ Lateral
III Inferior	aVF Inferior	V₃ Anterior	V₆ Lateral

C

Septal infarct

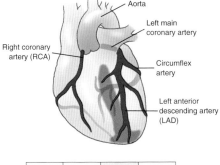

I Lateral	aVR	V₁ Septum	V₄ Anterior
II Inferior	aVL Lateral	V₂ Septum	V₅ Lateral
III Inferior	aVF Inferior	V₃ Anterior	V₆ Lateral

D

Posterior infarct

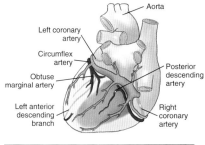

I Lateral	aVR	V₁ Septum	V₄ Anterior	V₇ Posterior
II Inferior	aVL Lateral	V₂ Septum	V₅ Lateral	V₈ Posterior
III Inferior	aVF Inferior	V₃ Anterior	V₆ Lateral	V₉ Posterior

E

Fig. 1.14 (A–E) The leads and arteries corresponding to the main regions of the heart. (Source: Aehlert, B. (2009) Introduction to the 12-lead ECG. In: *ECGs Made Easy*, 4th ed. Maryland Heights, MO: Elsevier.)

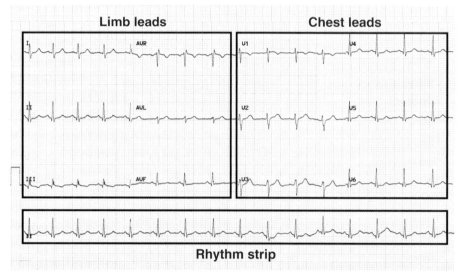

Fig. 1.15 A conventional ECG tracing. In most standard recordings, the limb leads are displayed on the left-hand side while the chest leads are on the right-hand side of the page. The bottom of the page displays the rhythm strip, which is usually lead II.

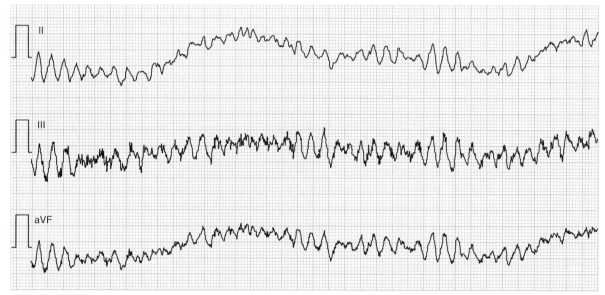

Fig. 1.16 Example of three-lead ECG. Three-lead ECGs are commonly done in pre-hospital settings as only three electrodes are required to obtain a recording. This ECG shows torsades de pointes (see Chapter 2). (Source: An unusual presentation of asymptomatic type 2 Brugada pattern 1561-8811.)

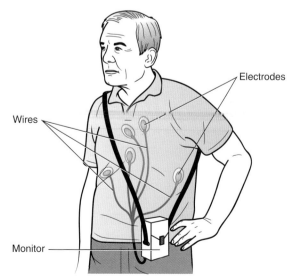

Fig. 1.17 Holter monitor. (Source: Deska Pagana, K., Pagana, T., Pagana, T. N. (2016). *Mosby's Diagnostic and Laboratory Test Reference*, 13th ed. Elsevier.)

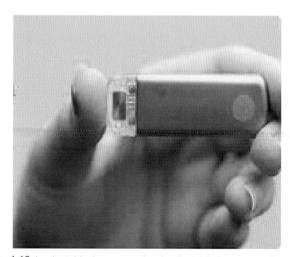

Fig. 1.18 Implantable loop recorder. Implantable loop recorders are devices that are inserted underneath the skin in the chest to record the ECG over long periods of time. They can record up to 3 years of data. (Source: Srinivasan, P., Shanmugam, T., Chokkalingam, L., Bakthavachalam, P. (2020). Cardiology. In: *Toxicological Aspects of Medical Device Implants*. Elsevier.)

of ischaemia on the ECG can guide which region(s) and vessel(s) are involved.

SMARTPHONE APPS

Several apps are available on smartphones and smartwatches that allow an ECG to be recorded. This can be achieved through the device itself or through a separate electrode attachment (Fig. 1.19). Advantages of this approach include ease of use and portability.

PRESENTING AN ECG

There are several ways to approach an ECG. Box 1.2 presents a fairly standard order and makes sure you find all the important aspects of the ECG. Each of these aspects will be discussed in the upcoming chapters.

This approach is also the order you should use to present your findings, as it ensures that you do not forget to mention any information. Of course, if there is a glaring abnormality, then it may make sense to present this first, but even when there is one obvious unusual feature, it is still important to run through the whole system to ensure that a more subtle problem is not missed. Remember to look at all leads, and if something is present in some leads but not in others, then specify which leads and consider the areas of the heart that these leads are looking at. Finally, always summarise your findings by listing any important positive (and negative) findings, and consider offering a differential diagnosis.

An example ECG presentation is described below (Fig. 1.20). You can practise with the cases later in this book after learning about the components needed to interpret ECGs in the next chapters. The cases will also

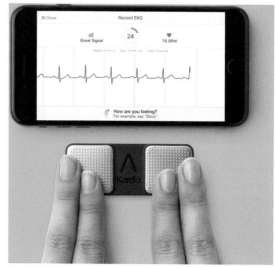

Fig. 1.19 Smartphones can be used to record ECGs. (Source: Al'Aref, S., Singh, G., Baskaran, L., Metaxas, D. (2020). Technological advances within digital medicine. In: *Machine Learning in Cardiovascular Medicine.* Elsevier.)

Box 1.2 **Structure for analysing ECGs**

- Basic details (whose ECG it is, how old they are, where it was recorded, calibration)
- Key features
- Rate and rhythm
- Cardiac axis
- PR and QT interval
- Wave morphology – P wave, QRS complex, ST segment, T waves
- Summary of findings
- Management

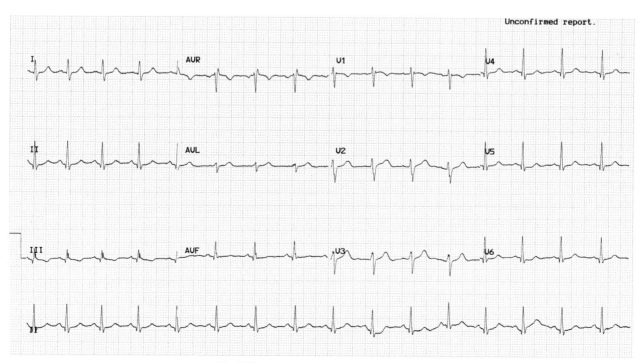

Fig. 1.20 Normal sinus rhythm at rate 96 bpm.

teach you to present ECGs in the context of clinical scenarios and as part of formulating management plans.

Basic details

This is an anonymised ECG recorded at an unknown date and time. I would like to ensure that this is calibrated to the usual 25 mm/s paper speed and 1 mV/cm gain.

Key features

There are no obvious abnormalities in this ECG.

Heart rate and rhythm

The heart rate is 96 bpm with a sinus rhythm.

Cardiac axis

The axis is normal (−30° to +90°)

PR and QT interval

The PR interval is normal (between 120 and 200 ms) and the QT interval is normal (between 400 and 440 ms).

Wave morphology

The P waves are normal. The QRS complexes are narrow and of normal amplitude. The ST segments and T waves are normal.

In summary

This is a normal ECG. There is normal sinus rhythm and no abnormal features are present.

---

¹₂₃ Key Points

1. ECGs are a non-invasive investigation that measures the electrical activity of the heart
2. Normally, electrical activity is initiated in the SAN in the right atrium to depolarise the atria. This is conducted to the AVN and then through the His–Purkinje fibres to depolarise the ventricles
3. ECG recordings are made over a minimum period of 10 s. The horizontal axis represents time, while the vertical axis represents electrical activity (voltage)
4. Leads measure electrical activity between two electrodes. A positive deflection indicates electrical activity travelling in the direction of the lead
5. Limb leads display activity in the frontal (coronal) plane, while precordial leads represent the horizontal (transverse) plane

---

6. The important ECG waves and intervals in a heart beat include:
   (a) P wave: represents atrial depolarisation
   (b) QRS complex: represents ventricular depolarisation
   (c) T wave: represents ventricular repolarisation
   (d) PR interval: represents time from atrial to ventricular depolarisation
   (e) ST segment: represents beginning of ventricular repolarisation
   (f) QT interval: represents time taken for ventricles to depolarise and repolarise
7. Analysing and presenting an ECG can be systematically done in the following order:
   (a) Technical aspects (whose ECG it is, how old they are, where it was recorded)
   (b) Rate and rhythm
   (c) Cardiac axis
   (d) Intervals – PR interval, QT interval
   (e) Wave morphology – P wave, QRS complex, ST segment, T waves
   (f) Summary of findings

FURTHER READING

Becker, D.E., 2006. Fundamentals of electrocardiography interpretation. Anesth. Prog. 53 (2), 53–63; quiz p. 64.

Edhouse, J., Thakur, R.K., Khalil, J.M., 2002. Conditions affecting the left side of the heart. BMJ. 324 (7348), 1264–1267.

Harrigan, R.A., Jones, K., 2002. Conditions affecting the right side of the heart. BMJ. 324 (7347), 1201–1204.

Mangi, M.A., et al., 2022. Atrioventricular block second-degree. In: StatPearls. Treasure Island, Florida.

Mattu, A., Brady, W.J., 2013. ECGs for the Emergency Physician 1. Wiley, London.

Mond, H.G., 2019. Interpreting the normal pacemaker electrocardiograph. Heart. Lung. Circ. 28 (2), 223–236.

Oldroyd, S.H., Quintanilla Rodriguez, B.S., Makaryus, A.N., 2022. First degree heart block. In: StatPearls. Treasure Island, Florida.

Rate and Rhythm

2

OVERVIEW

DEFINITION

Rate

The heart rate describes the frequency of the depolarisations of the cardiac muscle, and therefore the frequency of the heart beat. It is usually measured as 'beats per minute' (bpm).

- Normal heart rate: between 60 and 100 bpm
- Bradycardia: less than 60 bpm
- Tachycardia: greater than 100 bpm

Bradycardias and tachycardias may be physiological or the result of abnormal rhythms (arrhythmias).

Rhythm

The rhythm of the heart describes the pattern of electrical activity. In a normal heart, the pattern is described as sinus rhythm (Fig. 2.1). On the ECG, sinus rhythm (a rhythm originating from the sinoatrial node (SAN)) is a regular rhythm characterised by a normal P wave, followed by a QRS complex and a T wave. Sinus rhythm reflects the normal passage of electrical activity through the conduction system.

Electrophysiology

Cardiac cells normally undergo cycles of depolarisation (initiating contraction) and repolarisation (initiating relaxation). Most cells require a trigger to initiate action potential and depolarisation. Once an area of the heart is triggered to depolarise, this rapidly spreads like a wave to adjacent areas to depolarise the rest of the organ. This is automatically followed by repolarisation, which returns the cells to their resting membrane potential (and additionally resists repeat depolarisation because of the refractory period until repolarisation is completed). As long as depolarisation is triggered by a single area, waves of depolarisation are followed by repolarisation throughout the heart in a synchronised fashion. If this is disrupted, depolarisation in different areas may overlap with repolarisation, introducing the potential for dyssynchronous and inefficient muscle contraction and relaxation.

Many cells in the heart can depolarise spontaneously without an external trigger; this property is known as automaticity. The overall heart rate is determined by the group of cells that depolarise most frequently. This is normally the SAN, which acts as a pacemaker by depolarising regularly at an intrinsic rate of between 70 and 130

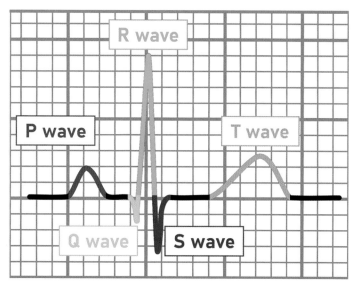

Fig. 2.1 Normal ECG waves in a heart beat. Sinus rhythm refers to signals originating from the sinoatrial node, so a P wave and narrow QRS complex would be observed.

bpm. This rate can be increased by the effect of circulating catecholamines (such as adrenaline) and the sympathetic nervous system, and can be decreased by the vagus nerve as part of the parasympathetic nervous system.

Abnormal rhythms (arrhythmias) arise due to three major mechanisms:

- Altered automaticity: the most rapidly depolarising group of cells determines the overall heart rate. Therefore, an ectopic group of cells that begins to depolarise at a greater rate than the SAN will take over the rhythm of the heart. This can be caused by an increase in automaticity at an abnormal location (an ectopic pacemaker site), causing a faster rhythm (automatic tachyarrhythmia), or a decrease in automaticity of the SAN due to disease of the sinus node, usually causing a slower rhythm (bradyarrhythmia).
- Triggered activity: small 'afterdepolarisations' of cardiac cells can occur during or after the main depolarisation event. If they reach sufficient magnitude to trigger an action potential, they are referred to as triggered activity and cause tachyarrhythmias.
- Re-entry: re-entrant arrhythmias are caused by loops of depolarisation around a non-excitable centre, such as a scar. If the wave of depolarisation loops around an area that was previously depolarised but is no longer refractory (i.e. is still excitable), it can 're-enter' this region, causing a repeating loop, or re-entrant tachyarrhythmia.

Interpretation

Calculating Heart Rate. At a normal paper speed of 25 mm/s, the rate of a regular rhythm can be calculated by dividing 300 by the number of large squares between R waves (the R–R interval) (Fig. 2.2), or (if the rate is very fast) by dividing 1500 by the number of small squares. Note that this method can only be used if the rhythm is regular.

Alternatively, at normal paper speed the rhythm strip represents 10 s of recording. Therefore, counting the number of QRS complexes in the rhythm strip and multiplying by 6 gives the average number of beats per minute (Fig. 2.3) (Box 2.1). This technique is especially useful when the rhythm is irregular.

Assessment of Cardiac Rhythm and Arrhythmias. Cardiac rhythms can be described in terms of the features on the ECG trace:

- Regular or irregular (Fig. 2.4)
- Narrow- or broad-complex (Fig. 2.5)
- Fast (tachycardia) (Fig. 2.6) or slow (bradycardia)

Box **2.1**	Rate can be Calculated from Standard (25 mm/s) ECG Tracings Using 2 Methods

1) 6 × number of peaks across rhythm strip in lead II.
2) 300 ÷ number of big squares between 2 QRS peaks (note: can only be used in regular rhythms).

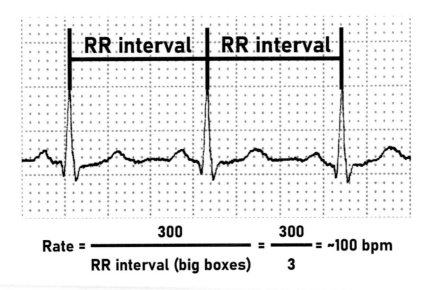

$$\text{Rate} = \frac{300}{\text{RR interval (big boxes)}} = \frac{300}{3} = \text{~100 bpm}$$

Fig. 2.2 The R–R interval is the interval between two QRS complexes. The rate in regular rhythms can be quickly calculated using the above equation (if the ECG tracing is done at 25 mm/s).

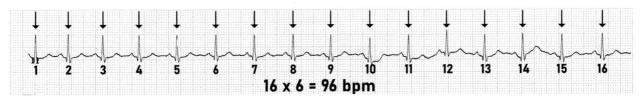

16 x 6 = 96 bpm

Fig. 2.3 Most ECG recordings display recordings over 10 s. An accurate method to calculate the rate is to count the QRS complexes across the ECG recording (which is ordinarily over 10 s) and multiply by 6.

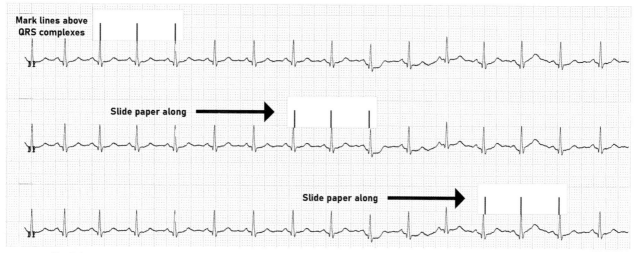

Mark lines above QRS complexes

Slide paper along ⟶

Slide paper along ⟶

Fig. 2.4 A practical method to check regularity. Place a small piece of paper above three QRS complexes and draw lines above the peaks. Move the paper along the rhythm strip (lead II) and check if the QRS complexes approximately line up with the drawn lines.

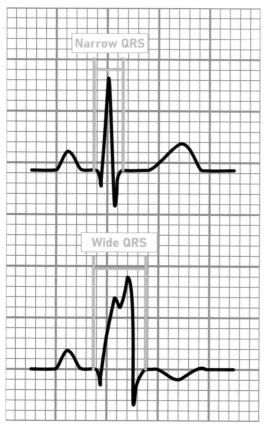

Narrow QRS

Wide QRS

Fig. 2.5 Narrow- and broad-complex rhythms. Note that the T wave can be inverted in broad-complex rhythms as both depolarisation and repolarisation of the ventricles are abnormal.

The regularity of rhythms can be determined by eyeballing the ECG tracing, although this is difficult in tachycardias. A more reliable method involves placing a small piece of paper above two QRS complexes and moving the paper along the rhythm strip to check if the spacing between complexes remains similar (Fig. 2.4).

The rhythm may also be described by the location of the focus that produces the rhythm:
- Sinus rhythms: arise at the SAN
- Junctional rhythms: arise at the junction between the atria and ventricles, including the atrioventricular node (AVN)
- Ventricular rhythms: arise within the ventricles (Box 2.2)

NORMAL VARIANTS

SINUS ARRHYTHMIA
Definition
Sinus arrhythmia is a phenomenon where the R–R interval (and therefore heart rate) varies in a regular manner, usually with the respiratory cycle.

ECG Findings
The ECG will show an increase in heart rate during inspiration and a decrease during expiration on both a 12-lead tracing and the rhythm strip (Fig. 2.7). The shape of the P wave and length of the P–R interval are constant throughout the respiratory cycle and there is a QRS complex after each P wave.

Clinical Significance
Sinus arrhythmia is a common and normal ECG finding, especially in children, young adults, and those with a high vagal tone (such as athletes). It is usually of no clinical significance.

Management
No management is necessary for sinus arrhythmia.

REGULAR NARROW-COMPLEX TACHYCARDIA

It is important to have a systematic approach to reviewing ECGs, particularly for abnormal heart rhythms.

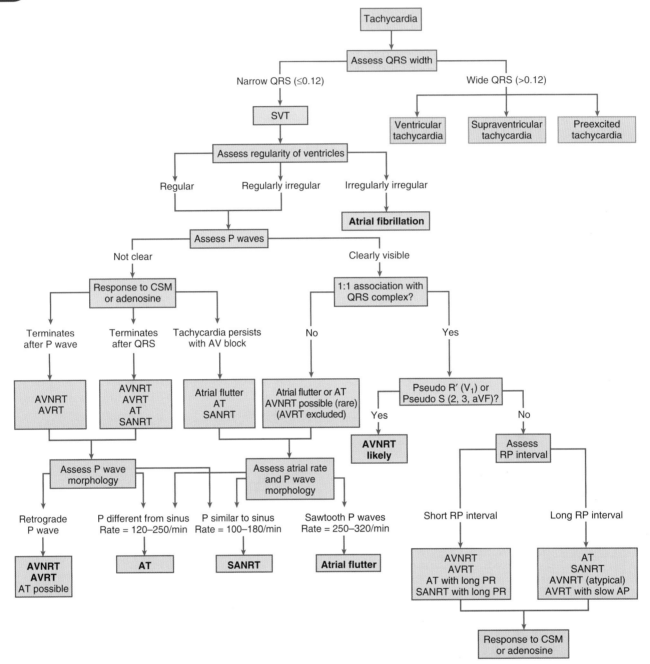

Fig. 2.6 Flowchart of tachycardia interpretation. Tachycardias can be divided according to QRS width and then further subdivided in terms of regularity. AP, accessory pathway; AT, atrial tachycardia; AV, atrioventricular; AVNRT, atrioventricular nodal re-entrant tachycardia; AVRT, atrioventricular reciprocating tachycardia; CSM, carotid sinus massage; SANRT, sinoatrial nodal re-entry tachycardia; SVT, supraventricular tachycardia. (Source: Zipes, D. P., Libby, P. (2018). *Braunwald's Heart Disease: A Textbook of Cardiovascular Medicine*, 11th ed. Elsevier.)

When reviewing the rhythm on an ECG, it is best initially to review the rhythm strip at the bottom of the ECG (usually of lead II).

When reviewing an ECG of a tachycardia, the following questions will help differentiate the type of tachycardia:

1. Is it a narrow or broad complex tachycardia?
2. Is the ventricular rhythm regular or irregular?
3. Are there visible 'P' waves? If so:
   a. Is the P wave morphology and axis normal?
   b. Where is the P wave seen in relation to the QRS?
      i. Before the QRS complex
      ii. Immediately after the QRS (short R-P)
      iii. Further away after the QRS (long R-P)
      iv. Not related to the QRS – VA dissociation

In order for the QRS to be narrow, cardiac conduction has to proceed normally through the AV node, through the Bundle of His and into the Purkinje system. Therefore, any tachycardia with a narrow complex must be arising before or above the AV node (see Fig. 2.8).

SINUS TACHYCARDIA

Definition

Sinus tachycardia is defined as a sinus rhythm with a rate greater than 100 bpm.

ECG Findings

Sinus tachycardia will show a P wave with normal morphology and axis followed by a QRS complex (Fig. 2.9). The R–R interval will be shorter than three large squares in length. PR and QT intervals may appear short (due to sympathetic nervous stimulation increasing the rate of impulse conduction through the AVN and increased rate of repolarisation, respectively).

Clinical Significance

Sinus tachycardia is extremely common and is almost always due to physiological stress. This can be physiological, such as in exercise and anxiety, or can reflect significant underlying pathology, such as hypotension, hypoxia, hyperthyroidism, sepsis or blood loss. It may also be due to increased sympathetic stimulation of the heart in response to reduced stroke volume, such as decompensated heart failure, pulmonary embolism and pericardial tamponade. Other causes include anxiety, medical or recreational drugs such as β_2 agonists (such as salbutamol), and sympathomimetics, including cocaine.

Management

Abnormal physiology and underlying illness are major causes of sinus tachycardia. As such your history, examination and investigations should focus on identifying and treating an underlying cause.

ATRIAL TACHYCARDIA

Definition

An atrial tachycardia (AT) is caused by an abnormal focus (or several abnormal foci (automatic or triggered)) within the atria.

Box **2.2**	Supraventricular Versus Ventricular Rhythms

Supraventricular rhythms conduct via the His–Purkinje system in the same way as sinus rhythm. As a result, they will have a normal QRS complex and T wave (unless there is other pathology present, such as bundle branch block). Sinus, atrial and junctional rhythms can be grouped together as supraventricular rhythms.

In contrast, ventricular rhythms begin from a focus below the His–Purkinje system and are transmitted across the ventricles much more slowly. Consequently, ventricular rhythms will have a broad QRS complex and abnormal T wave.

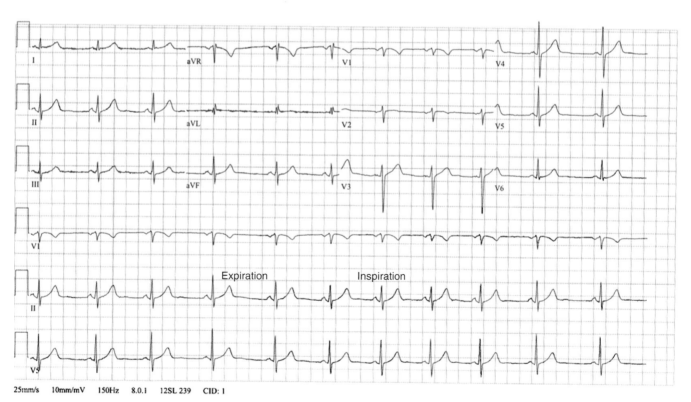

25mm/s   10mm/mV   150Hz   8.0.1   12SL 239   CID: 1

Fig. 2.7 Sinus arrhythmia. ECG showing sinus arrhythmia and a heart rate averaging 65 bpm. The heart rate increases with inspiration and slows down on expiration. This finding, a key aspect of heart rate variability, is physiological. (Source: Tokarev, J., Benditt, J. G. (2015). 'Sinus bradycardia and chronotropic incompetence associated with single-agent itraconazole antifungal therapy: A case report', *HeartRhythm Case Reports*, 1(1), pp. 6–9.)

TACHYCARDIA HR > 100 bpm

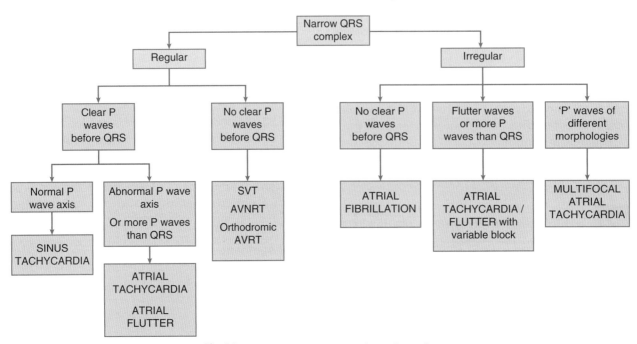

Fig. 2.8 Differential for narrow complex tachycardia.

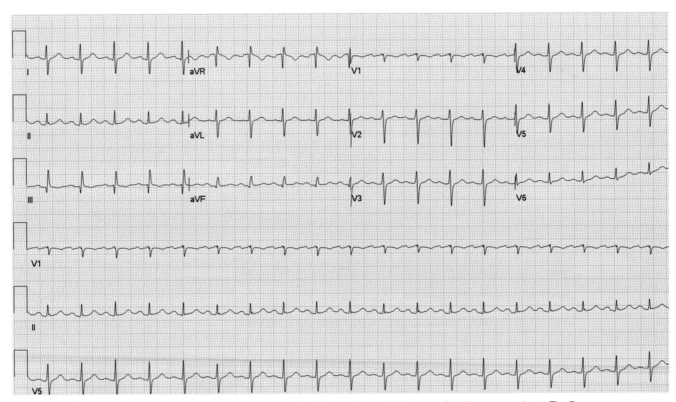

Fig. 2.9 Sinus tachycardia. ECG of sinus tachycardia with a regular ventricular rate of 114 beats per minute. The P waves are normal, suggesting the origin of atrial depolarisation is from the sinus node, and are followed by a narrow QRS complex. (Source: Naccarelli, G. V. (2012). 'Electrocardiography of arrhythmias: a comprehensive review,' *Circulation* 126: p. e198.)

AT may be a result of scarring of the atria due to myocardial infarction, cardiomyopathies or previous cardiac surgery. AT may also be precipitated by catecholamine excess, metabolic disturbances, alcohol intoxication and digoxin toxicity.

ECG Findings

Focal AT is characterised by a regular, narrow-complex rhythm of greater than 100 bpm. Atrial depolarisation arises from an abnormal focus, which may lead to P waves of abnormal morphology and axis (Fig. 2.10);

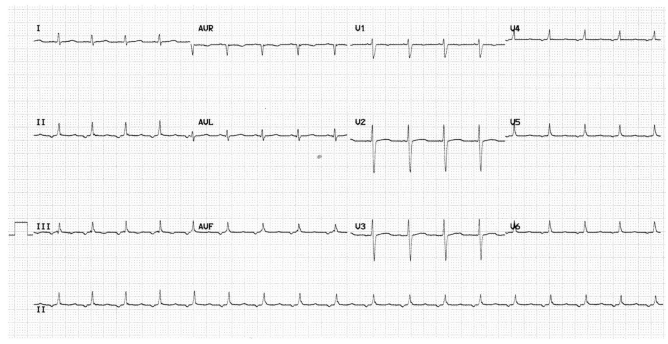

Fig. 2.10 Atrial tachycardia. The rate is slightly tachycardic at 108 bpm, regular and with a narrow QRS complex (<120ms/3 small squares). The P waves are visible before the QRS complex but with abnormal morphology and axis (inverted in leads II, III, aVF and V$_4$-V$_6$) suggesting depolarisation is away from the sinus node.

comparison with old ECGs may be helpful if the diagnosis is uncertain.

Management
Management is dependent on the aetiology, underlying precipitant and associated symptoms. Options include treating the underlying precipitant, drugs or catheter ablation.

ATRIAL FLUTTER

Definition
Atrial flutter is a re-entrant AT. Typical flutter is characterised by an anticlockwise re-entrant circuit within the right atrium. Atypical flutter includes other re-entrant circuits involving the left or right atria.

Atrial flutter commonly arises due to scarring or dilatation of the atria, which can be due to cardiac disease such as hypertensive heart disease, valvular dysfunction or ischaemia or secondary to previous catheter ablation. It can also be due to metabolic disturbances or antiarrhythmic treatment. Flutter often coexists with atrial fibrillation (AF).

ECG Findings
Typical atrial flutter is characterised by a 'sawtooth' baseline pattern (known as 'flutter' waves) of P waves due to cyclic activation of the atria (Figs 2.11 and 2.12), usually most visible in inferior leads and in V$_1$.

Classically, the atrial rate is around 300 bpm with only one in two impulses conducted to the ventricles

(2:1 atrioventricular block), resulting in regular ventricular complexes at a rate of 150 bpm. Other ratios are also possible (Fig. 2.13).

It should be noted that variable atrioventricular block can occur, whereby the ratio of P waves to QRS complexes changes across the ECG; this produces an irregular rhythm with narrow QRS complexes.

Management
Haemodynamically unstable patients should be managed by synchronised electrical cardioversion. In stable patients, a clinical decision should be made to control their ventricular rate or restore sinus rhythm.

The risk of clot formation and stroke in atrial flutter is similar to that of AF; appropriate anticoagulation is therefore important.

Long-term control of recurrent typical atrial flutter is usually achieved by catheter ablation.

ATRIOVENTRICULAR NODAL RE-ENTRANT TACHYCARDIA

Definition
Atrioventricular nodal re-entrant tachycardia (AVNRT) is caused by the presence of fast and slow conduction pathways within the AVN (Fig. 2.14). The presence of these pathways with different conduction speeds provides the opportunity for re-entry circuits to develop, especially in the presence of atrial ectopic beats (extra heart beats arising from the atria but outside the SAN).

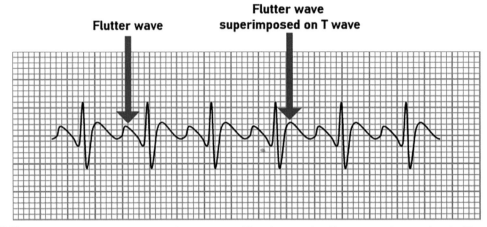

Flutter wave   **Flutter wave superimposed on T wave**

Fig. 2.11 Atrial flutter waves have a sawtooth appearance. There is normally a P wave superimposed on the T wave, so they are hidden. This example shows atrial flutter with 2:1 block (two P waves for every QRS complex) despite only one P wave being clearly visible.

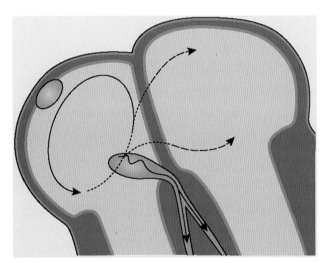

Fig. 2.12 Typical atrial flutter occurs as a result of a re-entry circuit forming in the right atrium. (Source: Crawford, M. H., DiMarco, J. P., Paulus, W. J. (2009). *Cardiology E-Book*. Elsevier Health Sciences.)

ECG Findings

AVNRT will present as a regular, narrow-complex tachycardia, usually of >150 bpm. There are no P waves before each QRS complex, although there may be a small negative deflection after the QRS complex in inferior leads or a small positive deflection in V_1, which represents retrograde conduction through the atria (Fig. 2.15).

Clinical Significance

AVNRT usually affects younger people with otherwise healthy hearts and is more common in women. It normally presents with palpitations with an abrupt onset, and usually an abrupt termination.

Management

AVNRT may be terminated acutely by performing vagal manoeuvres, such as Valsalva (Fig. 2.16). If this fails, intravenous adenosine is highly effective, with escalating medical treatment as needed, such as beta-blockers and calcium channel blockers. These measures attempt to terminate AVNRT by blocking AVN conduction (as the circuit relies on AVN). Catheter ablation of the slow pathway provides definitive management.

ATRIOVENTRICULAR RE-ENTRANT TACHYCARDIA

Definition

Atrioventricular re-entrant tachycardia (AVRT) is caused by the existence of an additional (accessory) pathway between the atria and ventricles aside from the AVN (see Chapter 10: Delta waves). AVRT occurs when the AVN and accessory pathway form a macroscopic re-entry circuit. This arrhythmia is usually triggered by an atrial ectopic beat that allows the re-entry circuit to form.

ECG Findings

AVRT is characterised by a regular narrow QRS tachycardia with no P waves before each QRS complex. Retrograde (inverted) P waves may be seen (Fig. 2.17); in comparison to AVNRT, the retrograde P waves are seen slightly later after the QRS and are therefore more likely to be visible within the ST segment (Figs 2.18 and 2.19). Delta waves (see Chapter 10: Delta waves), a slurred upstroke on the QRS complex, may be seen depending on the re-entry circuit formed (see antidromic circuit, below).

Normally, circuit formation in pre-excitation is prevented by the refractory period of the accessory pathway and AVN; both pathways depolarise at the same time, so impulses reach the ventricles during the refractory period of both pathways. Some patients have AVRT without pre-excitation in sinus rhythm due to accessory pathways that only conduct in the 'backwards' direction, called concealed accessory pathways. AVRT can be triggered by an ectopic beat, usually of atrial origin. This introduces the possibility of impulses travelling through the accessory pathway and AVN at different times and, consequently, outside their refractory period. Impulses can travel in a

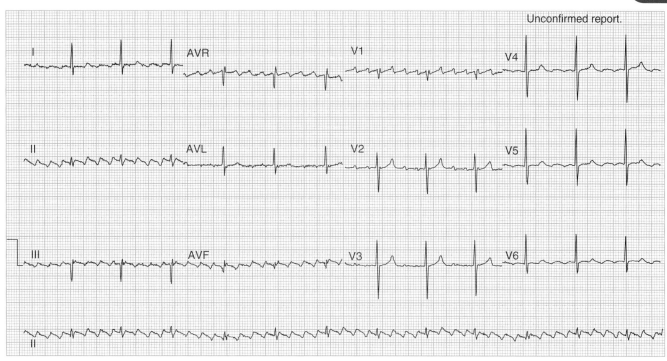

Fig. 2.13 ECG of atrial flutter with 4:1 conduction. Note that the ventricular rate is ~75 bpm as would be expected – an atrial rate of 300 bpm with four P waves for every QRS complex results in a ventricular rate of 75 bpm. P wave morphology and axis is abnormal – the morphology is suggestive of typical atrial flutter.

retrograde fashion through the accessory pathway and AVN.

Depolarisation can then circulate around the atria and ventricles, producing tachycardia. AVRT can be classified as orthodromic or antidromic depending on the direction of re-entry circuit (Fig. 2.20):

- Orthodromic circuit: atrial to ventricular conduction occurs via the AVN, while the accessory pathway permits retrograde conduction from the ventricle to the atria. As conduction to the ventricles occurs via the normal His–Purkinje fibres, QRS complexes are narrow and without a delta wave present; identifying preexcitation would involve examining a previous resting ECG. P waves are inverted and occur after the QRS complex. Orthodromic circuits represent the majority of AVRTs (90%).
- Antidromic circuit: the AVN conducts in a retrograde fashion from the ventricles up to the atria, while the accessory pathway conducts impulses from the atria down to the ventricles. The QRS complex is wide with delta waves present as ventricular depolarisation occurs outside the His–Purkinje system. Antidromic circuits represent a minority of AVRTs (10%).

Clinical Significance
AVRT usually affects younger people with otherwise structurally healthy hearts.

Management
AVRT can be managed as AVNRT in the acute setting, and catheter ablation of the accessory pathway has high success rates for long-term management.

IRREGULAR NARROW-COMPLEX TACHYCARDIA

ATRIAL FIBRILLATION
Definition
AF is a common atrial arrhythmia characterised by chaotic and irregular depolarisation of the atria, leading to a loss of atrial contractility (Fig. 2.21).

ECG Findings
In AF, P waves are absent due to the lack of co-ordinated atrial activity. Instead, erratic atrial activity is represented by an irregular baseline. The AVN intermittently conducts a small proportion of the impulses it receives, leading to classical 'irregularly irregular' QRS complexes (Fig. 2.22).

Clinical Significance
AF has a lifetime risk of around 25% over the age of 40, and a prevalence that rises rapidly with age. It is strongly associated with a history of hypertension, obesity, obstructive sleep apnoea, cardiac disease, especially heart failure, and valvular heart disease. It is also associated with diabetes, hyperthyroidism, previous cardiac surgery, alcohol excess and respiratory disease.

Loss of atrial contractility causes stagnation of blood in the atria and may lead to subsequent clot formation. These clots can be dislodged and enter the circulation, where they may cause thromboembolism. Up to 30% of strokes may be caused by AF.

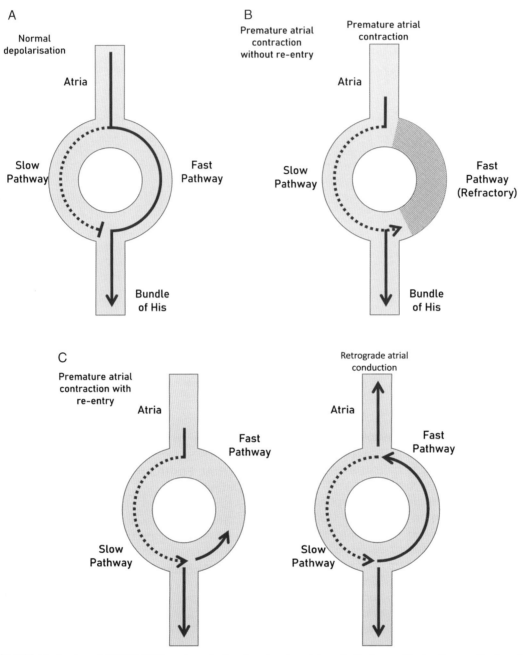

Fig. 2.14 Mechanism of AVNRT. (A) Normal conduction. Impulses travel down both slow and fast pathways. The bundle of His is activated by the fast pathway first, and re-entry from the slow pathway is blocked by the still refractory fast pathway. (B) Atrial ectopic beat without re-entry. The fast pathway has a long refractory period, while the slow pathway has a shorter refractory period. When atrial ectopic signals reach the AVN, the slow pathway is functional but the fast pathway is still refractory, so the impulse travels only via the slow pathway. (C) Atrial ectopic beat with re-entry. If the fast pathway is no longer refractory when the ectopic impulse reaches the bundle of His, the impulse can travel backwards (retrograde) up the fast pathway. The impulse cycles up the fast pathway and down the slow pathway, activating both the atria and ventricles as it does so, causing a re-entrant arrhythmia.

Management

Clinical decision should be made to control the ventricular rate or restore sinus rhythm.

The CHA_2DS_2-VASc score (Fig. 2.23) can be used to assess the need for anticoagulation, usually with direct oral anticoagulants or warfarin.

Catheter ablation could be considered in those with symptomatic AF.

REGULAR BROAD-COMPLEX TACHYCARDIA

Broad-complex tachycardias occur due to either (Fig. 2.24):
- Abnormal rhythms not passing through the His-Purkinje System
  - Ventricular Arrhythmias
  - Pre-excited Arrhythmias

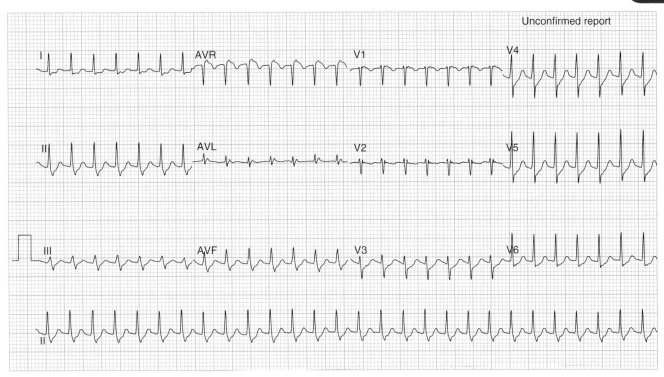

Unconfirmed report

Fig. 2.15 AVNRT. The heart rate is 168 bpm without preceding P waves – there are some P waves visible just after the QRS complex (short R-P tachycardia), most easily seen in lead V_1. The rate is regular with narrow QRS complexes.

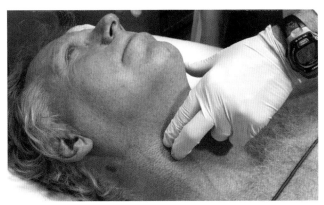

Fig. 2.16 Vagal manoeuvres can be used to terminate supraventricular tachycardia. Carotid massage is a vagal manoeuvre that can be used in supraventricular tachycardia. With the patient's head tilted backward and slightly to the opposite side, palpate the carotid pulse just below the angle of the mandible at the upper level of the thyroid cartilage and anterior to the sternocleidomastoid muscle. Once the pulsation is identified, use the fingertips to administer carotid sinus massage for 5 seconds in a posteromedial direction, aiming toward the vertebral column. (Source: Roberts, J. R. (2017). Techniques for supraventricular tachycardias. *Roberts and Hedges' Clinical Procedures in Emergency Medicine and Acute Care*, 7th ed. Elsevier.)

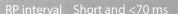

RP interval   Short and <70 ms

Typical AVNRT. AVRT is unusual.

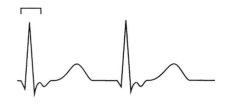

RP interval   Short but >70 ms

In most cases AVRT. Occasionally atypical AVNRT or AT.

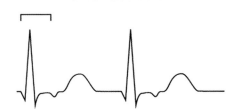

Fig. 2.17 RP intervals in AVRT and AVNRT. AVRT tends to have longer RP interval compared to AVNRT, so the P wave is more likely to be seen in the ST segment rather than immediately next to or within the QRS complex. (Source: https://ecgwaves.com/wp-content/uploads/2016/09/ecg-rp-interval-tachycardia-tachyarrhythmia-avnrt-avrt-p-wave.jpg)

- Abnormal rhythms passing through a diseased His-Purkinje System, such as in bundle branch block.

VENTRICULAR TACHYCARDIA
Definition
Ventricular tachycardia (monomorphic VT) is a regular tachycardia arising from the ventricles. It can be classified as:

- Non-sustained VT: lasts for at least 3 beats and resolves spontaneously in less than 30 s
- Sustained VT: lasts for longer than 30 s

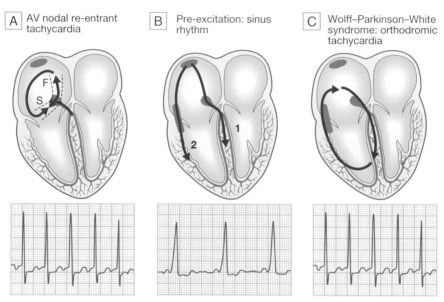

Fig. 2.18 AVNRT compared to accessory pathways and AVRTs.

(A) AVNRT occurs via two right atrial AV nodal input pathways: the slow (S) and fast (F) pathways. Antegrade conduction occurs via the slow pathway; the wavefront enters the AV node and passes into the ventricles, at the same time re-entering the atria via the fast pathway.

(B) In sinus rhythm with accessory pathways, the ventricles are depolarised through (1) the AV node and (2) the accessory pathway, producing an ECG with a short PR interval and broadened QRS complexes; the characteristic slurring of the upstroke of the QRS complex is known as a delta wave. The degree of pre-excitation (the proportion of activation passing down the accessory pathway) and therefore the ECG appearances may vary a lot, and at times the ECG can look normal.

(C) Orthodromic tachycardia is the most common form of tachycardia in Wolff-Parkinson-White syndrome (symptomatic AVRT). The re-entry circuit passes retrogradely through the accessory pathway and then antegradely through the AV node. The ventricles are therefore depolarised in the normal way, producing a narrow-complex tachycardia that is indistinguishable from other forms of supraventricular tachycardia.

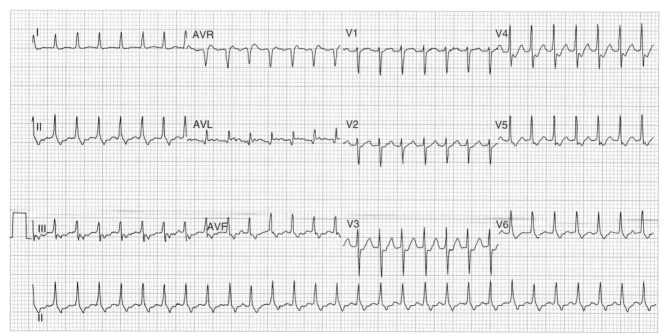

Fig. 2.19 AVRT. The rate is 174bpm and regular. There are no visible P waves. The QRS complex is narrow, and T wave is normal in morphology. There is a negative deflection after the QRS complex in the inferior leads (II, III, aVF) and in V4-V6, suggestive of retrograde P waves.

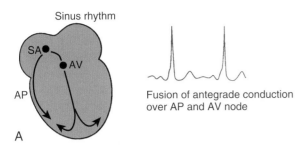

Sinus rhythm

Fusion of antegrade conduction over AP and AV node

A

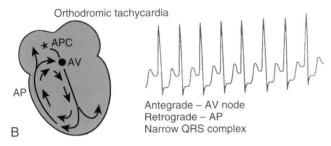

Orthodromic tachycardia

Antegrade – AV node
Retrograde – AP
Narrow QRS complex

B

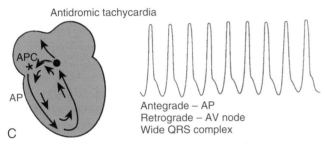

Antidromic tachycardia

Antegrade – AP
Retrograde – AV node
Wide QRS complex

C

Fig. 2.20 Orthodromic and antidromic circuits in AVRT. Schematic representation of possible rhythms in a patient with an accessory atrioventricular (AV) bypass tract.

(A) During sinus rhythm, the ventricles are activated by conduction over the accessory pathway (AP) and through the normal AV conduction system. This produces a short PR interval and delta waves (the slurred upstroke at the beginning of the QRS complex; see Chapter 10).
(B) During orthodromic re-entrant tachycardia, antegrade conduction occurs through the AVN and normal conduction system, whereas retrograde conduction occurs via the accessory pathway. The resulting tachycardia has a narrow QRS morphology. Retrograde P waves may be seen after the QRS complex.
(C) During antidromic re-entrant tachycardia, retrograde conduction occurs through the AVN and normal conduction system, whereas antegrade conduction occurs via the accessory pathway. The resulting tachycardia has a wide QRS complex because the normal conduction system is not used to initiate ventricular depolarisation (Source: Kern, M. J., Sorajja, P., Lim, M. J. (2015). The electrophysiology laboratory and electrophysiologic procedures. In: *The Cardiac Catheterization Handbook*, 6th ed. Elsevier.)

ECG Findings

VT is characterised by regular, broad QRS complexes, usually lasting longer than 140 ms (Fig. 2.25). P and T waves are usually difficult to distinguish in VT. P waves, if visible, will be dissociated from the QRS complexes (atrioventricular dissociation) in most situations.

VT can be difficult to distinguish from a supraventricular tachycardia with conduction abnormality (such as bundle branch block) or pre-excitation (such as Wolff–Parkinson–White syndrome) by ECG alone (Box 2.3). In these cases, it may be helpful to compare the current ECG to a previous trace in sinus

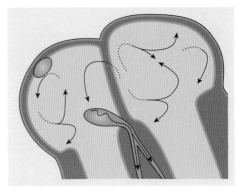

Fig. 2.21 AF has multiple activation wavelets propagating chaotically in the atria, leading to loss of organised contraction. (Source: Atrial tachycardias and atrial flutter. In: *Cardiology*, 3rd ed.)

rhythm to look for pre-existing bundle branch block or pre-excitation.

Clinical Significance

In most cases VT is due to ischaemic heart disease, although it can also be due to cardiomyopathies, inherited conditions, electrolyte disturbance or without a known cause (idiopathic VT). It is a cause of cardiac arrest and sudden cardiac death.

Management

The management of VT in an acute situation depends on if a patient has a pulse and is haemodynamically stable. Occasionally, VT can be well tolerated; if so, intravenous antiarrhythmics could be used. These patients could be considered for an implantable cardioverter defibrillator.

VT associated with haemodynamic compromise should undergo an emergency cardioversion. Pulseless VT is a form of cardiac arrest and should be managed as per advanced life support algorithm.

IRREGULAR BROAD-COMPLEX TACHYCARDIA

VENTRICULAR FIBRILLATION
Definition

Ventricular fibrillation (VF) is chaotic and irregular depolarisation of the ventricles that leads to cardiac arrest.

ECG Findings

There is no coordinated depolarisation of the ventricles. This results in a highly irregular baseline with no clear QRS complex and no identifiable pattern (Fig. 2.27).

Clinical Significance

VF is most commonly associated with ischaemic heart disease, including acute myocardial infarction, but may also be secondary to other cardiac diseases (such as heart failure and channelopathies) or metabolic disturbances.

Management

VF, along with pulseless VT, are shockable rhythms and should be managed by early cardiopulmonary

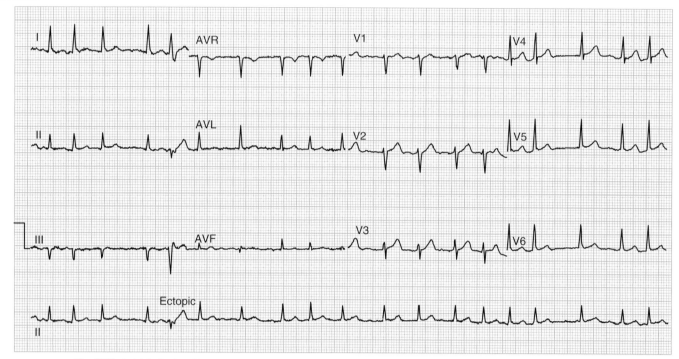

Fig. 2.22 Atrial fibrillation. The rhythm is irregular and no clear P waves are visible. The fifth ventricular beat seen on this ECG is an ectopic beat (see later in this chapter, Ectopic Beats).

resuscitation and defibrillation according to basic and advanced life support protocols. Survivors of a cardiac arrest due to VF should be considered for emergency coronary angiography and, depending on the aetiology, an implantable cardioverter defibrillator.

TORSADES DE POINTES VENTRICULAR TACHYCARDIA

Definition

Torsades de pointes is an uncommon type of VT (also referred to as polymorphic VT) that usually occurs in the context of a prolonged QT interval.

ECG Findings

Torsades de pointes ('twisting of points') is named for the characteristic appearance on ECG of an increasing and decreasing QRS complex amplitude, which may appear to be 'twisting' around the isoelectric line. There is a variable QRS morphology and complexes may appear to change from pointing upwards to pointing downwards (Fig. 2.28). Previous ECGs may show evidence of a prolonged QT interval or signs of electrolyte disturbance.

Clinical Significance

Although uncommon, it is important to recognise torsades de pointes as the acute treatment differs from that of other forms of VT. Although torsades de pointes is seen in the context of inherited long QT syndrome, it most commonly occurs due to drugs that prolong the QT interval, including antiarrhythmic drugs, antipsychotics, macrolide antibiotics (e.g. erythromycin) and tricyclic antidepressants.

Risk factors	Score	CHADS2-VASc score and annual stroke risk (%)
Congestive heart failure	1	Score 1 = 1.3
Hypertension	1	2 = 2.2
Age > 75 years	2	3 = 3.2
Diabetes mellitus	1	4 = 4
Stroke/TIA/systemic embolism	2	5 = 6.7
Vascular disease	1	6 = 9.8
Age 65 to 74 years	1	7 = 9.6
Sex (female)	1	8 = 6.7
		9 = 15.2

Fig. 2.23 CHA_2DS_2-VASc score and associated annual stroke risk. TIA, transient ischaemic attack.

Management

Torsades de pointes should be treated with emergency cardioversion. Antiarrhythmics should not be given for this as most prolong the QT interval. Further options include intravenous magnesium and rapid atrial/ventricular pacing. In addition, drugs that may prolong the QT interval should be stopped and electrolyte disturbances, if present, should be treated rapidly.

BRADYCARDIAS

Bradycardias can be physiological, such as in sinus bradycardia, or pathological. Pathological bradycardias are principally divided into 2 types:
- Disease of the sinus node (not generating impulses) – Sinus Node disease
- Disease of the atrioventricular node (not conducting impulses from atria to the ventricles) – Atrioventricular Node disease (see Chapter 5).

ECG clues suggestive of VT vs other rhythms with BBB (see Box 2.3):
- Atrioventricular dissociation
- Fusion or capture beats
- Positive and negative chest lead concordance

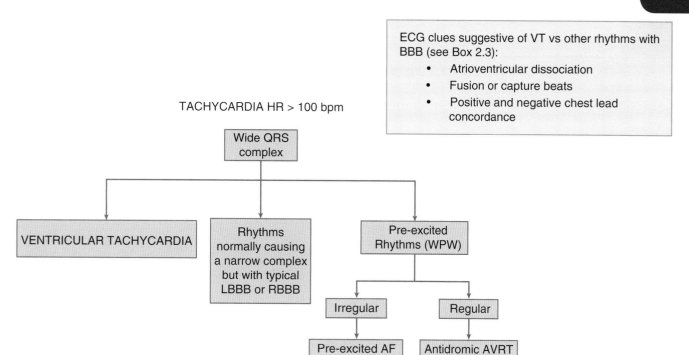

TACHYCARDIA HR > 100 bpm

Wide QRS complex

VENTRICULAR TACHYCARDIA

Rhythms normally causing a narrow complex but with typical LBBB or RBBB

Pre-excited Rhythms (WPW)

Irregular

Regular

Pre-excited AF

Antidromic AVRT

Fig. 2.24 Differential diagnosis for broad complex tachycardia.

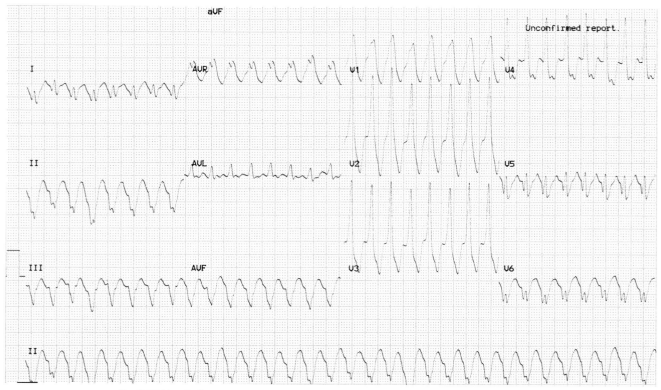

Fig. 2.25 Ventricular tachycardia. There is regular rapid tachycardia with wide QRS complexes.

SINUS BRADYCARDIA
Definition
Sinus bradycardia is defined as a sinus rhythm with a heart rate less than 60 bpm.

ECG Findings
Sinus bradycardia is characterised by a sinus rhythm (normal morphology and axis of P wave, QRS complex and T wave with normal intervals) with an R–R interval greater than five large squares in length (Fig. 2.29).

Clinical Significance
Sinus bradycardia can be physiological, especially among healthy young people and athletes. It may also occur during sleep.

Alternatively, sinus bradycardia can manifest secondary to systemic pathology, such as hypothyroidism. More

Box **2.3** How to Differentiate Supraventricular Tachycardia (SVT) with Aberrant Conduction from VT

Differentiating SVT with aberrant conduction (e.g. bundle branch block, AVRT) from VT can be difficult as they both produce wide-complex tachycardias.

There are several clues that suggest ventricular tachycardia:

- Compare ECG with previous ECGs in sinus rhythm to check for aberrant conduction
- Absence of left bundle branch block (notched R waves in V_4–V_6 and deep S waves in V_1–V_3) or right bundle branch block (RSR' pattern in V_1–V_3 and slurred S wave in V_5–V_6) characteristics (see Chapter 6)
- Extreme axis deviation (see Chapter 3)
- Very broad QRS complexes (longer than 160 ms width; >4 small squares)
- Concordance in the precordial leads. This refers to the presence of only dominant positive (positive concordance) or negative (negative concordance) QRS complexes in all the chest leads, rather than having the normal gradual transition from negative to positive QRS complexes from V_1 to V_6
- Presence of capture beats (Fig. 2.26). These are beats from a supraventricular source that have depolarised ("captured") the ventricles, producing narrow QRS complexes

Capture beat:

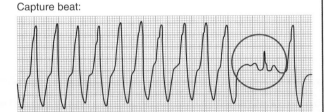

Fusion beat:

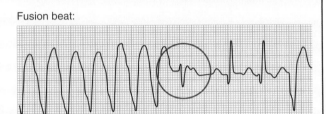

Fig. 2.26 Capture beats and fusion beats in VT. (Source: Ventricular arrhythmias and sudden cardiac death 2058-5349)

- Presence of fusion beats. These are P waves that occur at the same time as the QRS complex, producing a hybrid complex

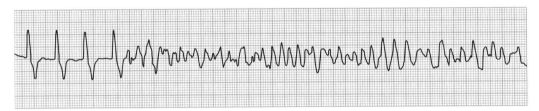

Fig. 2.27 Ventricular fibrillation. VT (on the left of the ECG) suddenly degenerates into VF (on the right of the ECG). (Source: Bassert, J. M. (2022). Emergency nursing. In: *McCurnin's Clinical Textbook for Veterinary Technicians*, 7th ed. Elsevier.)

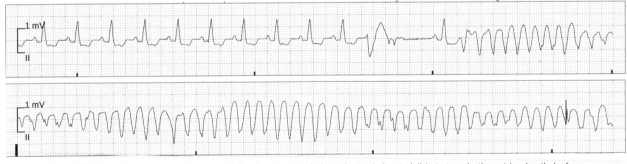

Fig. 2.28 Torsades de pointes triggered following an ectopic beat (ectopic beat visible in top rhythm strip shortly before rhythm changes to wide QRS complexes).

commonly, sinus bradycardia arises due to treatment with negatively chronotropic drugs, such as beta-blockers.

It is important to consider damage or degeneration of the SAN as a cause of bradycardia (see sick sinus syndrome, below).

Management

Treatment for sinus bradycardia is usually unnecessary unless the patient is symptomatic.

If symptoms such as dizziness, syncope or shortness of breath are present, the first step should be to identify and manage the cause of the bradycardia; for example, by stopping the offending medication or treating the underlying pathology. Administration of atropine or pacing may be necessary if the bradycardia does not respond to treatment.

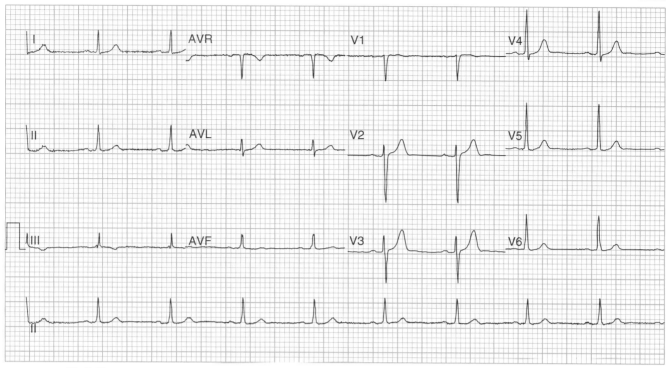

Fig. 2.29 Sinus bradycardia. The heart rate is ~54 bpm. The rhythm is regular with normal P waves and narrow QRS complexes.

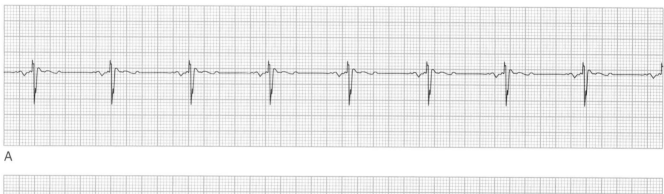

A

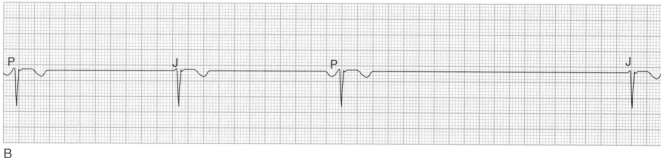

B

Fig. 2.30 Sick sinus syndrome – sinus arrest. (A) ECG showing normal sinus rhythm, where a P wave precedes each QRS complex. (B) A patient with sick sinus syndrome. The ECG shows sinus arrest with only occasional sinus P waves (labelled P). Due to the absence of P waves, a junctional escape rhythm (labelled J) can be observed. (Source: Kumar, P., Clark, M. (2017). Cardiovascular disease. In: *Kumar & Clark's Clinical Medicine*, 9th ed. Elsevier.)

SINUS NODE DISEASE

Definition

Also known as sick sinus syndrome, sinus node disease describes aberrant function of the SAN which may manifest as sinus bradycardia, sinus arrest (pauses of ≥3 s), sinus node exit block (failure of the SAN impulse to enter the atria) or tachycardia–bradycardia syndrome.

ECG Findings

Sick sinus syndrome may manifest on ECG as sinus bradycardia with a normal morphology but a rate of <60 bpm; the sinus bradycardia in sick sinus syndrome is one that is inappropriate (e.g. in a patient who is not athletic without hypothyroidism) and not caused by medication. Sinus arrest and exit block will be visible as pauses with no P waves present (Fig. 2.30). Tachycardia–bradycardia syndrome is a manifestation of sick sinus syndrome that refers to alternate runs of atrial tachyarrhythmia (such as AF) and bradycardia, often with sinus pauses in between (Fig. 2.31).

Clinical Significance

Sick sinus syndrome is most frequently caused by idiopathic fibrosis of the SAN but it can also be precipitated by ischaemia, metabolic disturbances or medications, including beta-blockers, calcium channel blockers and digoxin. The risk of sick sinus syndrome increases with age.

Management

If patients are asymptomatic, treatment is usually unnecessary.

Symptomatic, haemodynamically unstable patients must be managed as an emergency using atropine, adrenaline or temporary pacing. For definitive management, the first-line management of sick sinus syndrome is correcting reversible causes; if no reversible cause is identified, permanent pacing is necessary.

ESCAPE RHYTHMS

Definition

An escape rhythm occurs when an ectopic site in the atria, AVN or ventricles takes control of the heart rate from the SAN (due to either decreased SAN automaticity or AVN block).

ECG Findings

ECG findings depend on the origin of the escape rhythm, which may be atrial, junctional or ventricular.

Atrial Escape Rhythm. Atrial escape rhythms arise from the atria but not from the SAN itself. This will produce a narrow QRS complex with a preceding P wave, albeit of a different shape to the usual P waves produced by the SAN (Fig. 2.32).

Junctional Escape Rhythm. Junctional escape rhythms arise around the AVN and will normally have a narrow QRS complex (as signals pass through the His–Purkinje system) without a preceding P wave. The P wave may be absent, occur after the QRS complex or be completely dissociated from the QRS complex (Fig. 2.33). The rate is usually around 40–50 bpm.

Ventricular Escape Rhythm. Ventricular escape rhythms are characterised by broad QRS complexes (as ventricular

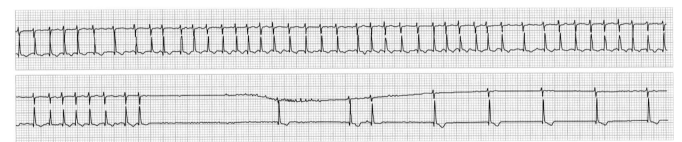

Fig. 2.31 (A, B) Tachycardia–bradycardia syndrome. The rhythm strip shows AF that terminates in a prolonged pause followed by a slow junctional rhythm. (Source: Das, M., Zipes, D. (2021). Sinus node dysfunction. In: *Electrocardiography of Arrhythmias: A Comprehensive Review.* Elsevier.)

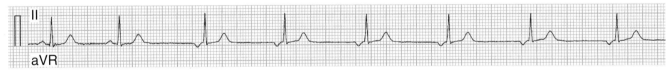

Fig. 2.32 Atrial escape rhythm. Note the change in P-wave polarity from positive to negative in lead II after the second beat. This shift from sinus bradycardia here to an atrial escape rhythm may occur as a normal (physiologic) variant. (Source: Goldberger, A., Goldberger, Z., Shvilkin, A. (2017). ECG basics. In: *Goldberger's Clinical Electrocardiography: A Simplified Approach*, 9th ed. Elsevier.)

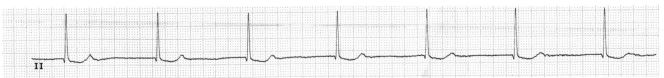

Fig. 2.33 Junctional escape rhythm. P waves are not clearly visible on this rhythm strip.

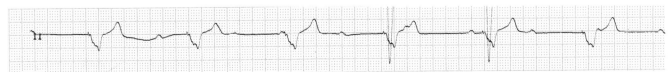

Fig. 2.34 Third-degree heart block with a ventricular escape rhythm. There is no electrical connection between the atria and ventricles, so ventricular escape rhythms initiate ventricular depolarisation. There is no relation between the P waves and QRS complexes.

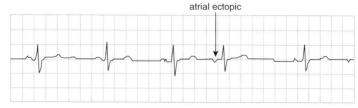

Fig. 2.35 Atrial ectopic beat. A premature atrial beat fires an abnormally shaped P wave (with arrow) and a normal QRS complex. A compensatory pause follows. (Source: Churchhouse, A., Ormerod, J. O. M., Horton-Szar, D. (2018). Supraventricular tachyarrhythmias. In: *Crash Course: Cardiology*, 4th ed. Elsevier.)

depolarisation occurs without the use of the rapid and efficient His–Purkinje pathway) with abnormal T waves. P waves may be absent or dissociated from QRS complexes (Fig. 2.34). The ventricular rate is usually around 30 bpm. Ventricular escape rhythms usually occur due to AVN block (third-degree heart block).

Clinical Significance

Escape rhythms most commonly arise due to dysfunction of either the SAN or AVN. In these scenarios (such as in third-degree heart block), the escape rhythm is generally vital to prevent fatal asystole.

Management

Escape rhythms are a manifestation of significant bradycardias. This requires treatment similar to sick sinus syndrome – manage haemodynamically unstable patients as an emergency, and definitive treatment is permanent pacing if no reversible cause is identified.

ECTOPIC BEATS

Definition

An ectopic beat is an early beat caused by depolarisation of an ectopic pacemaker site before the next SAN depolarisation. They are sometimes referred to as extrasystoles or premature complexes.

ECG Findings

The characteristics of the ectopic beat will depend on its origin:

Atrial Ectopic. The P wave (which may manifest as a peaked T wave) will typically have an abnormal morphology (Fig. 2.35). The ectopic beat usually conducts to the ventricles with normal QRS morphology, although may sometimes fail to conduct (or does so with a broad QRS complex) if the conduction system is still refractory. This beat will also depolarise the SAN, causing the next beat to be delayed.

Junctional Ectopic. These ectopics arise from around the AVN. There will be a narrow QRS complex that is not preceded by a P wave (although a P wave may be

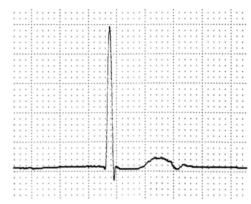

Fig. 2.36 Junctional ectopic beat. Junctional beat with a retrograde P wave visible just after the T wave.

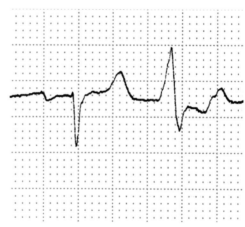

Fig. 2.37 Ventricular ectopic beat. A normal sinus beat is followed by a ventricular ectopic beat.

visible after the QRS) (Fig. 2.36). As with atrial ectopics, depolarisation of the SAN causes the next beat to be delayed.

Ventricular Ectopic. The QRS complex will be broad and followed by an abnormal T wave, and there is no preceding P wave (Fig. 2.37).

Atrial and ventricular ectopics may occur in isolation or may present in patterns. There may be two or three ectopics in a row (couplets or triplets, respectively) or they may occur in alternating beats. If every

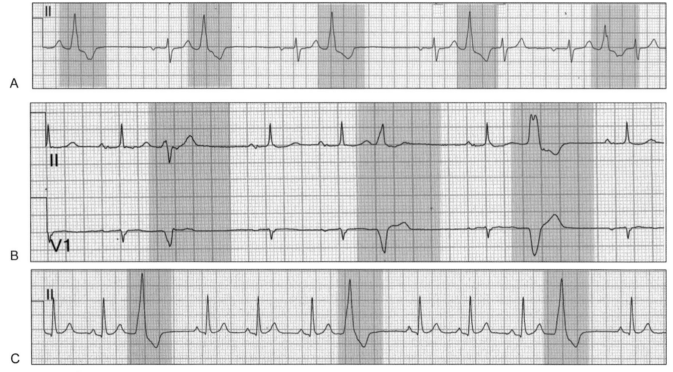

Fig. 2.38 Bigeminy, trigeminy and quadrigeminy. Ventricular ectopic beats are highlighted. (A) Bigeminy: a ventricular ectopic occurs after every sinus beat. (B) Trigeminy: a ventricular ectopic beat occurs after every two sinus beats. (C) Quadrigeminy: a ventricular ectopic beat occurs after every three sinus beats. (Source: The Electrocardiographic Footprints of Ventricular Ectopy. 1443-9506)

other beat is an ectopic, this is known as bigeminy; one in every three as trigeminy, or one in every four as quadrigeminy (Fig. 2.38).

Clinical Significance
Ectopic beats are common and of limited clinical significance, although they may cause the sensation of the heart skipping a beat. They tend to be more common following stimulation of the heart, such as by sympathomimetic drugs. They may also occur in the setting of cardiac diseases or electrolyte abnormalities.

The majority are benign and, in the absence of underlying cardiac disease, no specific treatment is required. However, if the ectopic burden is high or if there is evidence of structural heart disease then treatment could be considered.

Management
Symptomatic ectopics are common and are a cause of significant anxiety. Reassurance is usually all that is necessary. However, drugs could be considered if patients experience debilitating symptoms.

Key Points
1. Normal heart rate is 60–100 bpm
2. Normal rhythm is sinus, which refers to P waves followed by a QRS complex
3. Regular narrow-complex tachycardias include:
   (a) Sinus tachycardia
   (b) AT
   (c) Atrial flutter
   (d) AVNRT
   (e) AVRT
4. Irregular narrow-complex tachycardias include:
   (a) AF
   (b) Atrial flutter with variable atrioventricular block
5. Regular broad-complex tachycardias include:
   (a) VT
   (b) SVT with bundle branch block
6. Irregular broad-complex tachycardias include:
   (a) VF
   (b) Torsades de pointes VT
   (c) Any of the above irregular narrow-complex tachycardias in combination with bundle branch block
7. Bradycardias include:
   (a) Sinus bradycardia
   (b) Sick sinus syndrome
   (c) Escape rhythms
   (d) Atrioventricular node disease causing atrioventricular block

   Ectopic beats are a common finding and may be atrial, junctional or ventricular in origin.

FURTHER READING

Al-Khatib, S.M., et al., 2018. 2017 AHA/ACC/HRS guideline for management of patients with ventricular arrhythmias and the prevention of sudden cardiac death. Circulation 138 (13), e272–e391.

Hampton, J.R., Hampton, J., 2019. The ECG Made Easy. 2019.

January Craig, T., et al., 2014. 2014 AHA/ACC/HRS guideline for the management of patients with atrial fibrillation: executive summary. J. Am. Coll. Cardoil. 64 (21), 2246–2280.

Kim, D., et al., 2010. Calcium dynamics and the mechanisms of atrioventricular junctional rhythm. J. Am. Coll. Cardoil. 56 (10), 805–812.

Kirchhof, P., et al., 2016. 2016 ESC guidelines for the management of atrial fibrillation developed in collaboration with EACTS. Eur. Heart J. 37 (38), 2893–2962.

Kwaku, K.F., Josephson, M.E., 2002. Typical AVNRT – an update on mechanisms and therapy. Card. Electrophysiol. Rev. 6 (4), 414–421.

Lloyd-Jones, D.M., et al., 2004. Lifetime risk for development of atrial fibrillation: the framingham heart study. Circulation 110 (9), 1042–1046.

Olshansky, B., Sullivan, R.M., 2013. Inappropriate sinus tachycardia. J. Am. Coll. Cardoil. 61 (8), 793–801.

Page, R.L., et al., 2016. 2015 ACC/AHA/HRS guideline for the management of adult patients with supraventricular tachycardia. J. Am. Coll. Cardoil. 67 (13), e27–e115.

Yap, Y.G., Camm, A.J., 2003. Drug induced qt prolongation and torsades de pointes. Heart 89 (11), 1363–1372.

3

The Cardiac Axis

OVERVIEW

DEFINITION

The cardiac axis describes the average direction of the wave of depolarisation of the atria and ventricles as viewed in the coronal plane (i.e. as viewed from the front). It should be noted that the cardiac axis by convention usually refers to the directions of the QRS complexes. The direction of the cardiac axis can be affected by various pathologies.

ELECTROPHYSIOLOGY

The principle is that a wave of depolarisation travelling in the same direction as the ECG lead will cause a positive deflection on the ECG, while a wave travelling in the opposite direction to the direction of the lead will produce a negative deflection (Fig. 3.1). A wave travelling perpendicular to the lead will produce a deflection that is equally positive and negative (a biphasic deflection) or will produce a very small deflection.

The direction of the wave of depolarisation, like the amplitude, can be affected by the mass of depolarising tissue. An increase in muscle mass, such as hypertrophy, will pull the cardiac axis towards the affected side as more electrical potential is being generated on that

side of the heart. On the other hand, a loss of mass, such as myocardial scarring, will push the axis away from the affected side. The anatomical position of the heart can also affect the direction of depolarisation and, therefore, the axis.

INTERPRETATION

The cardiac axis can be determined by reviewing the limb leads. When viewing the heart face on, the direction that each of the limb leads 'looks at' the heart can be described by the angle they make to lead I (Fig. 3.2). Lead I is therefore considered to be at an angle of 0°. Lead II is at 60° and lead III 120°. This system of identifying the angle of ECG leads is referred to as the hexaxial reference system.

The normal cardiac axis is between −30° and +90° (Figs 3.3 and 3.4). A cardiac axis less than −30° is referred to as left-axis deviation, while an axis greater than +90° is considered right-axis deviation. A cardiac axis of between −90° and 180° is considered extreme axis deviation (also known as a northwest axis).

To determine the cardiac axis, the QRS complexes of the limb leads need to be reviewed. Positive QRS complexes (R dominant) indicate that the direction of

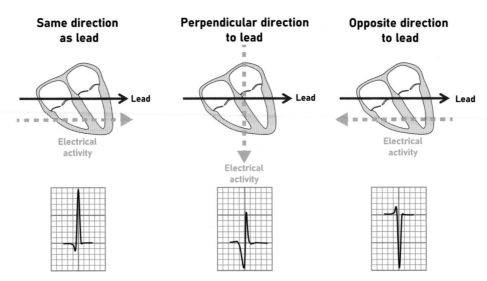

Fig. 3.1 The direction of impulse relative to the lead affects the direction and size of the ECG tracing deflection.

depolarisation is in the direction of the lead, while negative QRS complexes (S dominant) suggest depolarisation is in the opposite direction to the lead. For example, as shown in Fig. 3.5, if the QRS complex is more positive than negative in lead I, the cardiac axis must be somewhere in the blue semicircle (i.e. in the direction of the lead). This is true of any lead: if the QRS complex is more positive than negative, the direction of electrical activity must be in the direction of the lead. If the QRS complex in a lead is predominantly negative, the direction of the QRS complex must be in the opposite direction to the lead.

Any of the limb leads can be used to determine the cardiac axis, although using a combination of leads I and II is the quickest way of checking if it is normal (Table 3.1) as they cover the normal range (−30 to +90°). If both leads I and II are positive, the cardiac axis falls within the −30° to +90° bracket and is, therefore, a normal axis. If one or both of leads I and II are negative, the axis must be abnormal as it would be outside the normal −30 to +90° range. If both are negative, lead aVF should be reviewed to differentiate between right-axis deviation and extreme axis deviation.

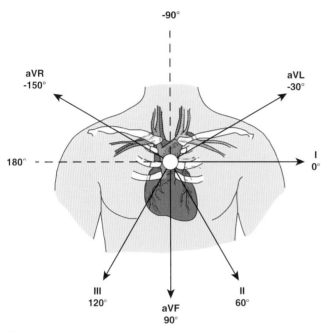

Fig. 3.2 Cardiac axis. The cardiac axis conventionally refers to the direction of depolarisation in the coronal plane. This can be determined using the limb leads. (Source: Adapted from Griffin Perry, A., Potter, P. A., Ostendorf, W., Laplante, N. (2021). Health assessment. In: *Clinical Nursing Skills & Techniques*, 10th ed. Elsevier.)

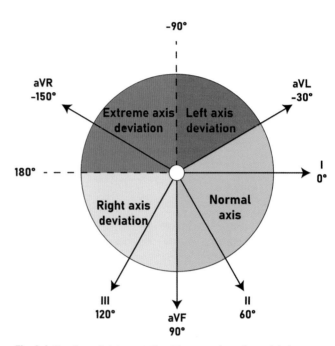

Fig. 3.4 Cardiac axis interpretation. The normal cardiac axis is between −30° and +90°.

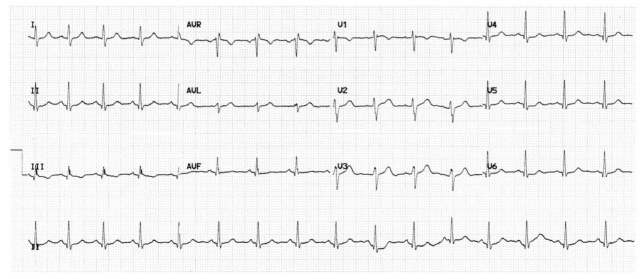

Fig. 3.3 Normal sinus rhythm with a normal cardiac axis. QRS complexes in lead II and aVF are both positive, indicating a cardiac axis that is between −30° and +90°.

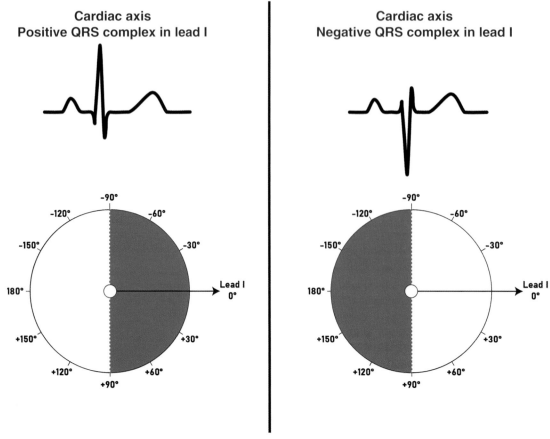

Fig. 3.5 An example of interpreting direction in lead I. A positive QRS complex in lead I means that the overall electrical activity is between –90° and +90° (left image). On the other hand, a negative QRS complex means that electrical activity lies between +90° and –90° (right image).

| Table **3.1** | Summary of possible cardiac axes when reviewing if QRS complexes are positive or negative in leads I and II[a] |

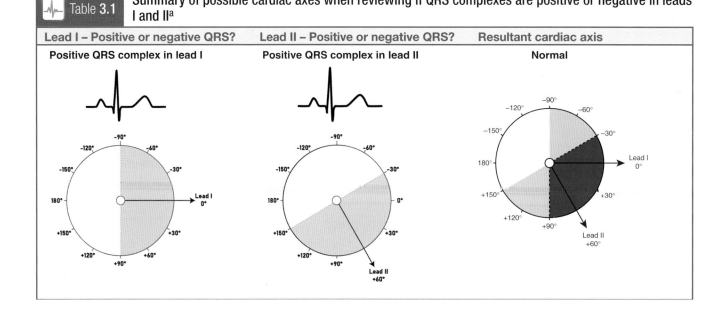

Table 3.1 Summary of possible cardiac axes when reviewing if QRS complexes are positive or negative in leads I and II[a]—con'd

Lead I – Positive or negative QRS?	Lead II – Positive or negative QRS?	Resultant cardiac axis
Positive QRS complex in lead I	Negative QRS complex in lead II	Left-axis deviation
Negative QRS complex in lead I	Positive QRS complex in lead II	Right-axis deviation
Negative QRS complex in lead I	Negative QRS complex in lead II	Right-axis deviation/extreme axis deviation

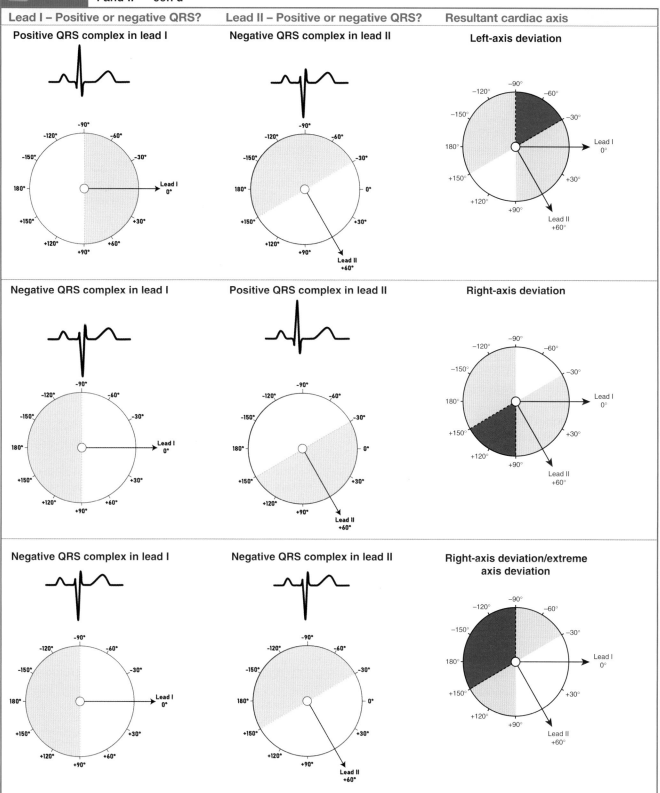

[a]Note that if both leads I and II have negative QRS complexes, the cardiac axis may be either right-axis deviation or extreme axis deviation; to differentiate, review lead aVF: positive QRS complexes indicate right-axis deviation, while negative complexes suggest extreme axis deviation.

AXIS DEVIATION

LEFT-AXIS DEVIATION

Definition
Left-axis deviation occurs when the cardiac axis is between –30° and –90°.

ECG Findings
The QRS complex will be positive in lead I but more negative than positive in lead II, and negative in lead III and aVF (Fig. 3.6). The ECG may otherwise be normal or there may be other abnormalities present that give an indication of the underlying pathology.

Clinical Significance
Left-axis deviation may be a normal variant in an otherwise normal ECG. However, it may also be associated with several underlying conditions:
- Hypertensive heart disease
- Defects of the conduction system: left anterior fascicular block and left bundle branch block (see Chapter 6) are common causes of left-axis deviation
- Left ventricular hypertrophy: this can be associated with other ECG changes, such as left ventricular strain pattern (see Chapter 6)
- Inferior myocardial infarction may cause left-axis deviation due to loss of electrical activity of the inferior myocardium
- Wolff–Parkinson–White syndrome may cause left-axis deviation if there is a right-sided accessory pathway (see Chapter 10)
- Ventricular pacing: a ventricular pacing lead in the inferior right ventricle will cause a left-axis deviation (see Chapter 10)

Management
Although there is no specific treatment for left-axis deviation, an incidental finding on ECG may prompt further investigation, particularly if there are signs or symptoms of cardiac pathology.

RIGHT-AXIS DEVIATION

Definition
Right-axis deviation occurs when the cardiac axis is between +90° and 180°.

ECG Findings
The QRS complex in right-axis deviation will be negative in lead I and positive in leads II and aVF (Fig. 3.7). The ECG may otherwise be normal or demonstrate additional pathology.

Clinical Significance
As with left-axis deviation, right-axis deviation may be a normal variant (especially in infants) or may be the result of an underlying pathology:
- Acute right-axis deviation may be a sign of a pulmonary embolism or other acute lung disease.
- Right ventricular hypertrophy, usually due to chronic lung pathology or congenital heart disorders, is a common cause of right-axis deviation.
- Left posterior fascicular block may cause the cardiac axis to deviate to the right (see Chapter 6).
- Lateral myocardial infarction due to loss of viable cardiac muscle in the left ventricle may cause right-axis deviation.
- Wolff–Parkinson–White syndrome may cause right-axis deviation if there is a left-sided accessory pathway (see Chapter 10).

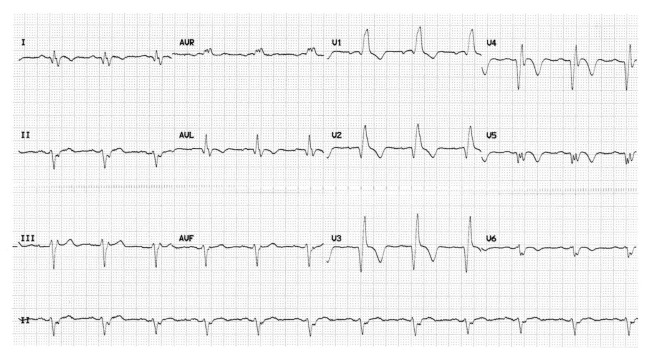

Fig. 3.6 Left-axis deviation as a result of bifascicular block. The QRS complex in lead I is predominantly positive while lead II has a negative QRS complex.

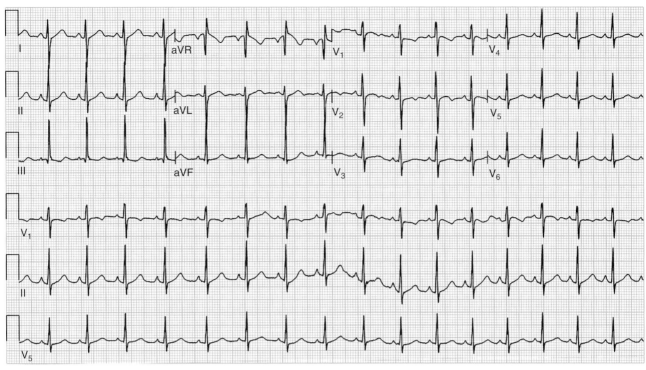

Fig. 3.7 Right-axis deviation. Right-axis deviation as a result of left posterior fascicular block. The QRS complex in lead I is negative while lead II has a positive QRS complex. (Source: Olshansky, B., et al. (2016). Bradyarrhythmias – conduction system abnormalities. In: *Arrhythmia Essentials*, 2nd ed. Elsevier.)

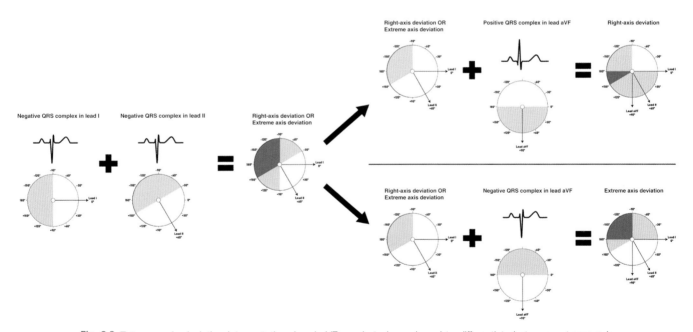

Fig. 3.8 Extreme axis deviation interpretation. Lead aVF needs to be reviewed to differentiate between extreme axis deviation and right-axis deviation if leads I and II are negative.

Management

As with left-axis deviation, there is no specific treatment for right-axis deviation but it may suggest an underlying pathology which could potentially be treated.

EXTREME AXIS DEVIATION

Definition

Also known as a 'northwest axis', extreme axis deviation is defined as a cardiac axis of –90° to 180° (Fig. 3.8).

ECG Findings

Negative QRS complexes in leads I, II and aVF indicate an extreme axis deviation (Fig. 3.9). Lead aVR will also be positive.

Clinical Significance

Extreme axis deviation is always abnormal and is usually caused by severe hyperkalaemia, ventricular tachycardia or cardiac pacing, although

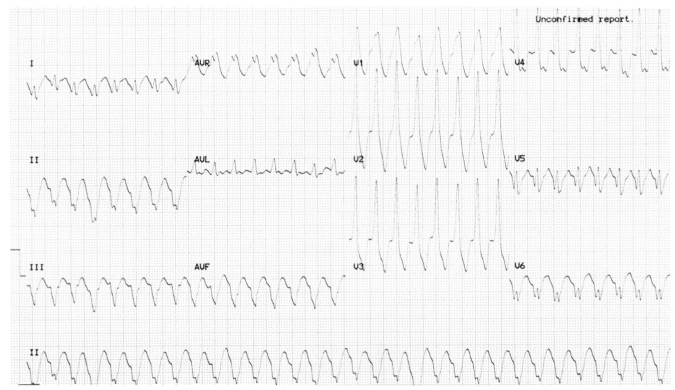

Fig. 3.9 Extreme axis deviation. Negative QRS complexes in leads I, II and aVF, and positive QRS complexes in lead aVR due to Ventricular Tachycardia.

it can also arise due to severe right ventricular hypertrophy.

In a broad-complex tachycardia, the presence of an extreme axis deviation is highly suggestive of a ventricular arrhythmia, as opposed to a supraventricular tachycardia with a conduction defect.

Management

There is no specific treatment for extreme axis deviation, although the underlying cause should be investigated and managed.

Key Points

1. The cardiac axis refers to the average direction of depolarisation in the coronal plane
2. A quick method of determining the cardiac axis is to review the QRS complexes in leads I, II and aVF. Positive QRS complexes in leads I and II indicate a normal cardiac axis
3. Normal cardiac axis: −30° to +90°
4. Left-axis deviation: −30° to −90°. Causes include:
   (a) Hypertensive heart disease
   (b) Left ventricular hypertrophy
   (c) Conduction defects, e.g. left anterior fascicular block, left bundle branch block
   (d) Inferior myocardial infarction
   (e) Wolff–Parkinson–White syndrome with right-sided accessory pathway
   (f) Ventricular pacing

5. Right-axis deviation: +90° to 180°. Causes include:
   (a) Acute lung disease, e.g. pulmonary embolism
   (b) Right ventricular hypertrophy
   (c) Left posterior fascicular block
   (d) Lateral myocardial infarction
   (e) Wolff–Parkinson–White syndrome with left-sided accessory pathway
6. Extreme axis deviation: −90° to 180°. Causes include:
   (a) Severe hyperkalaemia
   (b) Ventricular tachycardia
   (c) Cardiac pacing
   (d) Severe right ventricular hypertrophy

FURTHER READING

Aaronson, P.I., Ward, J.P.T., Connolly, M.J., 2020. The Cardiovascular System at a Glance. Wiley.

Grayzel, J., Neyshaboori, M., 1975. Left-axis deviation: etiologic factors in one-hundred patients. Am. Heart J. 89 (4), 419–427.

Hampton, J R., Hampton, J., 2019. The ECG Made Easy. Elsevier.

Steurer, G., et al., 1994. Cardiac depolarization and repolarization in Wolff–Parkinson–White syndrome. Am. Heart. J. 128 (5), 908–911.

P Wave

4

OVERVIEW

DEFINITION

The P wave corresponds to the depolarisation of the atria (Fig. 4.1).

ELECTROPHYSIOLOGY

Depolarisation of the heart begins at the sinoatrial node (SAN) in the right atrium and is rapidly conducted through atrial tissue to the atrioventricular node (AVN), where conduction is delayed.

The shape of the P wave is dependent on the muscle mass and size of the atria, and on the duration of the wave of depolarisation through the atria. Since there is much less muscle in the atria compared to the ventricles, the P wave appears much smaller on the ECG than on the QRS complex.

As the SAN is located in the right atrium, this begins depolarising before the left atrium. As a result, the first half of the P wave is mainly a measure of right atrial depolarisation, while the second half is a measure of the left atrium. The peak of the P wave represents the point where both left and right are depolarising simultaneously, therefore generating the strongest ECG signal (Fig. 4.2).

Note that although repolarisation of the atria occurs just as in the ventricles, it is usually not visible on ECG because of its low amplitude.

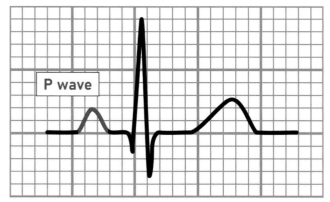

Fig. 4.1 Normal ECG waves in a heart beat. The P wave corresponds to atrial depolarisation.

INTERPRETATION

Normal

The normal P wave is less than 120 ms in duration (less than three small squares in length) and less than 2.5 mm in height (less than 2.5 small squares high).

Just like ventricular depolarisation, atrial depolarisation has a measurable axis, which is usually between −30° and +90°. As a result, the P wave is normally positive in all the limb leads except for aVR, where it is normally negative (Fig. 4.3).

The P wave is often biphasic in lead V_1. This is because the first half of atrial depolarisation (representing depolarisation of the right atrium) is directed anteriorly, while the second half (the left atrium) is directed posteriorly.

Absent P wave

An absent P wave (Fig. 4.4) suggests an abnormality of rhythm. This can either be atrial fibrillation or a defect of the SAN, such as sinus node arrest or exit block (see Chapter 2). The P wave may also appear absent in rapid tachycardias, where it may be concealed by the QRS complex.

Inverted P wave

An inverted P wave (Fig. 4.5) indicates that depolarisation of the atria originates from a focus outside the SAN. This may be an abnormal focus in the atria, such as atrial tachycardia (see Chapter 2), or due to retrograde conduction from the AVN or ventricles (which can lead to inverted P waves appearing after the QRS complex), such as in atrioventricular nodal re-entrant tachycardia (AVNRT) or a junctional rhythm (see Chapter 2).

Peaked P wave

A peaked P wave (more than 2.5 small squares in height) is indicative of prolonged conduction in the right atrium (Fig. 4.6), which is caused almost exclusively by right atrial enlargement, usually due to pulmonary hypertension (such as in cor

— Right atrium

— Left atrium

— ECG trace

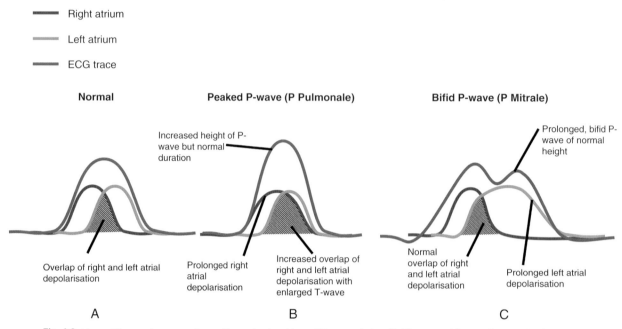

Normal

Peaked P-wave (P Pulmonale)

Bifid P-wave (P Mitrale)

Increased height of P-wave but normal duration

Prolonged, bifid P-wave of normal height

Overlap of right and left atrial depolarisation

Prolonged right atrial depolarisation

Increased overlap of right and left atrial depolarisation with enlarged T-wave

Normal overlap of right and left atrial depolarisation

Prolonged left atrial depolarisation

A   B   C

Fig. 4.2 Normal P wave in comparison with peaked and broad P waves in lead II. The normal P wave is a result of the left and right atrial signals partly overlapping (A). If the waves are closer together, the resultant P wave is shorter in duration but has a greater amplitude (peaked P wave; B). Conversely, if there is a delay in conduction, there is less overlap, producing a wave with longer width and shorter amplitude (prolonged P wave; image C).

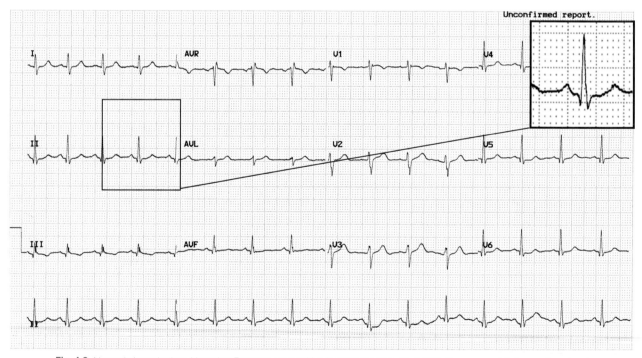

Fig. 4.3 Normal sinus rhythm. Note that P waves are positive in most leads except aVR. The zoomed-in image from lead II shows normal P-wave shape and duration.

pulmonale in chronic obstructive pulmonary disease). This sign is known as 'P pulmonale' and is due to a prolonged overlap of depolarisation in the left and right atria (Fig. 4.2) and is seen in lead II, III and aVF.

Prolonged or Bifid P Wave

A P wave of duration >120 ms, usually seen in lead II, is indicative of left atrial enlargement (Fig. 4.7). This is because of prolongation of the conduction through the left atrium causing a longer duration of the second

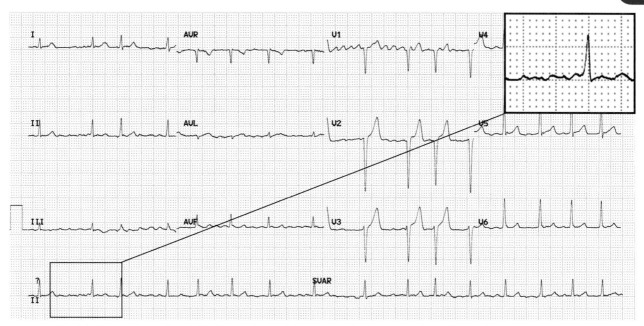

Fig. 4.4 Absent P wave in atrial fibrillation. Although there are deflections before the QRS complex, these are erratic in nature and do not form a clear P wave.

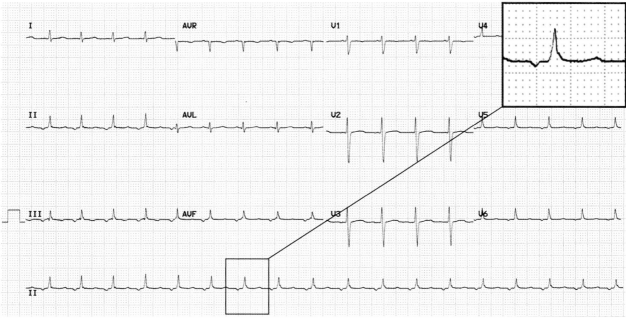

Fig. 4.5 Inverted P wave as seen in atrial tachycardia.

half of the P wave (Fig. 4.2). The depth of the second half of the P wave (reflecting left atrial activation) will also be greater in lead V_1. Often the P wave will become bifid, forming an M-shape. This sign is known as 'P mitrale' and can be due to hypertensive heart disease, heart failure and mitral valve disease.

Tall, Prolonged P Wave

Left and right atrial enlargement can coexist (bi-atrial enlargement), producing a tall and prolonged P wave (Fig. 4.8).

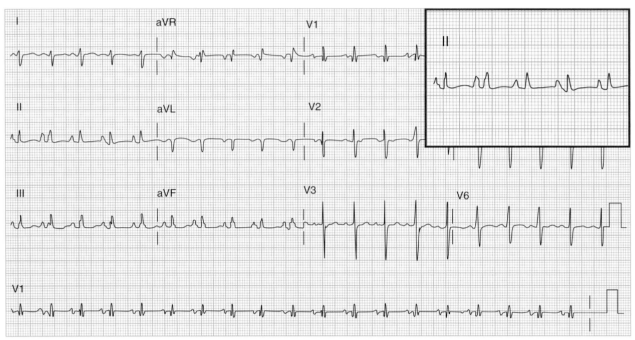

Fig. 4.6 Peaked P wave. Peaked P wave as seen in right atrial enlargement. (Source: Talley, N. J., O'Connor, S. (2016). The respiratory long case. In: *Examination Medicine: A Guide to Physician Training*, 8th ed. Elsevier.)

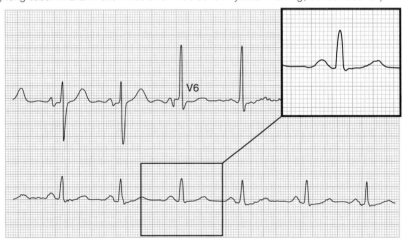

Fig. 4.7 Prolonged P wave as seen in left atrial enlargement.

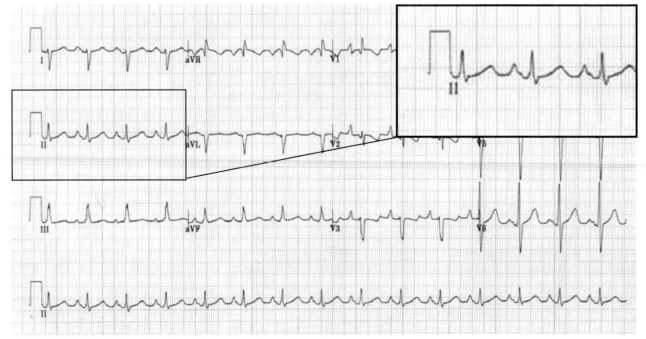

Fig. 4.8 Tall, prolonged P wave. ECG findings as seen in biatrial dilation. In this case, it is due to chronic heart disease with severe mitral regurgitation. (Source: Dougherty, S., et al. (2020). Clinical evaluation and diagnosis of rheumatic heart disease. In: *Acute Rheumatic Fever and Rheumatic Heart Disease*. Elsevier.)

Key Points

1. The P wave represents atrial depolarisation
2. Normal P waves are less than 120 ms (three small squares) in duration and less than 2.5 mm (2.5 small squares) in height
3. Absent P waves arise from: atrial fibrillation, sinus node arrest, exit block
4. Inverted P waves arise from: abnormal atrial focus (e.g. atrial tachycardia), retrograde conduction from AVN or ventricles (e.g. AVNRT)
5. Peaked P waves arise from right atrial enlargement
6. Prolonged or bifid P waves arise from left atrial enlargement
7. Peaked and prolonged P waves arise from bi-atrial enlargement

FURTHER READING

Camm, A.J., Lüscher, T.F., Serruys, P.W., 2009. The ESC Textbook of Cardiovascular Medicine. Oxford University Press, Oxford.

Meek, S., Morris, F., 2002. Introduction. II: Basic terminology. BMJ. 324 (7335), 470–473.

Thomas, J., Monaghan, T., 2014. Oxford Handbook of Clinical Examination and Practical Skills. Oxford University Press, Oxford.

OVERVIEW

DEFINITION

The PR interval is defined as the time interval between the start of the P wave and the beginning of the QRS complex (Fig. 5.1).

ELECTROPHYSIOLOGY

The PR interval represents the time taken for depolarisation to reach the ventricles from the sinoatrial node (SAN).

The SAN in the right atrium is the normal site of initiation of the heart beat. This depolarises the atria rapidly but not the ventricles, due to their separation by fibrous tissue (the cardiac skeleton).

Normally, the atrioventricular node (AVN) is the only electrical connection between the atria and ventricles. The AVN slows impulse conduction before activating the ventricles; this accounts for most of the delay between atrial and ventricular depolarisation, which is reflected in the PR interval (Figs 5.2 and 5.3).

INTERPRETATION

Normal PR Interval

The normal PR interval ranges from 120 to 200 ms (3–5 small squares). It is measured from the beginning of the P wave to the beginning of the QRS complex. The best leads for interpretation are where the P wave is clearest, which are usually leads II and V_1.

Long PR Interval

A PR interval longer than 200 ms is usually due to conduction delay in the AVN, termed 'first-degree AV block'.

Short PR Interval

A PR interval less than 120 ms is considered as short PR interval.

Causes include:
- Pre-excitation via an accessory pathway (see Chapter 10)
- Junctional rhythms, such as atrioventricular nodal re-entrant tachycardia (see Chapter 2)

PR Depression

PR depression, where the PR segment lies below the baseline, can be observed in cases of pericarditis (see Chapter 8).

ATRIOVENTRICULAR BLOCK

DEFINITION

Any interference in the conduction of impulses from the atria to the ventricles, particularly in the AVN or bundle of His, leads to AV block (also known as heart block), i.e. a PR interval longer than 200 ms. AV block can produce bradycardias. This results from either a delay or blockage of impulses and accounts for nearly 50% of all pacemaker implantations. It can be diagnosed by examining the relationship between the P waves and QRS complexes.

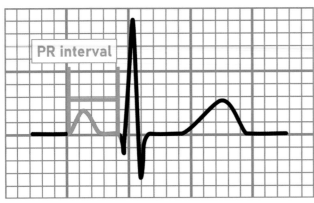

Fig. 5.1 Normal ECG waves in a heart beat. The PR interval is measured from the beginning of the P wave to the beginning of the QRS complex.

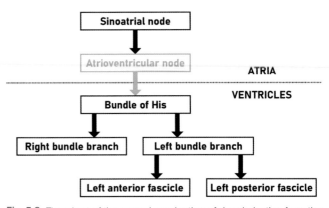

Fig. 5.2 Flowchart of the normal conduction of depolarisation from the SAN in the atria to the ventricles. The PR interval reflects the delay in conduction between the atria and ventricles caused by the AVN.

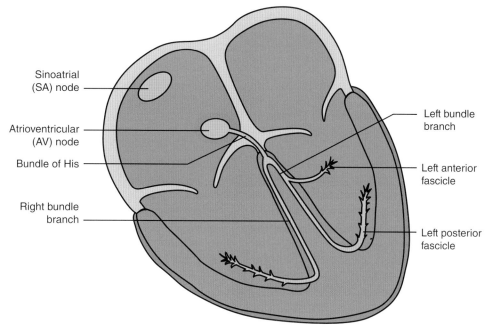

Fig. 5.3 Normal cardiac conduction from the SAN to the AVN (highlighted in purple) and His–Purkinje fibres. A conduction block between the atria and ventricles produces atrioventricular block. (Source: Adapted from Goldberger, A., Goldberger, Z., Shvilkin, A. (2017). Ventricular conduction disturbances. *Goldberger's Clinical Electrocardiography: A Simplified Approach*, 9th ed. Elsevier.)

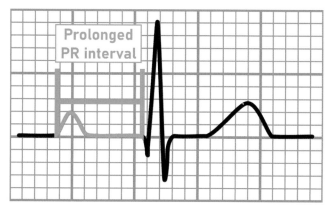

Fig. 5.4 First-degree heart block is a PR interval longer than 200 ms. In this image, the PR interval is 280 ms (seven small squares with each square representing 40 ms).

CLASSIFICATION

AV block is classified as:
1. First-degree heart block: consistently prolonged PR interval
2. Second-degree heart block: intermittent block of impulses
3. Third-degree heart block: complete block of impulses between atria and ventricles

FIRST-DEGREE HEART BLOCK

ECG FINDINGS

First-degree heart block has a PR interval consistently longer than 200 ms (Figs 5.4 and 5.5). This usually reflects slowing of conduction through the AVN.

However, the P wave and QRS complex have a normal morphology and there are no dropped beats.

CLINICAL FEATURES

First-degree heart block is a common finding, especially in the elderly. It is found in 1–2% of the general population. Individuals are usually asymptomatic.

MANAGEMENT

No treatment is usually required. However, in individuals where the PR interval is very long (>300 ms), regular monitoring of the PR interval is recommended. It can be a marker of underlying pathology, such as aortic root abscess, cardiac involvement in myotonic dystrophy and cardiac sarcoidosis.

SECOND-DEGREE HEART BLOCK

ECG FINDINGS

In second-degree heart block, there is intermittent failure of conduction. There are several types of second-degree heart block. Mobitz I and II blocks can be further classified according to the P wave-to-QRS wave ratio (Box 5.1).

Mobitz I (Wenckebach)

The PR interval gradually lengthens with each depolarisation until the AVN fails to conduct an impulse. The next beat then has a shorter PR interval. The cause of this finding is AVN conduction delay and block (Figs 5.6 and 5.7).

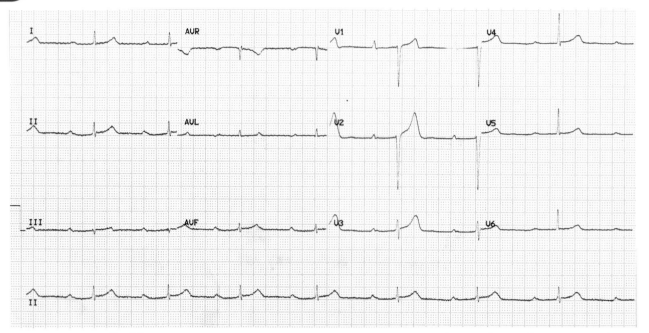

Fig. 5.5 First-degree heart block. The PR interval is approximately 360 ms (nine small squares).

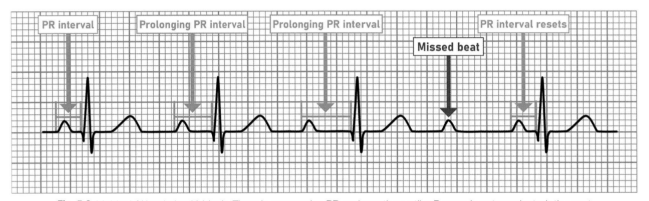

Fig. 5.6 Mobitz I (Wenckebach) block. There is progressive PR prolongation until a P wave is not conducted; the next beat then has a shorter PR interval.

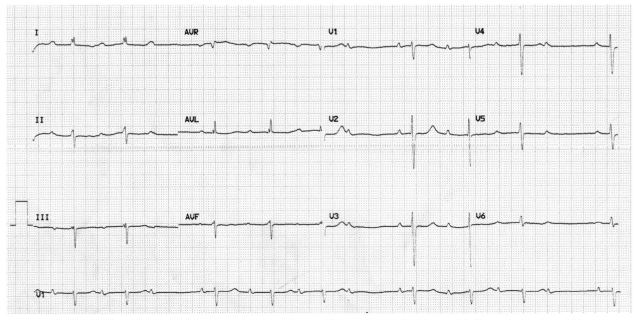

Fig. 5.7 Mobitz I (Wenckebach) block. PR interval prolongs with each beat until a P wave fails to conduct, upon which the next PR interval is shortened.

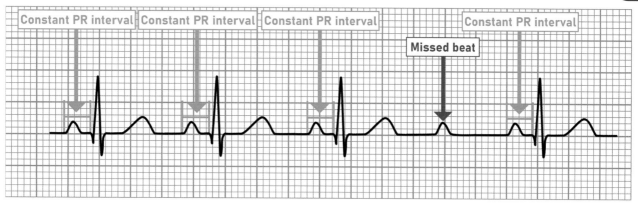

Fig. 5.8 Mobitz II block. The PR intervals are the same but there is intermittent failure of conduction of P waves.

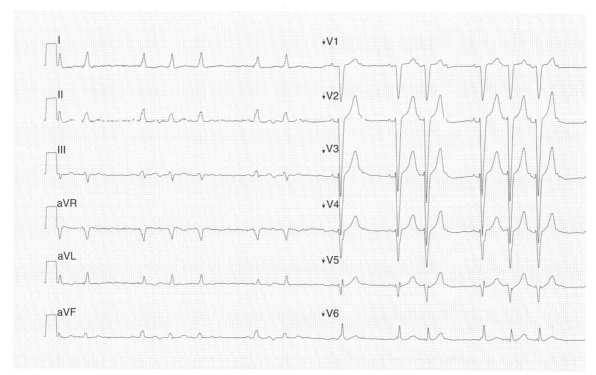

Fig. 5.9 Mobitz II block. There is intermittent failure to conduct signals to the ventricles. There is no PR interval prolongation before a non-conducted P wave. (Source: Maleki, M., Alizadehasai, A., Haghjoo, M. (2021). Bradyarrhythmias. In: *Practical Cardiology: Principles and Approaches*, 2nd ed. Elsevier.)

Mobitz II

PR interval is normal but with intermittent failure of conduction of a P wave (Figs 5.8 and 5.9). It usually occurs due to infranodal block, such as the bundle of His; therefore, there is a higher risk of it developing into complete heart block. Most Mobitz II blocks are fixed blocks (Box 5.1).

2:1 Atrioventricular Block

There are two P waves for every QRS complex, so beats are missed at regular intervals (Figs 5.10 and 5.11). This could be due to either block in the AVN or infranodal conducting tissue. It is considered a separate type of second-degree AV block to Mobitz I and II as it is particularly difficult to check if the PR interval is constant or prolonging.

CLINICAL FEATURES

Mobitz I (Wenckebach) is a common and often benign finding, especially in young individuals with high vagal tone. On the other hand, Mobitz II block reflects significant disease in the conduction system and can progress to complete heart block. Bradycardia can present with symptoms such as dizziness, lightheadedness and syncope.

MANAGEMENT

Reversible causes should be identified and treated (Box 5.2). However, most cases are due to intrinsic conduction disease; in cases of Mobitz II or symptomatic second-degree heart block, a pacemaker is indicated. In acute situations of symptomatic bradycardia, patients can be treated with atropine.

THIRD-DEGREE HEART BLOCK

ECG FINDINGS

In third-degree heart block (complete heart block), there is no conduction of impulses between the atria and ventricles. Therefore, there is no consistent PR relationship (Figs 5.12 and 5.13).

P waves are regularly spaced. QRS complexes have a slower rate, are regularly spaced and have no relation to the P waves. In addition, the QRS complexes can be broad if depolarisation originates from a ventricular focus (ventricular escape rhythm; see Chapter 2).

Atrial contraction remains under the control of the SAN. The ventricles depolarise using the His–Purkinje fibres, which have a slow and unreliable pacemaker activity termed 'ventricular escape rhythm'. Therefore, there is no relationship between the P wave and QRS complex (AV dissociation).

Escape rhythms originating in the AVN or bundle of His tend to have a narrower QRS complex; origins below the bundle of His will have a wider QRS and tend to be slower and more unstable.

CLINICAL FEATURES

Third-degree heart block reflects significant conduction disease. Individuals are usually symptomatic with dizziness, presyncope and/or syncope (Stokes–Adams attack).

MANAGEMENT

Most patients will require permanent pacing. The urgency of treatment depends on ECG and clinical

---

Box 5.1 **Describing atrioventricular blocks in P:QRS ratios**

Second-degree atrioventricular blocks can be further described according to the ratio of P waves to QRS complexes, e.g. 3:1, 4:1, 5:2 block.

For example, 3:1 block refers to requiring 3 atrial depolarisations for 1 impulse to conduct to the ventricles – 3 P waves are present for each QRS complex. If the PR length is prolonging between beats, it is referred to as 3:1 block with a Mobitz I pattern. If the PR length is constant, it is a 3:1 block with a Mobitz II pattern.

In terms of classifying ratios as Mobitz I or II, a notable exception is 2:1 atrioventricular block. Since it is extremely difficult to check if the PR interval is constant or prolonging, 2:1 blocks can be considered a separate type of second-degree AV block (see below).

If the ratio of P waves is consistent across the ECG, this can be further described as a fixed block, e.g. fixed 3:1 block if there are 3 P waves for every QRS complex across the whole ECG strip. Otherwise, it would be termed a variable block, whereby the ratio of P waves to QRS complexes varies across an ECG tracing, e.g. variable 3:1–4:1 block (the ratio of P:QRS varying from 3:1 to 4:1 across the ECG).

Box 5.2 **Risk factors for heart block**

- Ischaemic heart disease
- Antihypertensives, e.g. beta-blockers, calcium channel blockers
- Digoxin
- Electrolyte disturbance, e.g. hypokalaemia, hypomagnesaemia
- Rheumatic fever

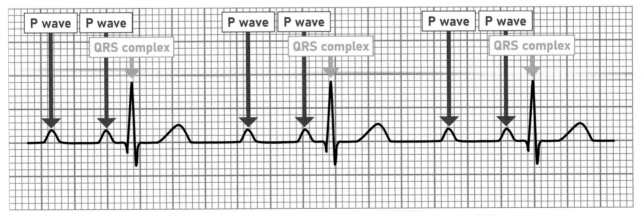

Fig. 5.10 2:1 atrioventricular block. There are two P waves (green arrows) for every QRS complex.

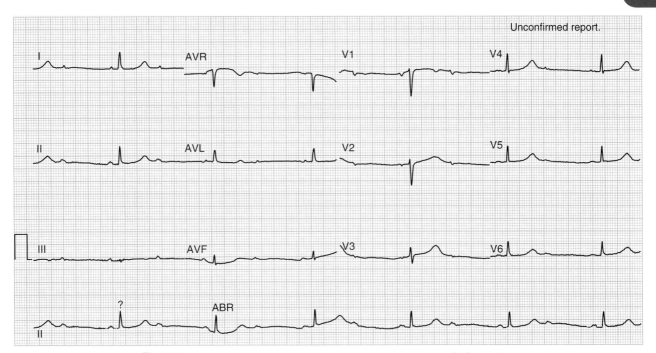

Unconfirmed report.

Fig. 5.11 2:1 atrioventricular block. There are two P waves for every QRS complex.

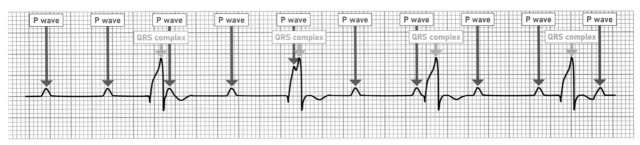

Fig. 5.12 Third-degree heart block. There is no relationship between the P waves (green arrows) and QRS complexes. Note that the QRS complexes are wide due to the ventricular escape rhythm with a rate of 40 bpm.

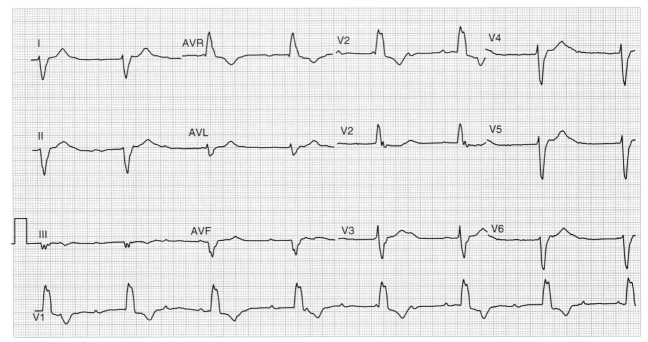

Fig. 5.13 Third-degree heart block. There is no relation between the P waves and QRS complexes. The ventricular rate is 48 bpm with broad QRS complexes, indicating a ventricular escape rhythm.

Box 5.3   **Assessment of risk – high-risk features that require urgent temporary pacing wires**

- Syncope
- Wide escape rhythm
- Haemodynamic compromise
- Low blood pressure (although cardiac output can be low with a normal blood pressure; look for other signs such as oliguria, confusion)
- Ventricular rhythms (ventricular ectopic/polymorphic ventricular tachycardia)

features (Box 5.3). Drugs that can be used in the acute setting for symptomatic patients include atropine and glucagon.

¹²₃ Key Points

1. Normal PR interval: 120–200 ms (3–5 small squares)
2. A prolonged PR interval suggests AV block. AV blocks can be:
   (a) First-degree AV block: PR interval >200 ms
   (b) Second-degree AV block (intermittent blockage of impulses):
      - Mobitz I (Wenckebach): Progressive PR prolongation until a P wave is not conducted
      - Mobitz II: Intermittent failure to conduct a P wave
      - 2:1 block: two P waves for every QRS complex
   (c) Third-degree AV block: No relation between P waves and QRS complexes
3. A short PR interval arises due to:
   (a) Pre-excitation, e.g. Wolff–Parkinson–White syndrome
   (b) Junctional rhythm

FURTHER READING

Barold, S.S., Herweg, B., 2012. Second-degree atrioventricular block revisited. Herzschrittmacherther Elektrophysiologie 23 (4), 296–304.

Barra, S.N., et al., 2012. A review on advanced atrioventricular block in young or middle-aged adults. Pacing Clin. Electrophysiol. 35 (11), 1395–1405.

Boron, W.F., Boulpaep, E.L., 2017. Medical Physiology. Elsevier, Philadelphia.

Hampton, J.R., Hampton, J., 2019. The ECG made easy. Elsevier.

Hayden, G.E., et al., 2004. Electrocardiographic manifestations: diagnosis of atrioventricular block in the emergency department. J. Emerg. Med. 26 (1), 95–106.

John, A.D., Fleisher, L.A., 2006. Electrocardiography: the ECG. Anesthesiol. Clin. North Am. 24 (4), 697–715.

Kumar, P., Clark, M., 2017. Kumar & Clark's Cases in Clinical Medicine, 9th ed. Elsevier.

6

QRS Complex

OVERVIEW

DEFINITION

The QRS complex corresponds to the depolarisation of the right and left ventricles of the heart occurring after the P wave. If the first deflection after the P wave is negative, it is termed the Q wave (Fig. 6.1). The R wave is the first upward deflection of the complex (even if there is no Q wave present) (Fig. 6.2). The negative deflection after the R wave is referred to as the S wave.

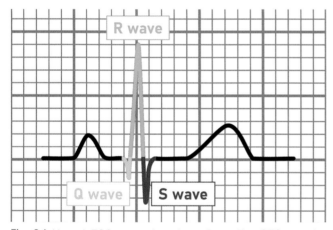

Fig. 6.1 Normal ECG waves in a heart beat. The QRS complex corresponds to ventricular depolarisation and is composed of up to three components: Q, R and S waves.

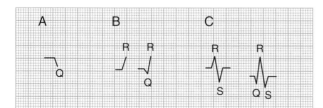

Fig. 6.2 Definitions of the individual waves in a QRS complex. Defining the parts of the QRS complex can be confusing as the nomenclature changes depending on whether the first deflection after the P wave is positive or negative. (A) If the wave following the P wave is negative, it is a Q wave. (B) If a positive deflection follows the P wave, it is called an R wave, whether it is preceded by a Q wave or not. (C) Any following negative deflection is known as an S wave, whether there has been a preceding Q wave or not.

ELECTROPHYSIOLOGY

In normal conduction, signals pass from the atria to the ventricles following the initial triggering of depolarisation by the sinoatrial node (SAN); these then conduct rapidly through the His-Bundle branch-Purkinje system, producing a narrow QRS complex due to simultaneous activation of both ventricles (Figs 6.3 and 6.4). The components of the QRS complex are produced by depolarisation of different parts of the ventricle:

- Small Q wave (if present): represents depolarisation of the interventricular septum. This starts on the left side of the septum and spreads to the right causing a small electrical current away from the lateral leads (I, aVL, V_5, V_6), creating small Q waves

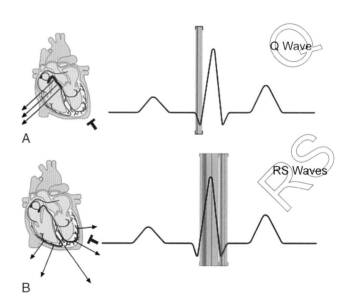

Fig. 6.3 The QRS complex is produced by depolarisation by different parts of the ventricle. Arrows represent the overall direction of depolarisation.
(A) Depolarisation of the interventricular complex produces the Q wave.
(B) Depolarisation of the main mass of ventricles produces the RS waves. ((A) Source: www.nottingham.ac.uk/nursing/practice/resources/cardiology/images/q_wave.gif. (B) Source: www.nottingham.ac.uk/nursing/practice/resources/cardiology/images/r_wave.gif.)

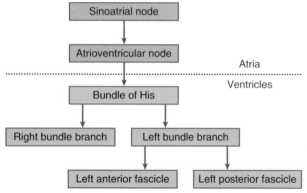

Fig. 6.4 Flowchart of the normal conduction of depolarisation from the SAN in the atria to the ventricles. The QRS complex reflects depolarisation of the heart, which involves the His–Purkinje system.

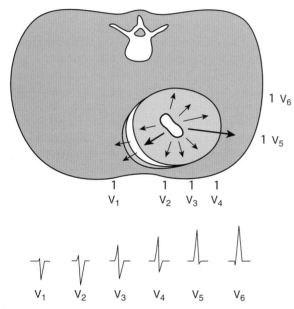

Fig. 6.5 Normal R-wave progression. Note that the transition zone, where the R and S waves are equal, is approximately at V_3. (Source: Aehlert, B. (2009) Introduction to the 12-lead ECG. In: *ECGs Made Easy*, 4th ed. Maryland Heights, MO: Elsevier.)

- RS wave: depolarisation of the main mass of the ventricles

Depolarisation starts on the endocardial surface and progresses to the epicardium of the ventricles.

INTERPRETATION

Q, R and S waves occur in rapid succession and reflect as a single depolarisation event. Thus, they are usually considered together during interpretation.

Normal

A normal QRS complex width is 80–120 ms (2–3 small squares).

R-wave progression should be noted in leads V_1–V_6 (Fig. 6.5). Normally, there should be a small R wave in V_1 which gets progressively larger when advancing laterally (towards V_6) due to the predominant muscle

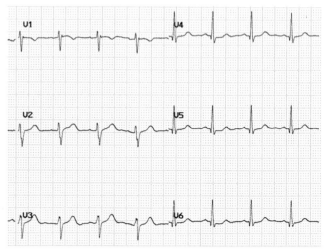

Fig. 6.6 Normal R-wave progression. Note that the transition zone, where the R and S waves are equal, is between V_3 and V_4.

mass and electrical activation of the left ventricle. In addition, the S wave gets smaller when moving from V_1 to V_6. Therefore, V_1 has a dominant S wave while V_6 has a dominant R wave.

The transition zone, the point where the R wave is equal to the S wave, should be in leads V_3–V_4 (Fig. 6.6); it indicates the position of the interventricular septum (Fig. 6.7) in a normal heart.

Wide QRS Complexes

QRS complexes are considered wide when they are longer than 120 ms (three small squares; Fig. 6.8).

Wide QRS complexes reflect slow conduction of electrical activity across the ventricles (Figs 6.9 and 6.10). Causes include:

- Disease of the His-Purkinje system, resulting in slow depolarisation of the ventricles. This causes ECG patterns termed 'Bundle Branch Block' or 'Non-specific intraventricular conduction delay' (Box 6.1)

Box **6.1**	Causes of wide QRS complexes

- Disease of the His–Purkinje system (bundle branch block)
- Ventricular rhythms: ventricular escape rhythm, ventricular ectopic beats, ventricular pacing (see Chapter 10), ventricular tachycardia
- Pre-excitation from an accessory pathway (see Chapter 10)
- Electrolyte and metabolic abnormalities, e.g. hyperkalaemia, hypothermia (see Chapter 10)

- Rhythms originating from the ventricle, which causes ventricular activation from myocyte to myocyte conduction instead of the usual rapid His-Purkinje system
- Pre-excitation where some of the electrical activation bypasses the His–Purkinje system via an accessory pathway

Ventricular repolarisation also tends to be affected in wide QRS complexes, so there may be T-wave changes.

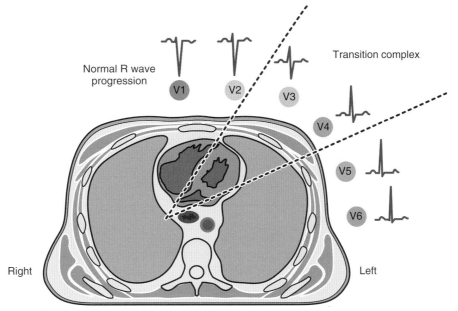

Fig. 6.7 Normal position of interventricular septum leads to a transition zone in V_3–V_4.

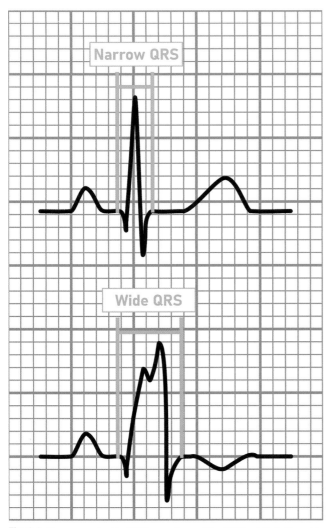

Fig. 6.8 Narrow and wide QRS complexes. The QRS width in the wide QRS complex is ~200 ms (five small squares) in this example.

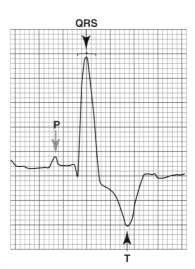

Fig. 6.9 Abnormal ventricular depolarisation leads to wide QRS complexes. This example shows wide QRS complex from a LBBB. The impulse first travels down the working right bundle to slowly travel and depolarise the left side of the heart, producing a wide QRS complex. The abnormal depolarisation pattern can also produce inverted T waves. (Source: Bassert, J. M. (2022). Emergency and critical care nursing. In: *McCurnin's Clinical Textbook for Veterinary Technicians*, 8th ed. Elsevier.)

High-Amplitude QRS Morphology

Larger electrical signals (Fig. 6.11) can be seen in individuals with larger ventricular muscle and a lower degree of tissue attenuation. This can be a normal finding in thin individuals or those with chest wall deformities. Physiological or pathological ventricular hypertrophy can also produce this (Box 6.2).

A

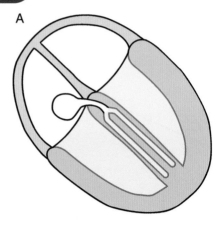

B

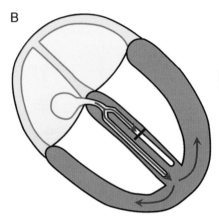

C

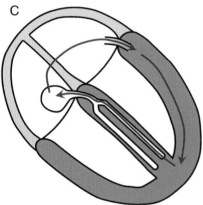

Origin below the bifurcation of the His bundle:
- VT
- Ventricular pacing

Origin above the bifurcation of the His bundle, with abnormal conduction:
- Pre-existing BBB
- Functional (rate-related) aberrancy
- Abnormal myocardial conduction, e.g. LVH, congenital heart disease, hyperkalaemia, Class 1A or 1C drugs

Pre-excited tachycardia:
- Antidromic AVRT, including conduction over a typical accessory pathway, or atypical pathways such as atriofascicular, nodoventricular or nodofascicular pathways
- Other supraventricular dysrhythmias (AVNRT, AT, AFL) with bystander conduction over an accessory pathway

Fig. 6.10 Schematic diagrams outlining potential mechanisms for producing wide (>120 ms) QRS complexes. (A) Rhythms originating below the bifurcation of the His bundle (yellow shading), e.g. ventricular tachycardia (VT), ventricular pacing.
(B) Abnormal conduction of a supraventricular rhythm, e.g. bundle branch block (BBB), abnormal myocardial conduction.
(C) Pre-excited tachycardia, where conduction to the ventricles occurs via an (additional) accessory pathway; in this case the impulses travel up from ventricles to the atria via the atrioventricular node and then back down through the accessory pathway. The accessory pathway conducts slower than the His bundle, producing wide QRS complexes. AFL, Atrial flutter; AT, atrial tachycardia; AVNRT, atrioventricular nodal re-entrant tachycardia; AVRT, atrioventricular re-entrant tachycardia; LVH, left ventricular hypertrophy. (Source: Vasan, R. S., Sawyer, D. B. (2017). Wide QRS complex tachycardia: what is the diagnosis? In: *Encyclopedia of Cardiovascular Research and Medicine.* Elsevier.)

Low-Amplitude QRS Morphology

The QRS amplitude is defined as low-voltage if it is 10 mm or less in all limb leads, or 5 mm or less in all precordial leads (Fig. 6.12). This can develop when there is an impedance to the electrical signals reaching recording the surface ECG electrodes, such as in cases of pericardial effusion, large body habitus and amyloidosis (infiltrative disease affecting the myocardium).

Pathological Q Waves

Q waves are considered pathological if they are longer than 40 ms (one small square), greater than 2 mm (two small squares) in height and >25% of the amplitude of the R wave (Fig. 6.13). Pathological Q wave can develop following myocardial infarction and can be a sign of an old infarct.

Poor R-Wave Progression

Poor R-wave progression refers to the absence of the normal increase in R-wave size from V_1 to V_6 (Fig. 6.14)

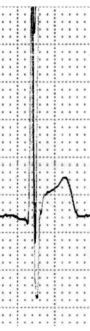

Fig. 6.11 High-amplitude QRS complex as seen in LVH.

| Box **6.2** | Causes of high-amplitude QRS complexes |

- Normal variant:
  - Thin individuals
  - Chest wall deformity
  - Athletic adaptation
- LVH:
  - Hypertension
  - Aortic valve stenosis
- RVH:
  - Severe lung disease and pulmonary hypertension
  - Pulmonary valve disease
  - Atrial septal defect
  - Ventricular septal defect
- Hypertrophic cardiomyopathy

and may be accompanied by a transition zone shift (the point where the R wave is equal to the S wave in the precordial leads). The most common cause is loss of muscle mass due to an old anterior myocardial infarction.

Transition Zone Rotation

The normal transition zone, where the R wave is equal to the S wave in the precordial leads, normally occurs in leads V_3 and V_4. A transition zone rotation refers to a change in the point where the R wave is equal to the S wave. This is not a sensitive marker of disease as it can be found in normal individuals.

A rightward rotation (also known as anticlockwise rotation) of the interventricular septum leads to a transition zone in V_1–V_2 (Fig. 6.15). Pathological causes include right ventricular hypertrophy (RVH) and posterior myocardial infarction.

A transition zone in V_5–V_6 indicates a leftward rotation (also known as clockwise rotation). Pathological

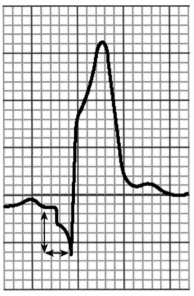

Fig. 6.13 Pathological Q waves are longer than 40 ms with an amplitude of more than 2 mm. (Source: Hampton, J. R. (2008). The ECG in patients with chest pain. In: *The ECG in Practice*, 5th ed. Churchill Livingstone.)

causes include chronic lung disease and dilated cardiomyopathy.

LEFT VENTRICULAR HYPERTROPHY

DEFINITION

Thickening of the walls of the left ventricle occurs in left ventricular hypertrophy (LVH). This can develop secondary to pressure overload, such as aortic stenosis and hypertension. It can also be a normal observation in young, athletic individuals.

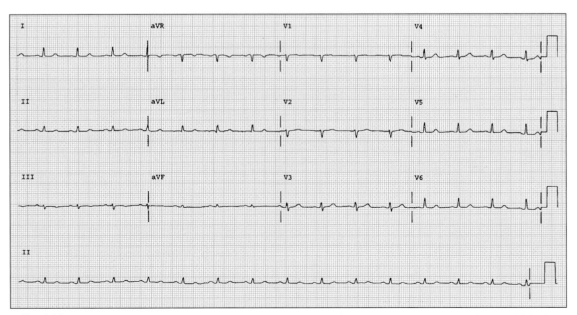

Fig. 6.12 Low-amplitude QRS complexes. There are low-voltage QRS complexes in both limb and precordial leads. Depending on the accompanying clinical situation, consider the following common diagnoses: pericardial effusion, chronic obstructive pulmonary disease and myxoedema. Other causes, such as morbid obesity and infiltrative myocardial diseases, are also possibilities. (Source: Koster, N. K. K. (2017). Electrocardiography. In: *Cardiovascular Imaging Review*. Elsevier.)

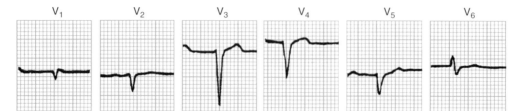

Fig. 6.14 Poor R-wave progression. There is poor R-wave progression and QS complexes in chest leads V_1–V_5. The transition zone is between V_5 and V_6. (Source: Goldberger, A., Goldberger, Z., Shvilkin, A. (2017). Myocardial infarction and ischemia. In: *Goldberger's Clinical Electrocardiography: A Simplified Approach*, 9th ed. Elsevier.)

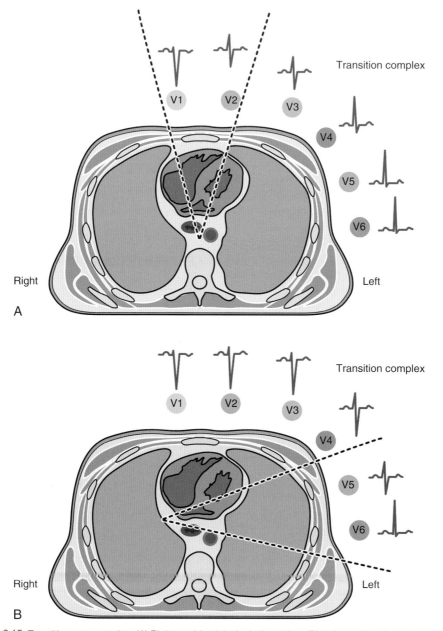

Fig. 6.15 Transition zone rotation. (A) Rightward (anticlockwise) rotation. (B) Leftward (clockwise) rotation.

ECG FINDINGS

Increased S-wave depth in V_1–V_3 and increased R-wave amplitude in V_4–V_6 (Fig. 6.16) are the most pertinent ECG findings in LVH. This reflects ventricular hypertrophy as an increase in muscle mass produces larger electrical signals (Fig. 6.17). An ECG fulfilling any of the voltage criteria of LVH suggests the presence of this pathology (Box 6.3).

Additional ECG findings suggestive of LVH include:
- Left 'strain' pattern in V_5–V_6, I and aVL: T-wave inversion and ST segment depression
- Left axis deviation

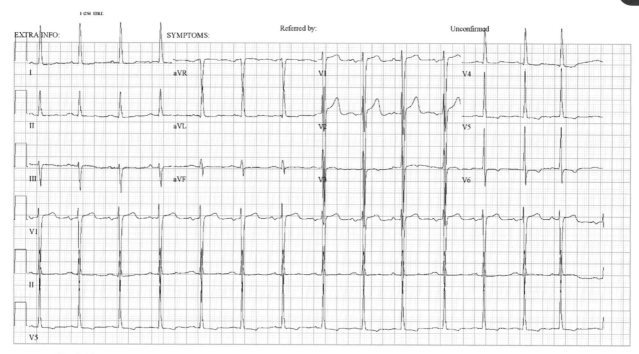

Fig. 6.16 LVH. This ECG fulfils both Sokolow–Lyon and Cornell criteria of LVH. T-wave inversion in the lateral leads is also present.

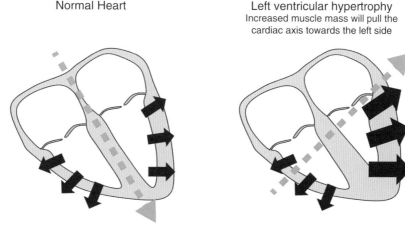

Normal Heart

Left ventricular hypertrophy
Increased muscle mass will pull the cardiac axis towards the left side

Green arrow = Cardiac axis
(AVERAGE direction of depolarisation)

Fig. 6.17 Effects of LVH on the cardiac axis. The increased muscle mass in LVH will pull the average direction of depolarisation, and thereby the cardiac axis, towards the left.

Box **6.3**	Voltage criteria for diagnosing left ventricular hypertrophy

- Sokolow–Lyon criteria: S-wave amplitude in V_1 plus R-wave amplitude in V_5/V_6 (whichever has the largest R wave) greater than 35 mm. This is the commonest criterion used during ECG interpretation of LVH
- Cornell criteria: R-wave amplitude in aVL plus S-wave amplitude in V_3 greater than 20 mm in women or greater than 28 mm in men

Note that ventricular hypertrophy cannot be accurately assessed if bundle branch block is present.

CLINICAL FEATURES

The clinical presentation of individuals with LVH depends on the underlying cause. If the voltage criteria described above are met, it is important to identify the aetiology; this will include assessment of the following:
- History:
  - Family history of cardiomyopathy (e.g. hypertrophic obstructive cardiomyopathy) – check for history of sudden death

- Hypertensive disease
- Examination:
  - Blood pressure – raised blood pressure and its complications, e.g. retinopathy
  - Cardiac murmurs – check for left ventricular outflow obstruction and murmur of aortic stenosis. Echocardiography can be used to assess valvular pathologies

MANAGEMENT

Management should be focused on treating the underlying cause of LVH. Echocardiography could be considered to confirm the presence of LVH and to identify the aetiology.

RIGHT VENTRICULAR HYPERTROPHY

DEFINITION

Thickening of the walls of the right ventricle following pressure overload occurs in RVH (Fig. 6.18). Causes include pulmonary hypertension, pulmonary valve problems and congenital heart defects (e.g. ventricular septal defect).

ECG FINDINGS

A dominant R wave, one that is larger than the S wave, in V_1 (which overlies the right ventricle) is the most pertinent finding in RVH (Fig. 6.19). However, in the presence of widened QRS complexes, consider the diagnosis of right bundle branch block (RBBB)

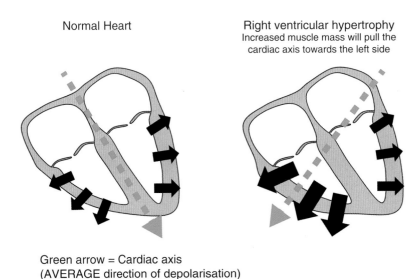

Normal Heart

Right ventricular hypertrophy
Increased muscle mass will pull the cardiac axis towards the left side

Green arrow = Cardiac axis
(AVERAGE direction of depolarisation)

Fig. 6.18 RVH. The increased muscle mass in RVH will pull the average direction of depolarisation, and thereby the cardiac axis, towards the right.

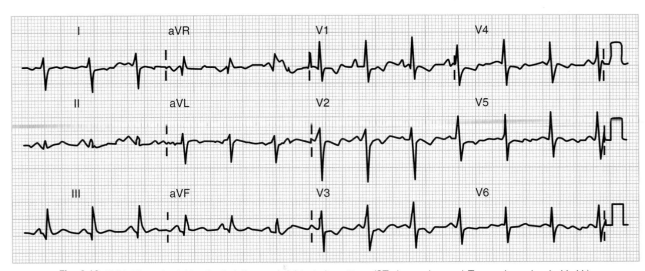

Fig. 6.19 RVH. There is right-axis deviation and right strain pattern (ST depression and T-wave inversion in V_1–V_4). Tall P waves can be seen in lead II consistent with right atrial dilation. (Source: Goldman, L., Ausiello, D. A. (2003). Electrocardiography. In: *Cecil Textbook of Medicine*, 22nd ed. Saunders.)

as it can also give positive QRS complexes in these leads.

Other ECG findings of RVH can include:
- Right-axis deviation
- Right 'strain' pattern in leads V_1–V_4 (right precordial) and/or leads II, III, aVF (inferior): T-wave inversion and ST segment depression
- P pulmonale (see Chapter 4) if there is coexisting right atrial dilatation

Note that ventricular hypertrophy cannot be accurately assessed if bundle branch block is present.

CLINICAL FEATURES

RVH is usually a manifestation of underlying disease and the presentation depends on the cause (Box 6.4).

MANAGEMENT

Management should be focused on treating the underlying cause of RVH. Echocardiography may not visualise the right heart well but may show valvular abnormalities and shunts.

PERICARDIAL EFFUSION

DEFINITION

A pericardial effusion is defined as an abnormal accumulation of fluid in the pericardial cavity leading to increased intrapericardial pressure. This can impair cardiac muscle contraction, producing a cardiac tamponade.

Although pericardial effusions are diagnosed on echocardiography, they can also lead to changes on the ECG.

ECG FINDINGS

Pericardial effusions can produce:
- Low-voltage QRS complexes
- Electrical alternans – alternating height of QRS with each beat (Fig. 6.20)
- Sinus tachycardia

The low QRS voltage reflects a damping effect by the fluid, reducing electrical signal conduction between the heart and recording electrode. Electrical alternans is due to the oscillating movement of the heart within the pericardial fluid.

CLINICAL FEATURES

The presentation of individuals with pericardial effusion depends on how quickly the fluid has accumulated and the compliance of the pericardium. A slowly accumulating pericardial effusion can be well tolerated, while rapidly developing effusions often lead to cardiac tamponade (Box 6.5).

MANAGEMENT

Most pericardial effusions can be effectively managed with bed rest, colchicine and non-steroidal anti-inflammatory drugs. More aggressive treatment, such as with pericardiocentesis, may be required if there are signs of tamponade and/or for diagnostic purposes.

BUNDLE BRANCH BLOCK

DEFINITION

Bundle branch blocks refer to a delay or block of the electrical impulses through the bundle branches.

From the atrioventricular node, the electrical impulse travels down the bundle of His into the left and right bundle branches (Fig. 6.21). The left bundle branch is further divided into anterior and posterior fascicles, whereas the right bundle branch has only one fascicle.

When there is an RBBB or left bundle branch block (LBBB), electrical impulses travelling from the atria to the ventricle will be delayed with a consequent change in travel pathways. This prolongs ventricular depolarisation and, therefore, widens the QRS complexes. As the direction of propagation of impulses changes, the morphology of QRS complexes also changes.

Box **6.4**   Causes of right ventricular hypertrophy
<ul><li>Pulmonary hypertension:<ul><li>Chronic obstructive pulmonary disease</li><li>Pulmonary embolism</li><li>Restrictive lung diseases</li></ul></li><li>Tetralogy of Fallot</li><li>Ventricular septal defect</li><li>Pulmonary valve stenosis</li></ul>

Box **6.5**   Symptoms and signs of pericardial effusion
<ul><li>Shortness of breath</li><li>Muffled heart sounds</li><li>Right-sided heart failure (e.g. peripheral oedema, hepatomegaly, ascites)</li><li>Beck's triad in tamponade:<ul><li>Hypotension</li><li>Raised jugular venous pressure</li><li>Muffled heart</li></ul></li></ul>

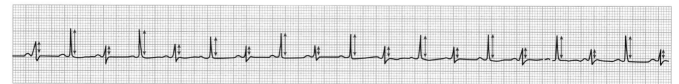

Fig. 6.20 The height of the QRS complex alternates with every beat. This was caused by pericardial effusion with tamponade. This finding, particularly in concert with sinus tachycardia and relatively low voltage, is a highly specific, although not sensitive, marker of cardiac tamponade.

A block in both right and left bundle branches produces third-degree heart block (see Chapter 5) as there is no communication between the atria and ventricles.

CLASSIFICATION

Bundle branch block is divided into:
- RBBB: rSR' in V_1, wide S waves in V_6
- LBBB: notched R wave in V_6, wide S waves in V_1 (Box 6.6 and Fig 6.23)

Interpretation of the left bundle branch can be further subdivided according to its anterior and posterior fascicles.

RIGHT BUNDLE BRANCH BLOCK

In RBBB, the impulses travel via the left bundle branch to the left ventricle, which then propagate slowly through the myocardium to the right ventricle (Fig. 6.22).

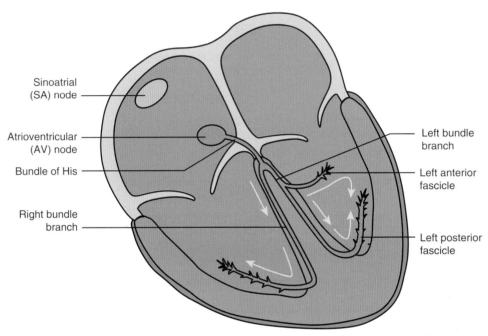

Fig. 6.21 Right and left bundle branches conduct electrical signals to the ventricles. The left bundle branch has two fascicles. (Source: Modified from Goldberger, A., Goldberger, Z., Shvilkin, A. (2017). Ventricular conduction disturbances. In: *Goldberger's Clinical Electrocardiography: A Simplified Approach*, 9th ed. Elsevier.)

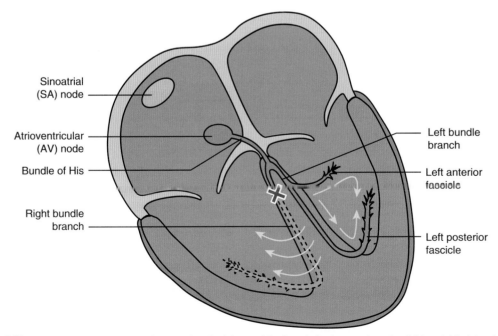

Fig. 6.22 RBBB. In RBBB, impulses first travel to the left ventricle. Depolarisation reaches the right ventricle later due to conduction through the myocardium. (Source: Modified from Goldberger, A., Goldberger, Z., Shvilkin, A. (2017). Ventricular conduction disturbances. In: *Goldberger's Clinical Electrocardiography: A Simplified Approach*, 9th ed. Elsevier.)

Box **6.6**   Bundle branch blocks made simple

An aide-mémoire for remembering the above is 'WiLLiaM MaRRoW', based on exaggerated appearances of the ECG changes. LBBBs produce QRS complexes resembling 'W' in V_1 and 'M' in V_6, while RBBBs produce 'M' in V_1 and 'W' in V_6 (Fig. 6.23).

ECG FINDINGS

Wide QRS (>120 ms), rSR' (M-shaped) pattern in V_1–V_3 and slurred S wave in V_5–V_6 (W-shaped) are the most pertinent findings in RBBB (Fig 6.24). In typical RBBB the first r wave is smaller than the second R' wave.

T-wave inversion may also occur, reflecting altered repolarisation through the ventricles.

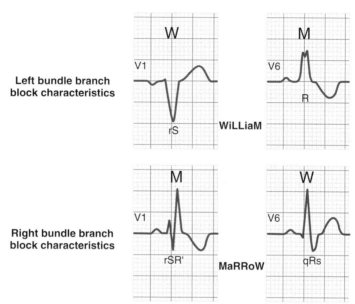

Left bundle branch block characteristics

Right bundle branch block characteristics

Fig. 6.23 Illustration of the 'M' and 'W' patterns of bundle branch blocks. 'WiLLiaM MaRRoW' can be used to remember which side is blocked.

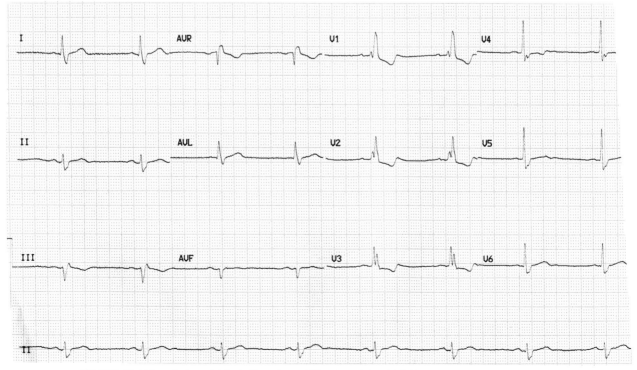

Fig. 6.24 Right bundle branch block. There is an rSR' pattern in leads V_1–V_2 and slurred S waves in V_5–V_6.

RBBB alone does not produce axis deviations as the left ventricle has a greater influence on cardiac axis due to its larger muscle mass.

CLINICAL FEATURES

RBBB is usually benign and can be a normal finding, although it may indicate underlying disease. It can develop as a result of primary pathologies affecting the right side of the heart or secondary effects from pulmonary disease (Box 6.7).

Most isolated RBBBs are asymptomatic. However, if present in conjunction with other conduction disease, symptoms can present due to symptoms of intermittent heart block.

MANAGEMENT

Treatment is not required unless the RBBB has developed due to a pathology. Management should be aimed towards the underlying cause.

Box **6.7**	Causes of right bundle branch block

- Normal variant
- Primary right ventricular disease (rare):
  - Right ventricular cardiomyopathies, e.g. arrhythmogenic right ventricular cardiomyopathy, sarcoidosis
  - Congenital heart disease
  - Atrial septal defect
- Secondary causes (more common):
  - Pulmonary embolism
  - Chronic pulmonary disease, e.g. chronic obstructive pulmonary disease, pulmonary fibrosis

---

LEFT BUNDLE BRANCH BLOCK

In individuals with LBBB, the left bundle does not conduct normally (either complete block or delayed conduction). Therefore, impulses travel via the right bundle branch to the right ventricle, and then propagate across the interventricular septum and then through the myocardium to the left ventricle (Fig. 6.25).

LBBB is abnormal and is caused by underlying conditions such as coronary heart disease, cardiomyopathy, thickening of the heart muscle (hypertension, aortic stenosis, left ventricular hypertrophic cardiomyopathy) or ageing of the electrical pathway in the heart (see Box 6.8). A new LBBB may indicate acute myocardial infarction (see Box 8.3 in Chapter 8).

The left bundle branch has two fascicles (left anterior and left posterior fascicle). A block in a single fascicle may also produce ECG changes.

ECG FINDINGS

Wide QRS (>120 ms), notched R waves (M-shaped) in V_4–V_6 and deep S waves in V_1–V_3 (W-shaped) are the most pertinent ECG findings in LBBB (Figs 6.23 and 6.26). These are consistent with the slow conduction of impulses through the myocardium from the right to the left ventricle. LBBB can also produce left axis deviation.

CLINICAL FEATURES

Unlike RBBB, LBBB usually indicates heart pathology and should be investigated further.

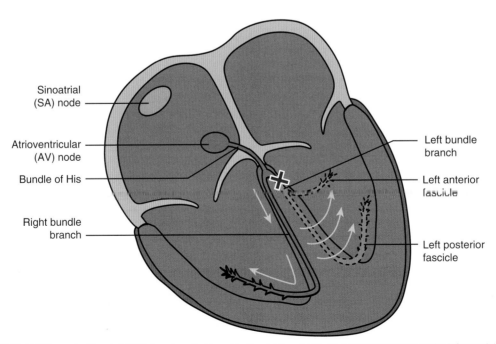

Fig. 6.25 LBBB conduction. In LBBB, impulses first travel to the right ventricle. Depolarisation reaches the left ventricle via myocardial conduction (Source: Modified from Goldberger, A., Goldberger, Z., Shvilkin, A. (2017). Ventricular conduction disturbances. In: *Goldberger's Clinical Electrocardiography: A Simplified Approach*, 9th ed. Elsevier.)

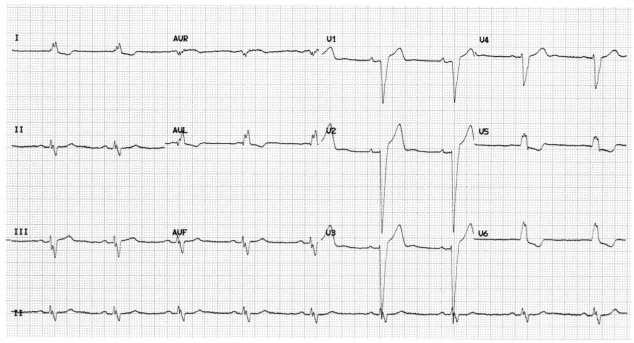

Fig. 6.26 Left bundle branch block. Note the left-axis deviation and the absence of Q waves in the lateral leads.

MANAGEMENT

Management depends on the underlying cause of the LBBB. Cardiac imaging, such as transthoracic echocardiography, is usually initially used to investigate potential causes.

LEFT ANTERIOR FASCICULAR BLOCK

A block in the left anterior fascicle (left anterior hemiblock) results in left ventricular depolarisation through only the left posterior fascicle, which activates the posterior and inferior left ventricular walls initially. The depolarisation then propagates superiorly to the rest of the left ventricle (Fig. 6.27).

ECG FINDINGS

Left-axis deviation is the most pertinent ECG finding in left anterior fascicular block. This is due to the change in direction of depolarisation as impulses travel superiorly from the posterior fascicle (Fig. 6.28). Other potential ECG findings include:
- qR complexes (small Q wave with large R wave) in lateral leads (I, aVL, V$_6$)
- rS complexes (small R wave with large S wave) in inferior leads (II, III, aVF)

Box **6.8**	Causes of left bundle branch block

- Systemic hypertension
- Cardiomyopathy
- Aortic stenosis
- Ischaemic heart disease
- Idiopathic conduction system fibrosis

Electrophysiologically, the initial depolarisation is directed downwards, producing the small R wave in inferior leads and small Q wave in lateral leads. This is followed by a major wave of depolarisation directed leftwards, producing the large S wave in inferior leads and large R wave in lateral leads.

The QRS width is usually normal, although it may occasionally be slightly prolonged.

CLINICAL FEATURES

Patients are usually asymptomatic. The commonest cause of left anterior fascicular block is hypertension.

MANAGEMENT

In practice, left anterior fascicular block can be difficult to differentiate from other conditions that cause left-axis deviation. If there are concerns about coexisting structural heart disease, cardiac imaging should be performed.

LEFT POSTERIOR FASCICULAR BLOCK

When there is a left posterior fascicular block (left posterior hemiblock), impulses initially travel through the left anterior fascicle to activate the anterior, superior and lateral left ventricular walls initially. Depolarisation then propagates inferiorly to the rest of the left ventricle (Fig. 6.29).

ECG FEATURES

Right-axis deviation is the most pertinent ECG finding in left posterior fascicular block. This is due to the change in direction of depolarisation as impulses travel inferiorly from the anterior fascicle (Fig. 6.30). Other potential ECG findings include:

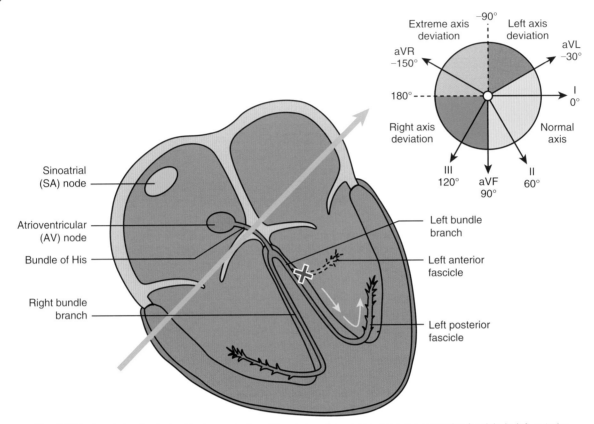

Fig. 6.27 Left anterior fascicular block conduction. Signals travel superiorly from the posterior fascicle in left anterior fascicular block, producing left-axis deviation. (Source: Modified from Goldberger, A., Goldberger, Z., Shvilkin, A. (2017). Ventricular conduction disturbances. In: *Goldberger's Clinical Electrocardiography: A Simplified Approach*, 9th ed. Elsevier.)

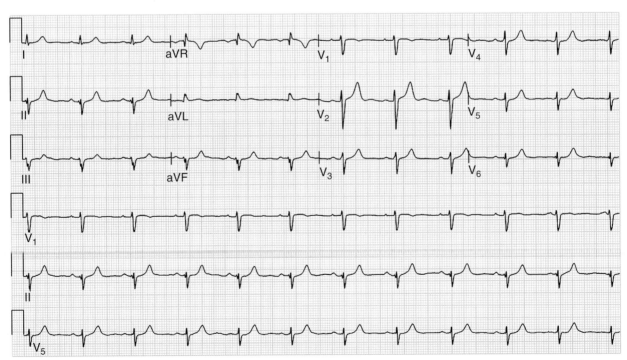

Fig. 6.28 Left anterior fascicular block. There is left-axis deviation with qR complexes in leads I and aVL, as well as rS complexes in lead II, III and aVF. (Source: Olshansky, B. et al. (2016). Bradyarrhythmias – conduction system abnormalities. In: *Arrhythmia Essentials*, 2d ed. Elsevier.)

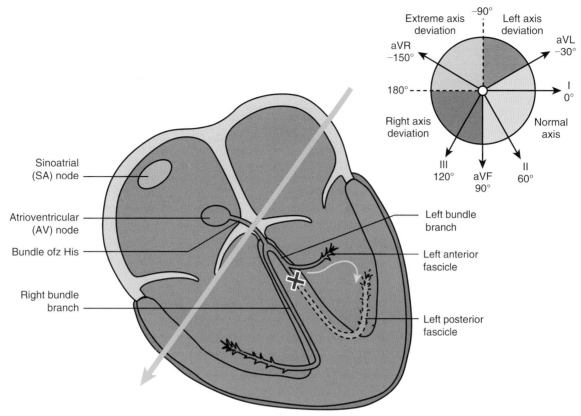

Fig. 6.29 Left posterior fascicular block conduction. Signals travel inferiorly from the anterior fascicle in left posterior fascicular block, producing right-axis deviation. (Source: Modified from Goldberger, A., Goldberger, Z., Shvilkin, A. (2017). *Ventricular conduction disturbances.* In: *Goldberger's Clinical Electrocardiography: A Simplified Approach*, 9th ed. Elsevier.)

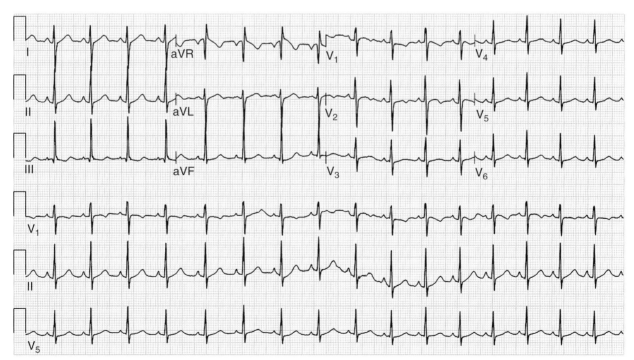

Fig. 6.30 Left posterior fascicular block. There is right-axis deviation with deep rS waves in lead I and qR waves in lead III. (Source: Olshansky, B. et al. (2016). *Bradyarrhythmias – conduction system abnormalities.* In: *Arrhythmia Essentials*, 2d ed. Edition. Elsevier.)

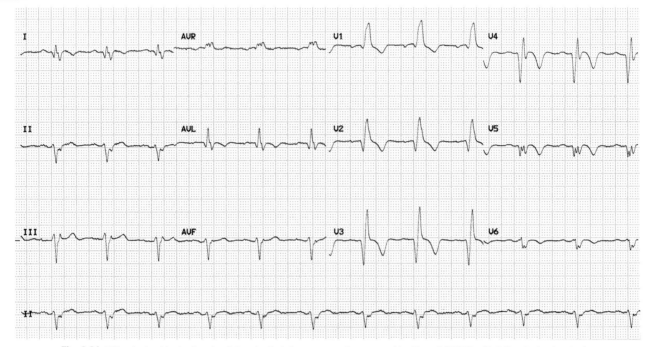

Fig. 6.31 Bifascicular block showing left-axis deviation, suggesting a combination of RBBB with left anterior fascicular block.

- rS complexes (small R wave with large S wave) in lateral leads (I, aVL, V$_6$)
- qR complexes (small Q wave with large R wave) in inferior leads (II, III, aVF)

Electrophysiologically, the initial depolarisation is directed leftwards, producing the small R wave in lateral leads and small Q wave in inferior leads. This is followed by a major wave of depolarisation directed downwards, producing the large S waves in lateral leads and large R waves in inferior leads.

The QRS width is usually normal, although it may occasionally be slightly prolonged.

CLINICAL FEATURES

Patients are usually asymptomatic.

MANAGEMENT

Isolated left posterior fascicular block is rare and difficult to differentiate from right ventricular disease (which also causes right-axis deviation). Therefore, cardiac image should be considered.

BIFASCICULAR BLOCK

ECG FINDINGS

Bifascicular block is the combination of RBBB with either left anterior fascicular block or left posterior fascicular block (Fig. 6.31).

The ECG shows a RBBB pattern in addition to either:
- Left-axis deviation (left anterior fascicular block)
- Right-axis deviation (left posterior fascicular block)

Box **6.9**	Indications for pacemaker insertion in bifascicular block

- Mobitz II heart block
- Third-degree heart block
- Recurrent syncope

CLINICAL FEATURES

Patients are usually asymptomatic. Some patients have intermittent high-degree atrioventricular block and present with dizziness, presyncope or syncope.

MANAGEMENT

For symptomatic patients, further cardiac monitoring (such as with internal loop recorders or ambulatory monitoring) may be required to assess whether permanent pacemaker insertion may be indicated (Box 6.9).

Asymptomatic patients should be treated conservatively.

TRIFASCICULAR BLOCK

ECG FINDINGS

Trifascicular block refers to the presence of the following three abnormalities on ECG (Fig. 6.32):
- RBBB
- Left anterior or left posterior fascicular block
- First-degree heart block

Note that the term 'trifascicular block' is a misnomer. Just like bifascicular block, two fascicles are blocked. However, there is an additional slowing of conduction in the atrioventricular node (which is notably not a

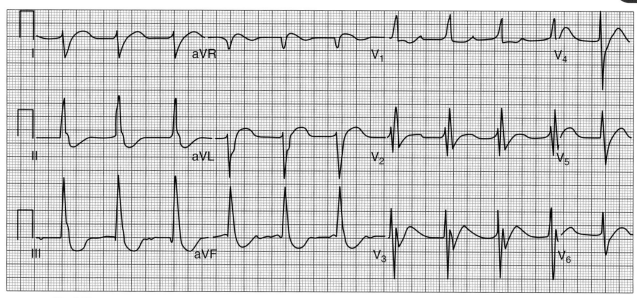

Fig. 6.32 Trifascicular block. There is both RBBB and left posterior fascicular block (right axis deviation) with prolonged PR interval. (Source: Raghawa Rao, B. N. V. (2012). Intraventricular conduction defects. In: *Clinical Examination in Cardiology*, 2nd ed. Elsevier.)

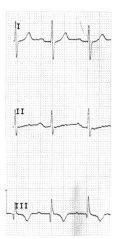

Fig. 6.33 $S_1Q_3T_3$ pattern is an uncommon finding in pulmonary embolus. It is a result of acute right heart strain. This refers to a pattern of ECG changes in leads I and III; there are S waves in lead I, Q waves in lead III and inverted T waves in lead III.

fascicle but has been included as such in this term) that produces first-degree heart block.

CLINICAL FEATURES

The presence of 'trifascicular block' increases the risk of developing complete heart block, which can subsequently present with dizziness, presyncope or syncope.

MANAGEMENT

A permanent pacemaker is indicated if the patient is symptomatic. If asymptomatic, the patient should be informed of the symptoms suggesting the development of intermittent atrioventricular conduction block.

PULMONARY EMBOLISM

Definition

A blockage of the pulmonary vasculature by a thromboembolus.

ECG FINDINGS

Most cases of pulmonary embolus present with an ECG showing no abnormality other than sinus tachycardia. Whilst ECGs are neither sensitive nor specific for the diagnosis of pulmonary embolism, the following ECG changes can suggest the presence of significant embolism (reflecting increased right heart pressure and strain):

- Sinus tachycardia: the commonest abnormality
- Right ventricular 'strain' pattern:
  - RBBB
  - T-wave inversion and ST depression in right ventricular leads (V_1–V_4) and/or inferiorly (II, III, aVF)
  - Right-axis deviation
  - A combination of the above is sometimes referred to as the $S_1Q_3T_3$ pattern (Fig. 6.33): an uncommon finding of deep S waves in lead I along with Q waves and T-wave inversion in lead III
- Right atrial enlargement – P pulmonale

CLINICAL FEATURES

Clinical features of pulmonary embolism are non-specific. The commonest presentation is sudden-onset dyspnoea and pleuritic chest pain, which may be accompanied by haemoptysis.

MANAGEMENT

Pulmonary embolism can be confirmed using computed tomography pulmonary angiography or a lung ventilation/perfusion (V/Q) scan. Treatment includes intravenous fluid resuscitation and anticoagulation, with thrombolysis or catheter-based therapies in cases of massive pulmonary embolism causing haemodynamic compromise.

₁₂₃ Key Points

1. Normal QRS complex width: 80–120 ms
2. LVH: amplitude of S wave in V_1 plus R wave in V_5/V_6 is greater than 35 mm
3. RVH: dominant R wave in V_1
4. Pericardial effusions: low QRS voltage and electrical alternans in massive effusions
5. ECG findings to localise bundle branch blocks:
    (a) LBBB: wide QRS, notched R wave in V_6 ('WiLLiaM')
    (b) RBBB: wide QRS, rSR' in V_1 ('MaRRoW')
    (c) Left anterior fascicular block: left-axis deviation
    (d) Left posterior fascicular block: right-axis deviation
    (e) Bifascicular block: RBBB and left/right-axis deviation
    (f) Trifascicular block: RBBB, left/right-axis deviation and first-degree heart block
6. Pulmonary embolus: sinus tachycardia is the commonest finding. Other findings include RBBB, right-axis deviation, right 'strain' pattern, P pulmonale, $S_1Q_3T_3$

FURTHER READING

Boron, W.F., Boulpaep, E.L., 2017. Medical Physiology. Elsevier, Philadelphia.

Hampton, J.R., Hampton, J., 2019. The ECG Made Easy. Elsevier.

John, A.D., Fleisher, L.A., 2006. Electrocardiography: the ECG. Anesthesiol. Clin. North Am. 24 (4), 697–715.

Patel, S., et al., 2017. Counterclockwise and clockwise rotation of QRS transitional zone: prospective correlates of change and time-varying associations with cardiovascular outcomes. J. Am. Heart Assoc. 6 (11).

Vecht, R.J., et al., 2009. ECG diagnosis in clinical practice. https://doi.org/10.1007/978-1-84800-312-5.

QT Interval

7

OVERVIEW

DEFINITION

The QT interval is defined as the time interval between the start of the Q wave and the end of the T wave (Fig. 7.1).

ELECTROPHYSIOLOGY

The time taken for ventricular depolarisation and completion of repolarisation is represented by the QT interval.

INTERPRETATION

The QT interval is best measured in either lead II or leads V_5–V_6. It is inversely proportional to heart rate; it shortens at faster heart rates and lengthens at slower heart rates.

The corrected QT interval (QTc) is the most accurate method of interpreting QT intervals. This allows comparison of QT values at different heart rates by including the R–R interval, which is the time between two consecutive R peaks.

The QTc is calculated using the following equation based on the Fridericia formula:

$$QTc = \frac{QT(s)}{\sqrt[3]{RR\ interval\ (s)}}$$

Normal

In a normal adult, the QTc interval should be 350–440 s (Fig. 7.2).

It is not always practical to calculate the QTc for every ECG interpreted. For practical purposes, when quickly viewing ECGs, a QT interval that measures less than half the R–R interval can be considered normal (Fig. 7.3). However, note that this crude method is only effective at normal heart rates.

Short QT Interval

The QTc is abnormally short if <350 ms. This rarely occurs and causes are shown in Box 7.1.

A short QT interval is a risk factor for ventricular arrhythmias and initial evaluation and treatment are aimed at identifying and treating secondary causes. If no secondary cause is identified, consider referral to a specialist for consideration of genetic testing.

Long QT Interval

The QTc is normal if <440 ms and prolonged if >470 ms. A value of 440–470 ms is considered 'borderline' QT prolongation. An abnormally prolonged QT is associated with an increased risk of ventricular arrhythmias, especially torsades de pointes.

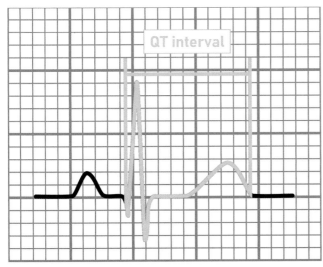

Fig. 7.1 The QT interval is measured from the beginning of the QRS complex to the end of the T wave.

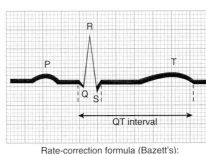

Rate-correction formula (Bazett's):

$$QTc\ (ms) = \frac{QT\ (s)}{\sqrt{RR\ (s)}}$$

Fig. 7.2 QT interval and calculating QTc. Since the QT interval is affected by heart rate, the corrected QT (QTc) interval should be calculated for more accurate interpretation. Crudely, a QT interval less than half the R–R interval could be considered normal when the heart rate is 60–100 bpm. (Source: Nussbaum, R., McInnes, R., Willard, H. (2015). Clinical case studies illustrating genetic principles. In: *Thompson & Thompson Genetics in Medicine*, 8th ed. Elsevier.)

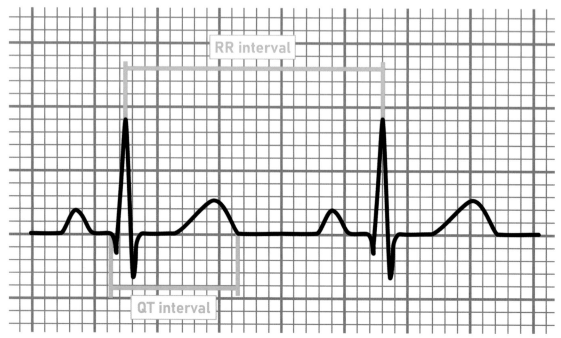

Fig. 7.3 In a regular rhythm at a normal heart rate, a QT interval less than half the R–R interval can crudely be considered normal.

Box 7.1 Causes of short QT interval

PRIMARY
- Short QT syndrome (genetic ion channelopathy)

SECONDARY
- Hypercalcaemia
- Acidosis
- Hyperthermia
- Drugs, e.g. digoxin

Important causes of long QT interval include:
- Hypocalcaemia
- Hypomagnesaemia
- Hypokalaemia
- Long QT syndromes
- Hypothermia

HYPERCALCAEMIA

DEFINITION

Hypercalcaemia is defined as a corrected serum calcium level greater than 2.6 mmol/L.

ECG FINDINGS

Shortening of the QT interval is the most important ECG change in hypercalcaemia (Fig. 7.4). In addition, severe hypercalcaemia can produce:
- Prolonged PR
- Wide QRS
- Osborn waves (positive elevation of the point at which the QRS complex meets the ST segment; see Chapter 10)
- Complete heart block

CLINICAL FEATURES

Hypercalcaemia produces a wide range of symptoms:
- *Stones*: Renal colic
- *Bones*: Osteolysis and fractures
- *Abdominal groans*: Constipation, nausea and vomiting
- *Psychic moans*: Depression

MANAGEMENT

Initially, resuscitate with intravenous fluids and offer bisphosphonates. Consider steroids, chemotherapy and diuretics according to the cause of hypercalcaemia. Haemodialysis should be used in cases of cardiovascular or renal compromise.

HYPOCALCAEMIA

DEFINITION

Hypocalcaemia is defined as a corrected serum calcium level of less than 2.1 mmol/L.

ECG FINDINGS

Prolongation of the QT interval is the most important ECG change in hypocalcaemia (Fig. 7.5). Consequently, severe hypercalcaemia can lead to ventricular tachycardia, including torsades de pointes, as it increases the likelihood of depolarisation occurring when ventricles have not fully repolarised. Other ECG changes include shortening of the PR interval and flattening or inversion of T waves.

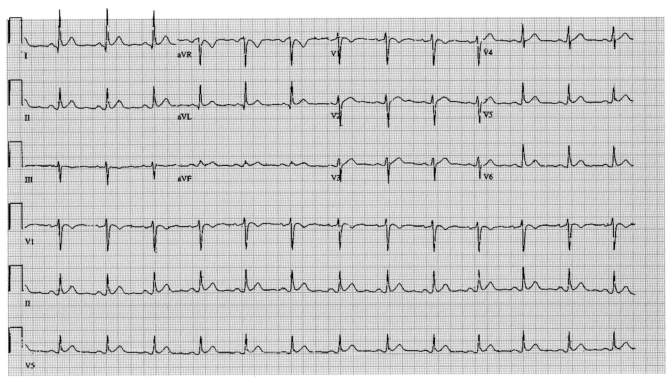

Fig. 7.4 Hypercalcaemia. ECG of a patient with hypercalcaemia (Ca+ level: 11.6 mmol/L). QT/QTc intervals are 320/368 ms. (Source: Das, M., Zipes, D. (2021). Polymorphic ventricular tachycardia and ventricular fibrillation in the absence of structural heart disease. In: *Electrocardiography of Arrhythmias: A Comprehensive Review*. Elsevier.)

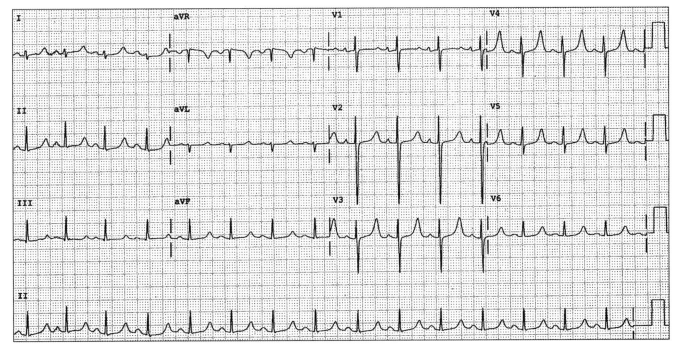

Fig. 7.5 Hypocalcaemia. ECG of a patient with hypocalcaemia. QT/QTc intervals are 420/500 ms. Peaked T waves can also be seen as there is concomitant hyperkalaemia. (Source: Baker, T., Nikolic, G., O'Connor, S. (2008). An overview of clinical electrocardiography. In: *Practical Cardiology: An Approach to the Management of Problems in Cardiology*, 2nd ed. Churchill Livingstone Australia.)

CLINICAL FEATURES

Hypocalcaemia mostly affects nerves and muscles, producing:

- Numbness and paraesthesia
- Tetany
- Chvostek sign (tapping on facial muscles produces contraction of the muscles)
- Trousseau sign (inflation of blood pressure cuff around the arm produces spasm of the muscles of the hand and wrist)
- Confusion
- Seizures
- Cardiac arrest

MANAGEMENT

Discontinue any drugs that can cause calcium depletion or prolongation of the QT interval. Depending on the severity of hypocalcaemia, provide oral or intravenous calcium supplementation and offer alfacalcidol in cases of chronic kidney disease.

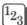 **Key Points**

1. The QT interval is measured from the start of the Q wave to the end of the T wave
2. QTc is the most accurate method for interpreting QT interval
3. At normal heart rates, the QT interval can be crudely considered normal if it is less than half the R–R interval
4. Hypercalcaemia produces shortening of the QT interval
5. Hypocalcaemia produces prolongation of the QT interval

FURTHER READING

Boron, W.F., Boulpaep, E.L., 2017. Medical Physiology. Elsevier, Philadelphia.

Douglas, P. S., Carmichael, K. A., Palevsky, P. M. Extreme hypercalcemia and electrocardiographic changes. Am. J. Cardiol. 54 (6), 674–675.

Hampton, J.R., Hampton, J., 2019. The ECG Made Easy. Elsevier.

John, A.D., Fleisher, L.A., 2006. Electrocardiography: the ECG. Anesthesiol. Clin. 24 (4), 697–715.

Kumar, P., Clark, M., 2021. Kumar & Clark's Cases in Clinical Medicine. Elsevier.

Thaler, M.S., 2017. The only EKG book you'll ever need. Lippincott Williams & Wilkins.

Vecht, R.J., et al., 2009. ECG Diagnosis in Clinical Practice. Springer.

Wang, K., 2012. Atlas of Electrocardiography. Jaypee Brothers Medical Publishers.

ST Segment

8

OVERVIEW

DEFINITION

The ST segment refers to the section between the end of the QRS complex (known as the J-point) and the start of the T wave (Fig. 8.1).

ELECTROPHYSIOLOGY

The ST segment represents the initial phase of ventricular repolarisation.

INTERPRETATION

The ST segment height should be interpreted in reference to the isoelectric line (Fig. 8.2). The isoelectric line is usually taken as the segment between the end of the T wave and the start of the next P wave (TP segment).

Normal

The ST segment lies at the same level as the isoelectric line in normal ECGs (Fig. 8.2).

ST Segment Elevation

The ST segment lies above the isoelectric line (Fig. 8.2) in ST elevation.

The most important cause of ST elevation is acute myocardial infarction (ST elevation myocardial infarction or STEMI). The leads that display ST elevation can be used to localise the site of infarction (Table 8.2).

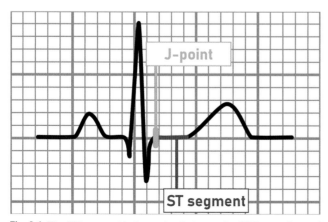

Fig. 8.1 The ST segment is the region between the QRS complex and the T wave. The junction between the end of the QRS complex and the start of the ST segment is termed the J-point.

STEMI is the commonest cause of ST elevation (Box 8.1) and is a medical emergency. Immediate referral for consideration for primary percutaneous coronary intervention (PCI) is the priority. Sometimes ECGs can be equivocal; if in doubt seek urgent cardiology opinion.

ST Segment Depression

The ST segment lies below the isoelectric line (Fig. 8.2) in ST depression.

Several pathologies can cause ST depression (Box 8.2), including myocardial ischaemia. ST segment depression due to coronary disease is associated with a poor outcome and should be managed as an emergency as per the STEMI pathway.

ACUTE CORONARY SYNDROME

DEFINITION

Acute coronary syndrome (ACS) is a syndrome encompassing a range of conditions that include unstable angina, NSTEMI and STEMI. These develop due to decreased blood flow in the coronary arteries, mostly occurring as a result of thrombosis, plaque rupture and inflammation.

CLASSIFICATION

ACS includes the following conditions:
- STEMI: transmural infarction (Fig. 8.3)
- NSTEMI: subendocardial infarction
- Unstable angina: ischaemia without infarction

These can be clinically differentiated according to the presence of ST elevation on ECG and raised serum cardiac enzymes (suggesting infarction) (Table 8.1).

STEMI

STEMI relates to a complete thrombotic occlusion of a main coronary artery or branch. A diagnosis of acute STEMI should be considered if any of the following changes are present on ECG:
- ≥2 mm ST elevation in at least two contiguous leads in leads V_2–V_3
- ≥1 mm ST elevation in at least two contiguous leads in all other precordial leads and limb leads

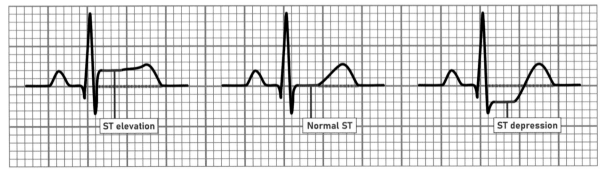

Fig. 8.2 ST segment height should be compared to the isoelectric point (where amplitude is 0).

Box 8.1 | **Causes of ST elevation**

- ST elevation myocardial infarction (STEMI)
- Pericarditis: widespread ST elevation (ECGs)
  - Saddle-shaped ST elevation not related to a single coronary territory
  - PR depression
- Ventricular aneurysm
- Brugada syndrome: coved ST elevation with RSR' pattern in V_1–V_3
- Young athletes ECGs – high-takeoff: widespread concave ST elevation with no reciprocal changes; a benign finding
- Subarachnoid haemorrhage

Box 8.2 | **Causes of ST depression**

- Posterior myocardial infarction – equivalent of posterior STEMI
- Non-ST elevation myocardial infarction (NSTEMI)
- Reciprocal changes of ST elevation (e.g. anterior STEMI with ST elevation in anterior leads and ST depression in inferior leads)
- Myocardial ischaemia: produces horizontal ST depression
- Digoxin: produces downsloping ST depression
- Ventricular hypertrophy with 'strain' pattern
- Altered repolarisation:
  - Bundle branch block
  - Ventricular hypertrophy
  - Hypokalaemia
  - Pre-excitation

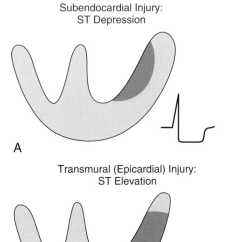

Fig. 8.3 Transmural and subendocardial infarcts. (A) Subendocardial infarction is necrosis of the inner surface of the myocardium, producing NSTEMI. (B) Transmural infarction is a full-thickness infarction of the myocardium, leading to STEMI. (Source: Zipes, D. P., Libby, P. (2019). *Braunwald's Heart Disease: A Textbook of Cardiovascular Medicine*, 12th ed. Elsevier.)

Table 8.1 | **Features used to differentiate STEMI, NSTEMI and unstable angina**

	STEMI	NSTEMI	Unstable angina
ST elevation	✓	✗	✗
Raised cardiac enzymes, e.g. troponin	✓	✓	✗

- Posterior myocardial infarction (ST depression and dominant R waves in V_1–V_3)

ECG FINDINGS

Hyperacute T waves and ST elevation are the earliest ECG changes in STEMI. Given its higher specificity for STEMIs, ST elevation is the most pertinent finding in this condition (Fig. 8.4) and develops within hours of infarction. Over a period of a few days, pathological Q waves and T-wave inversion occurs.

In the long term, the ECG normalises and the only remaining ECG change is the presence of pathological Q waves, which indicates scar formation. A persistently elevated ST segment in most chest leads is a sign of a ventricular aneurysm, an uncommon complication of myocardial infarction.

It should be noted that the interpretation of the ST segment is complicated if there is a previous, known LBBB (Box 8.3).

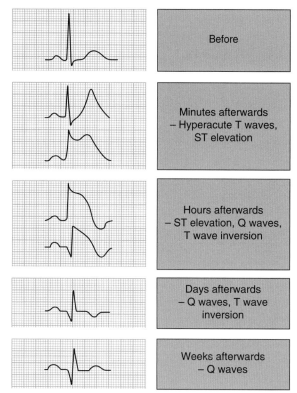

	Before
	Minutes afterwards – Hyperacute T waves, ST elevation
	Hours afterwards – ST elevation, Q waves, T wave inversion
	Days afterwards – Q waves, T wave inversion
	Weeks afterwards – Q waves

Fig. 8.4 ECG changes in STEMI according to time following infarction. After the first few minutes, the T waves become tall, pointed and upright and there is ST-segment elevation. After the first few hours, the T waves invert, the R-wave voltage is decreased and Q waves develop. After a few days, the ST segment returns to normal. After weeks or months, the T wave may return to upright but the Q wave remains. (Source: Hinds, C. J., Watson, J. D. (2008). Myocardial ischaemia, cardiopulmonary resuscitation and management of arrhythmias. In: *Intensive Care: A Concise Textbook*, 3rd ed. Saunders.)

The above ECG changes occur in specific leads according to the vessel occluded and region affected (Table 8.2 and Figs 8.5–8.9). Frequently, ST elevation in one region is associated with ST depression in leads on the opposite side of the heart; this is termed reciprocal ST depression. For example, an inferior STEMI produces ST elevation in the inferior leads (II, III, aVF) and ST depression in the superior leads (I, aVL).

Posterior infarctions can be easily missed: they initially present with ST depression and later dominant R waves (R wave larger than S wave) in V_1–V_3 (Fig. 8.10). Therefore, posterior infarcts are said to produce a mirror image of an anterior STEMI. There may be associated mild ST segment elevation in the inferior and/or lateral leads. ECG electrodes can be placed posteriorly to evaluate suspected posterior MI further (Figs 8.11 and 8.12).

If a posterior MI is suspected, the presence of ST elevation on leads placed on the posterior chest wall (Fig. 8.7) may be helpful.

Additional ECG findings of MI can include:

- Atrioventricular block and consequent bradycardia, particularly in inferior MIs

Box 8.3   LBBB and STEMI

Interpreting the ECG for signs of MI can be difficult in LBBB, given the abnormal depolarisation and repolarisation of the ventricles, particularly if no old ECGs are available for comparison.

LBBB is an uncommon ECG presentation for STEMI. The Sgarbossa criteria are a useful tool to diagnose acute MI in such situations. Points are given based on the following findings:

- ST segment elevation ≥1 mm in lead and in the same direction (concordant) as the QRS complex: 5 points
- ST segment depression ≥1 mm in leads V_1, V_2 or V_3: 3 points
- ST segment elevation ≥5 mm in lead and in the opposite direction (discordant) as the QRS complex: 2 points

A score of 3 or more is highly suggestive (with a high specificity but low sensitivity) of acute MI.

 Table 8.2   **Sites of infarction, their ECG changes and the most likely coronary arteries involved**

Site	ST segment changes	Coronary artery commonly involved
Septal	Elevation: V1–V2	Left anterior descending
Anterior	Elevation: V3–V4	Left anterior descending
Lateral	Elevation: I, aVL, V5–V6	Left circumflex; left anterior descending
Inferior	Elevation: II, III, aVF	Right coronary
Posterior	Depression: V1–V3 Elevation: V7–V9 (with dominant R wave and ST depression in V1–V3); see Fig. 8.11	Left circumflex

- Poor R-wave progression, particularly in old anterior MIs

CLINICAL FEATURES

Central, crushing chest pain is the commonest symptom of MI; the pain can radiate to the jaw, neck or shoulder. It may also be associated with nausea, vomiting and sweating. Note that atypical presentations of MIs also exist without the classic central chest pain, and are more likely in diabetics, women and the elderly.

MANAGEMENT

All patients presenting with STEMI should be considered for immediate emergency primary PCI. If PCI is not available, patients should receive fibrinolysis instead. While primary PCI should not be delayed, consideration should be given for treatment with aspirin 300 mg, a potent second antiplatelet agent (such as prasugrel 60 mg or ticagrelor 180 mg), opiate analgesia and antiemetics.

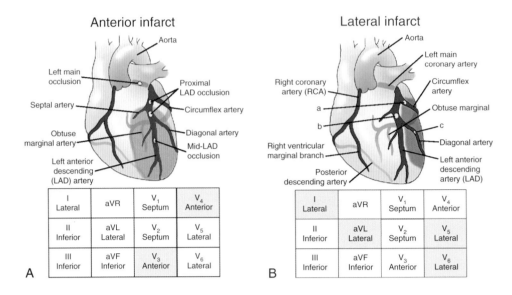

Anterior infarct

I Lateral	aVR	V₁ Septum	V₄ Anterior
II Inferior	aVL Lateral	V₂ Septum	V₅ Lateral
III Inferior	aVF Inferior	V₃ Anterior	V₆ Lateral

A

Lateral infarct

I Lateral	aVR	V₁ Septum	V₄ Anterior
II Inferior	aVL Lateral	V₂ Septum	V₅ Lateral
III Inferior	aVF Inferior	V₃ Anterior	V₆ Lateral

B

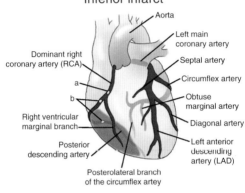

Inferior infarct

I Lateral	aVR	V₁ Septum	V₄ Anterior
II Inferior	aVL Lateral	V₂ Septum	V₅ Lateral
III Inferior	aVF Inferior	V₃ Anterior	V₆ Lateral

C

Septal infarct

I Lateral	aVR	V₁ Septum	V₄ Anterior
II Inferior	aVL Lateral	V₂ Septum	V₅ Lateral
III Inferior	aVF Inferior	V₃ Anterior	V₆ Lateral

D

Posterior infarct

I Lateral	aVR	V₁ Septum	V₄ Anterior	V₇ Posterior
II Inferior	aVL Lateral	V₂ Septum	V₅ Lateral	V₈ Posterior
III Inferior	aVF Inferior	V₃ Anterior	V₆ Lateral	V₉ Posterior

E

Fig. 8.5 (A–E) The leads and arteries corresponding to the main regions of the heart. (Source: Aehlert, B. (2009). Introduction to the 12-lead ECG. In: *ECGs Made Easy*, 4th ed. Maryland Heights: Elsevier.)

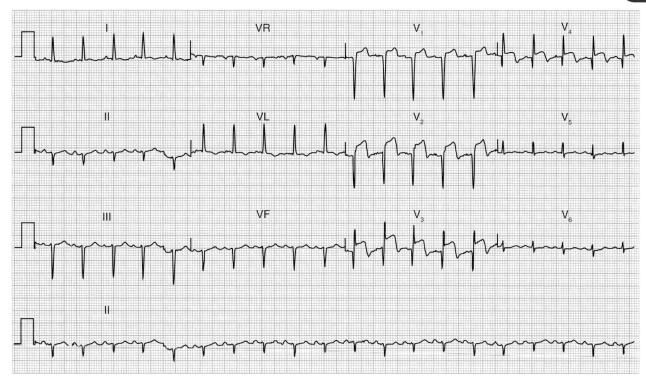

Fig. 8.6 Anterior STEMI. There is ST elevation in leads V_2–V_4. (Source: Wijaya, I. P., Salim, S. (2021). EKG pada pasien dengan nyeri dada dan sesak napas. In: *Membaca EKG Cara Mudah*, 9th ed. Elsevier.)

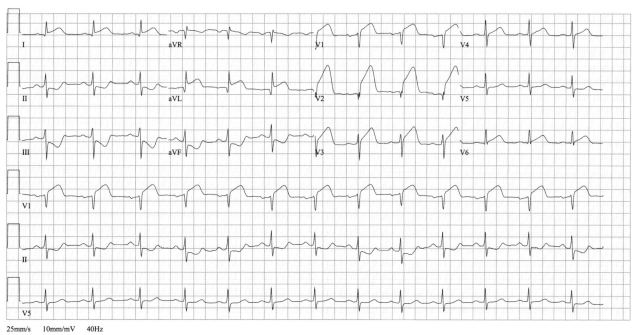

25mm/s   10mm/mV   40Hz

Fig. 8.7 Anterolateral STEMI. There is ST elevation in leads V_1–V_3 and I and aVL. (Source: De Bliek, E. C. (2018). ST elevation: differential diagnosis and caveats. A comprehensive review to help distinguish ST elevation myocardial infarction from non-ischemic etiologies of ST elevation. *Turkish Journal of Emergency Medicine*, 18(1): pp. 1–10.)

MYOCARDIAL ISCHAEMIA AND NSTEMI

Inadequate blood flow to cardiac muscle produces myocardial ischaemia. This can present as angina or, if there is partial obstruction to coronary blood flow or occlusion of a small vessel, NSTEMI.

ECG FINDINGS

ST depression and T-wave inversion are the most pertinent findings in myocardial ischaemia and NSTEMI (Figs 8.13–8.15). The ST segment depression may be horizontal or downsloping (Fig. 8.16). These findings are temporary in ischaemia; in cases of angina, these

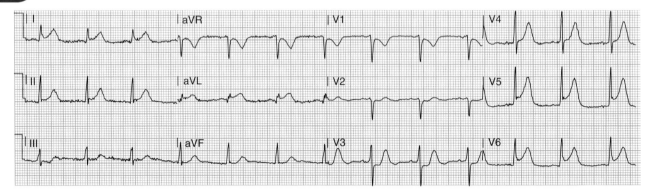

Fig. 8.8 Lateral STEMI. There is ST elevation in leads V$_5$–V$_6$ and I.

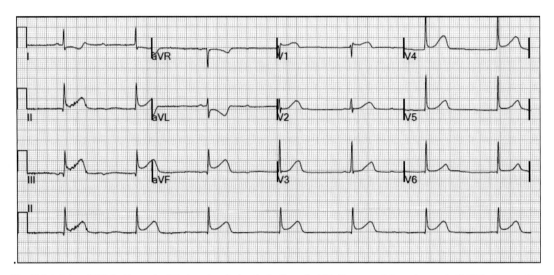

Fig. 8.9 Inferior STEMI. There is ST elevation in leads II, III and aVF. (Source: Crisp, J., et al. (2020). Supporting oxygenation and perfusion. In: *Potter & Perry's Fundamentals of Nursing*, 6th ed. Elsevier.)

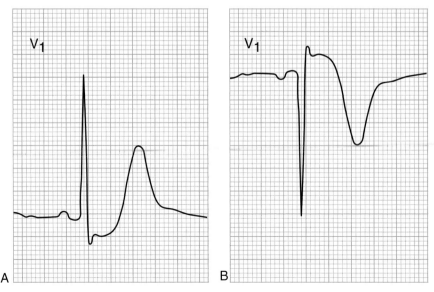

Fig. 8.10 Lead V$_1$ in posterior MI. (A) ST depression and dominant R wave can be seen. (B) Mirroring the tracing replicates the pattern of ST elevation and Q waves typically seen in other STEMIs. Practically, this can be seen by flipping the printed ECG paper over and viewing the trace from the unprinted side against a light source. (Source: Hampton, J. R. (2008). The ECG in patients with palpitations and syncope. In: *The ECG in Practice*, 5th ed. Churchill Livingstone.)

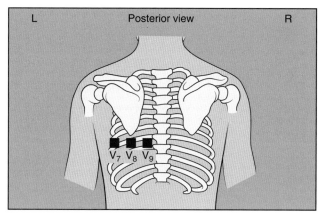

Fig. 8.11 Posterior lead positions. In a posterior MI, leads V_7–V_9 on the posterior chest wall will show ST elevation. (Source: Urden, L., Stacy, K., Lough, M. (2014). Cardiovascular diagnostic procedures. In: *Critical Care Nursing: Diagnosis and Management*, 7th ed. Mosby.)

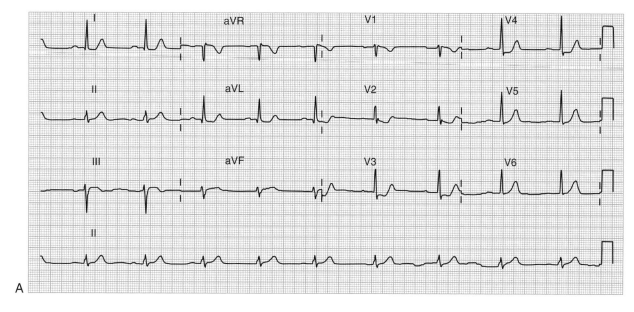

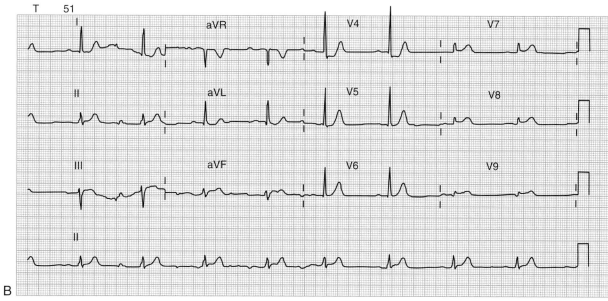

Fig. 8.12 Posterior MI in usual lead configuration (A) and with V_7–V_9 recorded (B). (Source: https://litfl.com/wp-content/uploads/2018/08/ECG-Posterior-AMI-2.jpg)

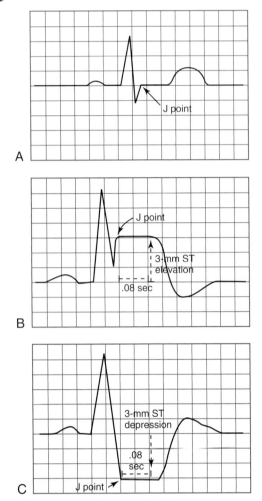

Fig. 8.13 The ST segment starts from the J-point (end of QRS complex). (A) Normal ST segment. (B) A 3-mm ST segment elevation, as could be seen in STEMI. (C) A 3-mm ST segment depression, as could be seen in NSTEMI. (Source: Urden, L., Stacy, K., Lough, M. (2014). Cardiovascular diagnostic procedures. In: *Critical Care Nursing: Diagnosis and Management*, 7th ed. Mosby.)

ECG changes occur on exercise and can be elicited through a stress ECG test. Persistent ECG changes are suggestive of ongoing infarction. As implied by the term, there is no ST elevation in an NSTEMI.

CLINICAL FEATURES

Myocardial ischaemia commonly produces chest pain. Unstable angina and NSTEMI present with the same symptoms and signs as STEMI; central, crushing chest pain, which may potentially radiate to the jaw or shoulders, is the commonest presenting symptom.

Unstable angina and NSTEMI are differentiated by the presence of an elevated troponin (indicating infarction). Given the widespread use of high-sensitivity troponin tests, a diagnosis of unstable angina is becoming increasingly rare.

MANAGEMENT

The acute management of NSTEMI and unstable angina is the same and includes:

- Analgesia (morphine with antiemetic)
- Glyceryl trinitrate
- Antiplatelets (aspirin with second antiplatelet agent, e.g. clopidogrel, ticagrelor)
- Antithrombotic agents, for example, low-molecular-weight heparin, fondaparinux
- Consider coronary angiography depending on clinical presentation:
    - Emergency (similar to STEMI):
        - Haemodynamic instability
        - Ventricular arrhythmias
        - Dynamic ST segment changes
        - Ongoing chest pain
    - Early (within 24 h):
        - Elevated troponin
        - ECG changes

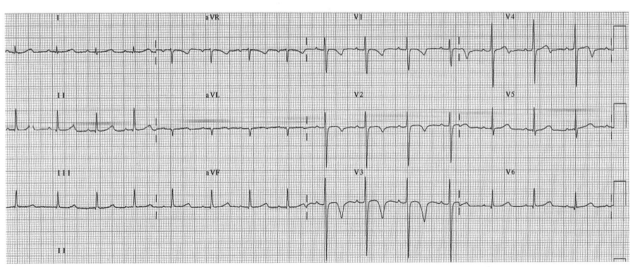

Fig. 8.14 NSTEMI with T-wave inversion that is most prominent in anteroseptal leads (V_1–V_4). (Source: Reed-Poysden, C., Gupta, K. J. (2015). Acute coronary syndromes. *BJA Education*, 15(6): pp. 286–293.)

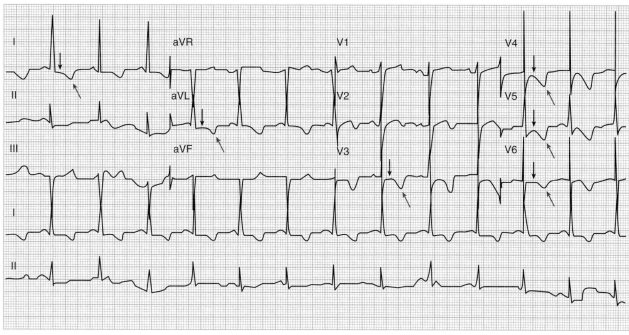

Fig. 8.15 NSTEMI with ST depression (black arrows) and T-wave inversion (red arrows) in anterior and lateral leads (V₃–V₆, aVL, I). (Source: Harding, M., et al. (2019). Coronary artery disease and acute coronary syndrome. In: *Lewis's Medical-Surgical Nursing: Assessment and Management of Clinical Problems*, 11th ed. Elsevier.)

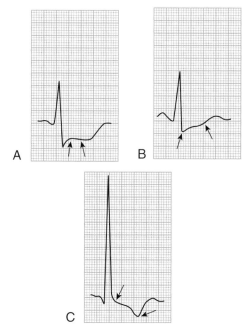

Fig. 8.16 ST depression. ST depression can be: (A) horizontal; (B) upsloping; (C) downsloping. (Source: Ehrenwerth, J., Eisenkraft, J. B., Berry, J. M. (2013). Electrocardiographic monitoring. In: *Anesthesia Equipment: Principles and Applications*, 2nd ed. Philadelphia: Elsevier.)

PERICARDITIS

DEFINITION

Pericarditis refers to inflammation of the pericardium. Most cases are viral in origin. However, any infection or inflammation of structures neighbouring the pericardium can cause pericarditis (Box 8.4).

Box 8.4	Causes of pericarditis

- Idiopathic
- Infection:
  - Viral, e.g. coxsackievirus, echovirus
  - Bacterial, e.g. tuberculosis, pneumococcus
  - Fungal, e.g. histoplasmosis
- Post-injury:
  - Cardiac surgery
  - Trauma
  - Radiation
  - MI – immediate or delayed (Dressler syndrome)
  - Post-catheter ablation for cardiac arrhythmias
- Neoplasms
- Metabolic disease:
  - Uraemia
  - Medication, e.g. hydralazine, isoniazid
- Autoimmunity:
  - Rheumatoid arthritis
  - Systemic lupus erythematosus
  - Sarcoidosis
  - Dermatomyositis
- Aortic dissection

Pericarditis can lead to the development of a pericardial effusion, which may impair ventricular contraction and produce haemodynamic compromise (tamponade).

ECG FINDINGS

Widespread saddle-shaped ST elevation is the most sensitive ECG finding of pericarditis (Figs 8.17 and 8.18). Other ECG findings are listed in Box 8.5.

CLINICAL FEATURES

Retrosternal, pleuritic chest pain that is relieved by sitting forward and worse by lying down is the characteristic presentation for pericarditis. Auscultation may reveal a pericardial friction rub.

Later, they may develop symptoms related to a pericardial effusion, such as breathlessness.

MANAGEMENT

Most patients can be managed conservatively with bed rest, colchicine and non-steroidal anti-inflammatory drugs. Investigations should be directed at excluding secondary causes and, in the presence of elevated troponins (suggesting cardiac muscle involvement), echocardiography should be arranged. If there is an associated large pericardial effusion, pericardiocentesis may be required for diagnostic and treatment purposes.

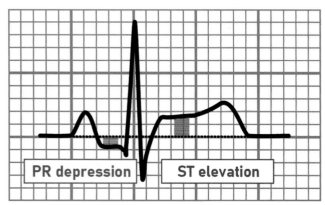

Fig. 8.17 Pericarditis has ST elevation with PR depression.

BRUGADA SYNDROME

DEFINITION

Brugada syndrome is a rare inherited condition that is characterised by a genetic abnormality (SCN5A) of the sodium channel that results in abnormal cardiac conduction. This is associated with an increased risk of ventricular arrhythmias and sudden cardiac death.

ECG FINDINGS

The diagnosis of Brugada syndrome is based on a characteristic ECG pattern in the absence of structural heart disease.

Coved ST elevation with a right bundle branch block appearance (RSR′ appearance of QRS complex) in V_1–V_3 with T-wave inversion is the most pertinent ECG finding (Fig. 8.19).

CLINICAL FEATURES

Many patients are asymptomatic. Symptomatic cases may present with syncope and palpitations. Brugada syndrome predisposes patients to develop sudden cardiac death due to ventricular fibrillation.

Box 8.5	ECG changes in pericarditis

- Saddle-shaped ST elevation not corresponding to a single coronary territory
- PR depression (very specific sign of pericarditis)
- Sinus tachycardia

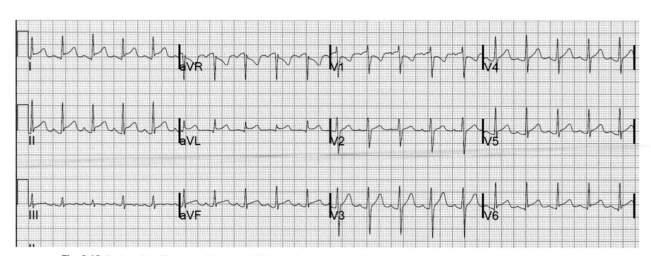

Fig. 8.18 Pericarditis. There is widespread ST elevation alongside PR depression. The rate is tachycardic at 120 bpm. (Source: Bischhof, J. E., et al. (2016). ST depression in lead aVL differentiates inferior ST-elevation myocardial infarction from pericarditis. *American Journal of Emergency Medicine*, 34(2): pp. 149–154.)

MANAGEMENT

There is no definitive treatment for Brugada syndrome. Individuals at high risk of ventricular arrhythmias should be considered for an implantable cardioverter defibrillator.

DIGOXIN

DEFINITION

Digoxin is a drug used to control ventricular rate in atrial fibrillation. Its electrophysiological effect includes slowing of atrioventricular conduction due to a parasympathetic effect.

Digoxin has a low therapeutic index and toxicity is common. This can occur acutely following an overdose or develop gradually over long-term treatment, particularly in the presence of renal disease.

ECG FINDINGS

Digoxin use produces downsloping ST depression that resembles a 'reverse tick' (Fig. 8.20).

Digoxin toxicity can produce any arrhythmia, which is usually due to increased automaticity and decreased atrioventricular conduction (Fig. 8.21). The most common ECG changes include:

- Atrial ectopic beats
- Ventricular ectopic beats
- Atrioventricular block
- Bigeminy
- Ventricular arrhythmias

CLINICAL FEATURES

Symptoms of digoxin toxicity are non-specific and may include:

- Nausea and vomiting
- Abdominal pain
- Confusion
- Yellow vision (xanthopsia)

MANAGEMENT

Digoxin toxicity can be treated with digoxin-specific antibody fragments (Digibind) if signs of haemodynamic instability or ventricular arrhythmias are present. If the patient is asymptomatic with no arrhythmias, s/he can be managed conservatively.

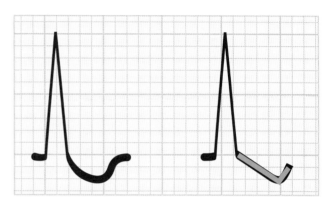

Fig. 8.20 Downsloping ST depression in therapeutic digoxin use. This is commonly referred to as the 'reverse tick' sign. (Source: Modified from Zipes, D. P., Libby, P. (2004). Electrocardiography. In: *Braunwald's Heart Disease: A Textbook of Cardiovascular Medicine*, 7th ed. Elsevier.)

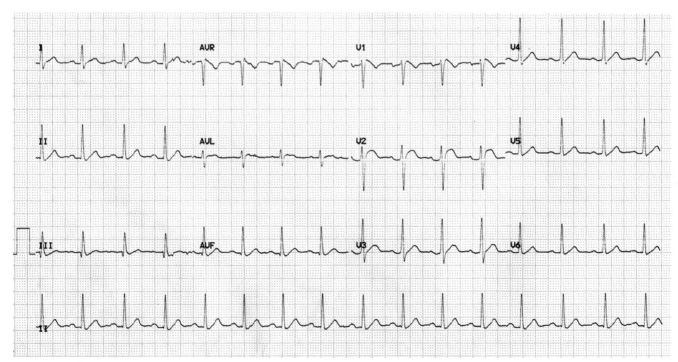

Fig. 8.19 Brugada syndrome. There is coved ST elevation with RSR' pattern in V_1–V_2.

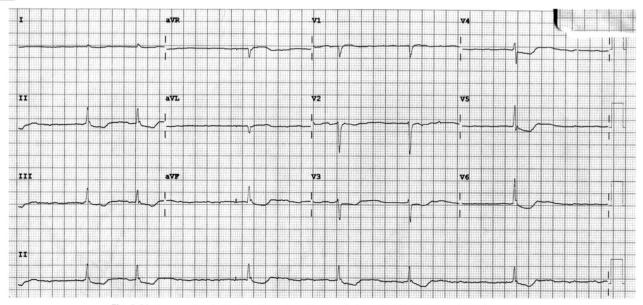

Fig. 8.21 Severe digoxin toxicity. There is evidence of slow atrial fibrillation and ST depression.

Key Points

1. ST segment height should be compared with the isoelectric line
2. ST elevation arises due to:
   (a) MI
   (b) Pericarditis
   (c) Brugada syndrome
3. ST depression arises due to:
   (a) NSTEMI
   (b) Myocardial ischaemia: produces horizontal ST depression
   (c) Posterior MI
   (d) Digoxin use: produces downsloping ST depression
   (e) Ventricular hypertrophy and 'strain' pattern
   (f) Altered repolarisation:
     - Bundle branch block
     - Ventricular hypertrophy
     - Hypokalaemia
     - Pre-excitation
4. STEMI:
   (a) ECG changes include:
     - ≥1 mm ST segment elevation in at least two contiguous limb leads
     - ≥2 mm ST segment elevation in at least two contiguous precordial leads
     - Posterior MI (ST depression and dominant R waves in V_1–V_3)
     - New LBBB

   (b) Sites of infarction:
     - Septal: ST elevation in V_1–V_2
     - Anterior: ST elevation in V_3–V_4
     - Lateral: ST elevation in I, aVL, V_5–V_6
     - Inferior: ST elevation in II, III, aVF
     - Posterior: dominant R wave and ST depression in V_1–V_3
5. Myocardial ischaemia and NSTEMI: ST depression and T-wave inversion
6. Pericarditis: widespread ST elevation
7. Brugada syndrome: coved ST elevation in V_1–V_3
8. Digoxin:
   (a) Therapeutic range: downsloping ST depression
   (b) Toxicity: arrhythmias

FURTHER READING

Boron, W.F., Boulpaep, E.L., 2017. Medical Physiology. Elsevier, Philadelphia.

Hampton, J.R., Hampton, J., 2019. The ECG Made Easy. Elsevier.

John, A. D., Fleisher, L. A. 'Electrocardiography: The ECG,' Anesthesiol. Clin. North Am. 24 (4), 697–715.

Pollehn, T., et al., 2002. The electrocardiographic differential diagnosis of ST segment depression. Emerg. Med. J. 19 (2), 129–135.

Rotondo, N., et al., 2004. Electrocardiographic manifestations: acute inferior wall myocardial infarction. J. Emerg. Med. 26 (4), 433–440.

Vecht, R.J., et al., 2009. ECG Diagnosis in Clinical Practice. Springer.

T Wave

9

OVERVIEW

DEFINITION

The T wave is the deflection following the QRS complex, which represents repolarisation of the ventricles (Fig. 9.1).

ELECTROPHYSIOLOGY

Repolarisation of the ventricles produces a current in the opposite direction to depolarisation. Therefore, one would expect it to produce a deflection in the opposite direction to the QRS complex. However, repolarisation starts in the epicardium (outer myocardial surface) and progresses to the endocardium, which is the opposite sequence to what occurs during depolarisation. Therefore, the T wave points upwards in most leads (like the QRS complex) due to the 'double negative' of charge and direction.

INTERPRETATION

Normal

T waves are upright in most leads. T-wave inversion (Fig. 9.2) is a normal finding in the following leads:
- aVR
- V_1
- V_2
- V_3 in athletes
- V_4 in children

Peaked T Waves

Tall, narrow and symmetrically peaked (also referred to as 'tented') T waves (Fig. 9.3) are characteristically seen in hyperkalaemia.

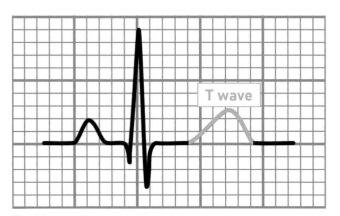

Fig. 9.1 The T wave is the deflection after the QRS complex. It represents ventricular repolarisation.

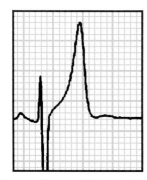

Fig. 9.3 Peaked T wave. (Source: Olshansky, B., et al. (2016). Drug effects and electrolyte disorders. In: *Arrhythmia Essentials*, 2nd ed. Elsevier.)

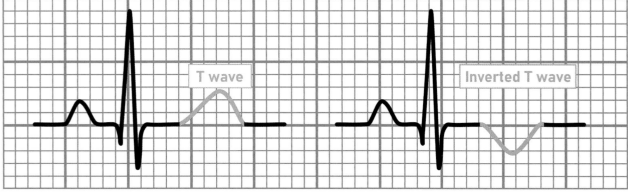

Fig. 9.2 Normal T wave and an inverted T wave.

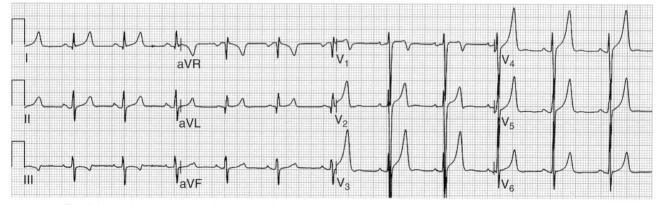

Fig. 9.4 Hyperkalaemia – tented T waves. Tented T waves are commonly seen in mild to moderate degrees of hyperkalaemia. (Source: Olshansky, B., et al. (2016). Drug effects and electrolyte disorders. In: *Arrhythmia Essentials*, 2nd ed. Elsevier.)

Box **9.1**   Causes of T-wave inversion
Myocardial ischaemia and infarction Bundle branch blocks Ventricular hypertrophy Pulmonary embolism Cardiomyopathy

T Wave Inversion

Various conditions can produce abnormal T wave inversion (Box 9.1).

HYPERKALAEMIA

DEFINITION

Hyperkalaemia is defined as a serum potassium level greater than 5.5 mmol/L.

ECG FINDINGS

Peaking or 'tenting' of T waves is usually the first ECG change seen in hyperkalaemia (Fig. 9.4).

As hyperkalaemia increases in magnitude, the following changes also develop in the following sequence (Fig. 9.5): flattened P wave, prolonged PR interval, depressed ST segment, atrial standstill, prolonged QRS duration, short QT and sinusoid wave pattern (Fig. 9.6). If untreated, these would lead to asystole, ventricular fibrillation or pulseless electrical activity.

ECG Changes in Hyperkalemia

QRS Complex	Approximate Serum Potassium (mmol/l)	ECG Change
P wave T wave	4-5	Normal
	6-7	Peaked T waves
	7-8	Flattened P wave, prolonged PR interval, depressed ST segment, peaked T wave
	8-9	Atrial standstill, prolonged QRS duration, further peaking T waves
	>9	Sinusoid wave pattern

Fig. 9.5 ECG changes in hyperkalaemia. Progressive hyperkalaemia results in identifiable changes in the ECG. These include peaking of the T wave, flattening of the P wave, prolongation of the PR interval, depression of the ST segment, prolongation of the QRS complex and, eventually, progression to a sine wave pattern. Ventricular fibrillation may occur at any time during this ECG progression. (Source: Johnson, R., et al. (2018). Disorders of potassium metabolism. In: *Comprehensive Clinical Nephrology*, 6th ed. Elsevier.)

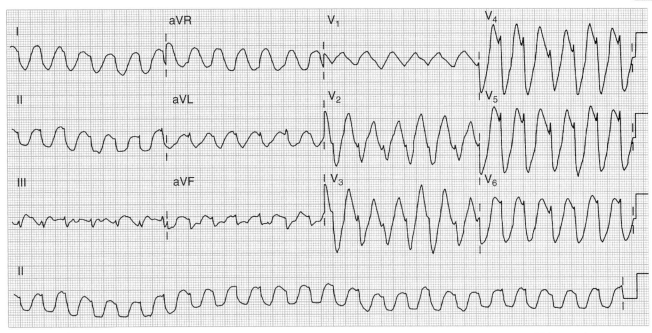

Fig. 9.6 Severe hyperkalaemia – sine wave appearance. This ECG shows a rapid, fairly regular wide QRS complex tachycardia (~150 bpm) with a sine wave pattern typical of severe hyperkalaemia. The patient's serum potassium level was 7.5 mmol/L (normal 3.5–5.1 mmol/L). (Source: Olshansky, B., et al. (2016). Drug effects and electrolyte disorders. In: *Arrhythmia Essentials*, 2nd ed. Elsevier.)

CLINICAL FEATURES

Mild hyperkalaemia is usually asymptomatic. When severe, it may result in palpitations, malaise, muscle aches, weakness and numbness.

MANAGEMENT

Hyperkalaemia that is symptomatic, greater than 6.5 mmol/L serum potassium or associated with ECG changes should be considered a medical emergency.
Management of hyperkalaemia includes:

- Cardiac protection: intravenous calcium gluconate or calcium chloride
- Intravenous insulin and dextrose
- Nebulised salbutamol (avoid in tachyarrhythmias)
- Selective potassium binder: sodium zirconium cyclosilicate
- Haemodialysis in resistant cases

Key Points

1. T waves are upright in most leads
2. T-wave inversions are normal in leads aVR and V_1. They can also be normally inverted in V_2 in young individuals.
3. Abnormal T-wave morphologies include:
   (a) Peaked or 'tented' T waves: hyperkalaemia
   (b) T-wave inversion: myocardial ischaemia, pulmonary embolism, bundle branch blocks, ventricular hypertrophy, hypertrophic cardiomyopathy
4. Hyperkalaemia produces:
   (a) Peaked T waves
   (b) Flat P waves
   (c) Prolonged PR interval
   (d) Wide QRS complex
   (e) ST segment depression
   (f) Atrial standstill
   (g) Sinusoidal waves

FURTHER READING

Boron, W.F., Boulpaep, E.L., 2017. Medical Physiology. Elsevier, Philadelphia.

Diercks, D.B., et al., 2004. Electrocardiographic manifestations: electrolyte abnormalities. J. Emerg. Med. 27 (2), 153–160.

Ettinger, P.O., Regan, T.J., Oldewurtel, H.A., 1974. Hyperkalemia, cardiac conduction, and the electrocardiogram: a review. Am. Heart J. 88 (3), 360–371.

John, A.D., Fleisher, L.A., 2006. Electrocardiography: the ECG. Anesthesiol. Clin. 24 (4), 697–715.

Marx, J.A., et al., 2014. Rosen's Emergency Medicine: Concepts and Clinical Practice. Elsevier, Philadelphia.

Vecht, R.J., et al., 2009. ECG Diagnosis in Clinical Practice. Springer.

U WAVE

DEFINITION

U waves are small waves occurring immediately following the T wave (Fig. 10.1). Their mechanism is unknown but is thought to relate to delayed repolarisation of the ventricles or Purkinje fibres.

ECG FINDINGS

U waves tend to be small and are not usually seen, although if present are usually seen in the anterior chest leads. Normal U waves, if present, should point in the same direction as the T wave; an inverted U wave is always abnormal.

HYPOKALAEMIA

Hypokalaemia is a common and important cause of prominent U waves among other ECG changes (Fig. 10.2). Low potassium initially causes flattening of the T wave.

At a potassium level of <3.0 mmol/L, the T wave becomes increasingly flattened and occasionally inverted. Prominent U waves that may exceed the size of the T wave can occur and prolongation of the QT interval may be seen. Other ECG changes in hypokalaemia include increased amplitude of the P wave, prolongation of the PR interval and mild ST depression.

Hypokalaemia

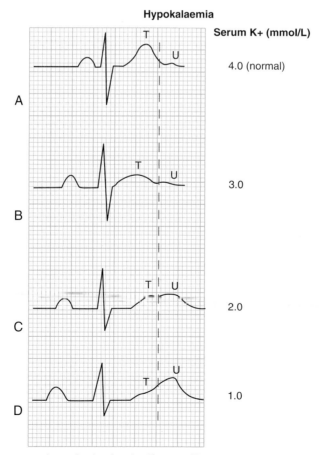

Serum K+ (mmol/L)

A — 4.0 (normal)

B — 3.0

C — 2.0

D — 1.0

Fig. 10.1 (A–D) U waves occur immediately after the T wave. They can be observed in hyperkalaemia. (Source: Urden, L., Stacy, K., Lough, M. (2021). Cardiovascular diagnostic procedures. In: *Critical Care Nursing: Diagnosis and Management*, 9th ed. Mosby.)

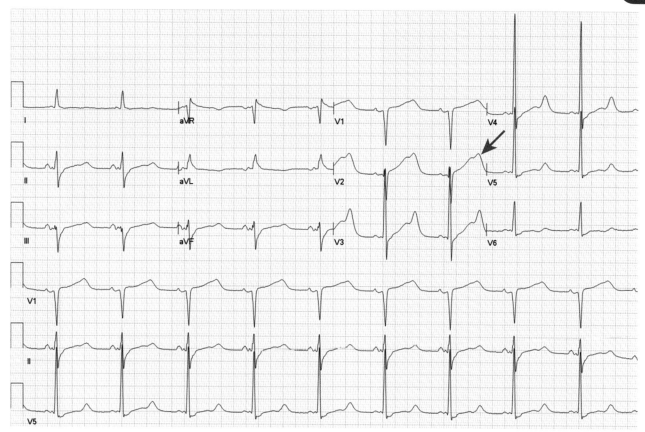

Fig. 10.2 Hypokalaemia. There are prominent U waves in the inferior leads (II, III, aVF) and leads V$_2$ to V$_5$ (blue arrow). The peak of the T wave is shown by the green arrow. There is also a prolonged QT-U interval (638 ms). (Source: Das, M., Zipes, D. (2021). Important concepts. In: *Electrocardiography of Arrhythmias: A Comprehensive Review*, 2nd ed. Elsevier.)

CLINICAL FEATURES

U waves can be a normal finding, particularly in bradycardic patients. Hypokalaemia should be suspected if prominent U waves are associated with other ECG changes consistent with low potassium. Severe hypokalaemia may predispose to ventricular tachyarrhythmias.

MANAGEMENT

Small U waves are not normally associated with an underlying cause. If hypokalaemia is present, an underlying cause should be sought and treated; this may include stopping offending medications such as diuretics. Intravenous (IV) or oral potassium supplementation may be required in severe symptomatic hypokalaemia.

DELTA WAVES AND PRE-EXCITATION

DEFINITION

Delta waves (slurred upstroke appearance on QRS complexes) occur due to the presence of a congenital accessory (additional) pathway. This allows impulses to cross from the atria to the ventricles (or vice versa) without passing through the atrioventricular node (AVN). The accessory pathway conducts impulses more rapidly than the AVN. This leads to early depolarisation of the ventricle, referred to as pre-excitation, that can predispose the patient to arrhythmias. Anatomically, the accessory pathway can be on the right or the left side of the heart.

Wolff-Parkinson-White (WPW) syndrome is diagnosed if there is pre-excitation on an ECG and the patient has a history of palpitations or arrhythmias.

ECG FINDINGS

Resting ECG

The ventricles receive impulses from both the AVN and the accessory pathway. Conduction through the accessory pathway occurs more rapidly than conduction through the AVN, producing an abnormally short PR interval. The QRS initially begins broad as ventricular depolarisation begins early and from an abnormal location, resulting in a slurred upstroke to the QRS or 'delta wave'; this is known as pre-excitation. However, the rapidly conducted impulse through the His-Purkinje system will 'catch up' with the broad QRS, causing the remainder of the QRS complex to be narrow (Figs 10.3–10.4 and Box 10.1). Pre-excitation may also cause axis deviation, depending on the location of the accessory pathway (see Chapter 3).

The location of the accessory pathway can be determined by assessing the direction of the delta wave on a 12-lead ECG (Box 10.2).

Tachycardias

Patients with pre-excitation tend to be more prone to the following arrhythmias:
- Atrioventricular re-entrant tachycardia (AVRT) (see Chapter 2)

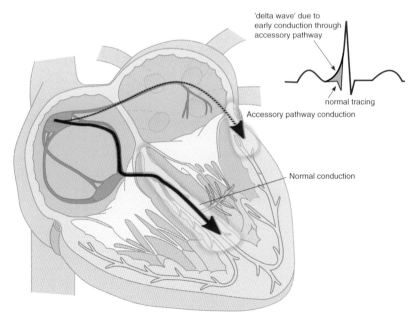

Fig. 10.3 Cause of delta wave in pre-excitation. In ventricular pre-excitation, a 'delta wave' is generated by early conduction through the accessory pathway. This conduction through the accessory pathway occurs through relatively slowly conducting, which is reflected in the relatively shallow, slurred upstroke of the delta wave. Conduction eventually progresses rapidly through the His–Purkinje system as usual (solid line), resulting in the remaining, steeply sloped QRS deflection. (Source: Kim, S. S., Knight, B. P. (2017). Long-term risk of Wolff–Parkinson–White pattern and syndrome. *Trends in Cardiovascular Medicine*, 27(4): pp. 260–268.)

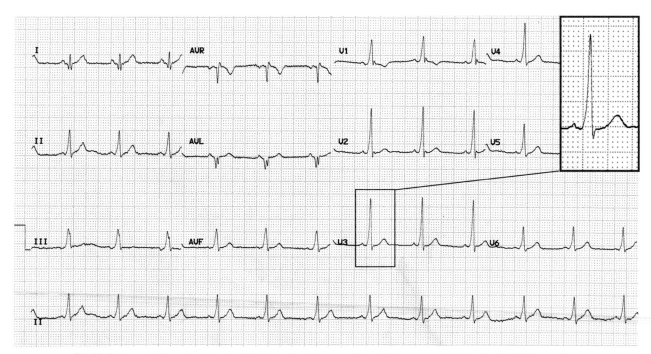

Fig. 10.4 Pre-excitation showing short PR interval, delta wave (slurred R-wave upstroke) and wide QRS complex.

Box **10.1**   Summary of ECG features of pre-excitation

- Short PR interval (<120 ms; <3 small squares)
- Wide QRS (>120 ms; >3 small squares)
- Presence of delta waves

- Pre-excited atrial fibrillation (AF). AF in Wolff–Parkinson–White syndrome predominantly conducts impulses from the atria to the ventricles via the accessory pathway. This produces a tachycardia

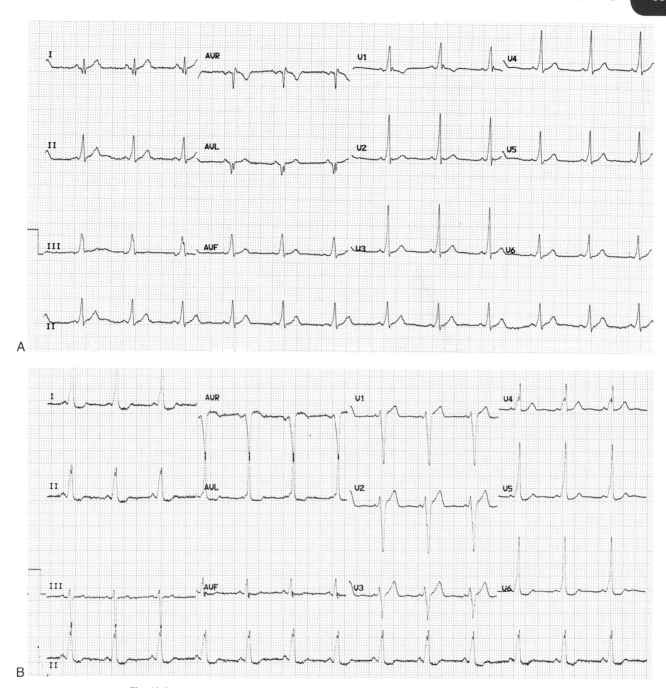

Fig. 10.5 ECGs of preexcitation from (A) left-sided and (B) right-sided accessory pathways.

Box 10.2	**Pre-excitation is classified into two types depending on the side of the accessory pathway and, consequently, ECG features (Fig. 10.5)**

- Type A (left-sided pathway): positive delta wave in V_1
- Type B (right-sided pathway): negative delta wave in V_1

with an irregular rhythm and wide QRS complexes (Fig. 10.6).

CLINICAL FINDINGS

The presence of an accessory pathway is congenital and is often identified in childhood or early adulthood. It may present as intermittent tachycardia as the accessory pathway allows for the occurrence of AVRT.

Pre-excitation is normally benign but can be associated with a risk of sudden death. This is often due to AF or atrial flutter: the accessory pathway allows rapid conduction of flutter or fibrillation waves into the ventricles without being delayed by the AVN. This can cause ventricular tachycardia or ventricular fibrillation, leading to sudden cardiac death.

MANAGEMENT

Definitive management of Wolff–Parkinson–White syndrome is catheter ablation of the accessory pathways; this treatment leads to a good prognosis.

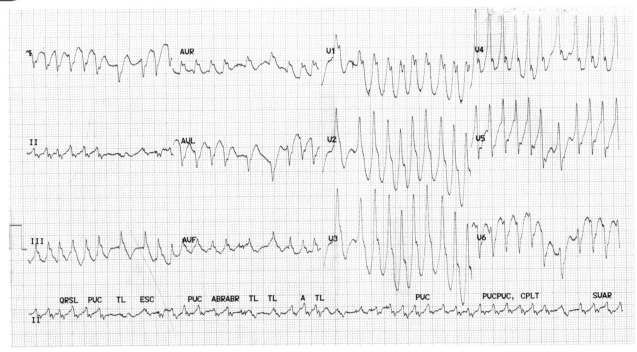

Fig. 10.6 ECG of pre-excited AF with an irregularly irregular wide-complex tachycardia.

OSBORN WAVE

DEFINITION

The Osborn wave (also known as J-wave) is a positive elevation of the point at which the QRS complex meets the ST segment (known as the J-point) (Fig. 10.7). It is a characteristic ECG feature in severe hypothermia but may also be seen in severe hypercalcaemia.

ECG FINDINGS

The presence of an elevated J-point tends to occur with moderate to severe hypothermia (temperature <32°C) and is thought to relate to repolarisation abnormalities. Hypothermia slows down metabolic processes and, therefore, will slow down all aspects of the ECG. Consequently, other ECG findings in hypothermia include sinus bradycardia, QRS complex widening and PR and QT prolongation (Fig. 10.8).

CLINICAL FEATURES

Osborn waves, if visible, are suggestive of severe hypothermia and warrant immediate attention. Changes to the J-point may also occur in hypercalcaemia and Brugada syndrome.

MANAGEMENT

Active rewarming is the definitive management for hypothermia. This may involve external rewarming with blankets and heated equipment. Internal rewarming, such as heated IV fluids, may also be used.

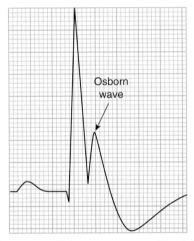

Fig. 10.7 Osborn waves. Osborn waves are positive deflections at the J-point. They can be seen in severe hypothermia. (Source: Williams, B., Ross, L. (2020). Hypothermia and hyperthermia. In: *Paramedic Principles and Practice: A Clinical Reasoning Approach*, 2nd ed. Elsevier.)

PACEMAKERS

DEFINITION

Pacemakers are implanted devices used for the treatment of sinus node and AVN disease. The function of these devices is to introduce a current to the heart to initiate depolarisation and subsequent contraction. This may include stimulating only one chamber (e.g. right atrium, right ventricle) or multiple chambers (e.g. dual-chamber pacemakers stimulate the right atrium and right ventricle) (Fig. 10.9). They can also be implanted in patients with symptomatic heart failure and evidence of ventricular dyssynchrony to improve the contraction efficiency of the right and left ventricles;

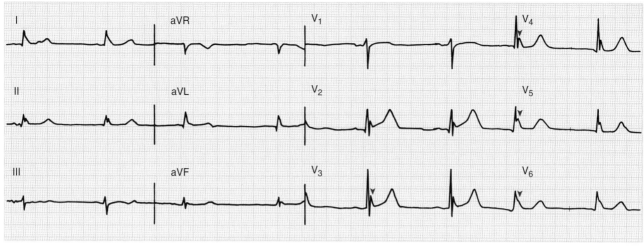

Fig. 10.8 Osborn waves in leads V_3–V_6 as seen in hypothermia. Sinus bradycardia and QT prolongation are also present. (Source: Zipes, D. P., Libby, P. (2018). Electrocardiography. In: *Braunwald's Heart Disease: A Textbook of Cardiovascular Medicine*, 11th ed. Elsevier.)

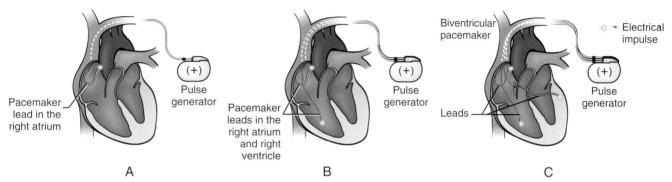

Fig. 10.9 Types of pacemakers. (A) Single chamber pacemaker. In this case, the lead is in the right atrium. (B) Dual chamber pacemaker. There are two leads – one in the right atrium and the other in the right ventricle. (C) Biventricular pacemaker. There are three leads; there is a lead in each ventricle as well as a lead in the right atrium. This can be used to synchronise right and left ventricular contraction. (Source: Koesterman, J. L. (2020). National codes. In: *Buck's 2020 HCPCS Level II*. Saunders.)

Table 10.1   Summary of the NBG code for describing pacemaker activity

Letter position	First-letter position	Second-letter position	Third-letter position	Fourth-letter position
Category	Chamber being paced	Chamber being sensed	The pacemaker's response to sensed activity	Rate modulation
Program setting	O = none A = atrium V = ventricle D = dual chamber (atrium and ventricle)	O = none A = atrium V = ventricle D = dual chamber (atrium and ventricle)	O = none (response generated without sensing) I = inhibits pacemaker T = triggers pacemaker D = dual action (inhibits and triggers)	O/absent letter = no rate modulation R = rate modulation present

this is referred to as cardiac resynchronisation therapy and has leads stimulating the left and right ventricles.

The placement and function of pacemakers are described by a five-letter code (the NBG code), with each letter describing a function (Table 10.1). Note that only the first four-letter positions of the code are commonly used when describing pacemaker settings; multi-site pacing (fifth-letter position) is rarely included in annotations, so has not been included in Table 10.1.

Commonly used modes include VVI (ventricular pacing that is inhibited by sensed ventricular activity) and DDDR (where both the atrium and ventricle are paced and sensed with the ability for the pacemaker to inhibit and trigger). An example of a dual (inhibition and triggering) response of a pacemaker is inhibition of pacing when a signal is sensed in the atrium but with subsequent triggering of stimulation of the ventricle if there is complete heart block

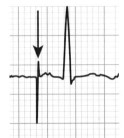

Fig. 10.10 Atrial pacing. There is a pacing spike (arrow) before the P wave, indicating atrial pacing. Note that the QRS complex is narrow as conduction to the ventricles occurs through the normal His–Purkinje system. (Source: Urden, L., Stacy, K., Lough, M. (2002). Cardiac rhythm assessment and management. In: *Critical Care Nursing: Diagnosis and Management*, 4th ed. Mosby.)

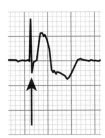

Fig. 10.11 Ventricular pacing. There is a pacing spike (arrow) before the QRS complex, indicating ventricular pacing. The QRS complex is wide as conduction to ventricles does not use the rapid His–Purkinje system. There is no discernible P wave. (Source: Urden, L., Stacy, K., Lough, M. (2002). Cardiac rhythm assessment and management. In: *Critical Care Nursing: Diagnosis and Management*, 4th ed. Mosby.)

(as the signal from the atrium fails to reach the ventricles).

ECG FINDINGS

Pacing spikes may be visible on ECG, although this is not always the case. Pacing spikes before the P wave indicate atrial pacing (Fig. 10.10) and before the QRS complex indicate ventricular pacing (Fig. 10.11). Pacing spikes occurring before the P wave and QRS complex suggest dual-chamber pacing (Figs 10.12 and 10.13).

Ventricular pacing typically produces broad QRS complexes, which may have a left bundle branch block morphology as the ventricular lead is often placed in the right ventricle; this depolarises the right ventricle first and the signal then propagates to the left ventricle, mimicking the spread of depolarisation seen in left bundle branch blocks. Right ventricular pacing also usually produces left-axis deviation of the cardiac axis.

CLINICAL FEATURES

Pacing is well tolerated. However, it is important to exclude pacemaker malfunction in patients with permanent pacemakers presenting with dizziness, presyncope or syncope.

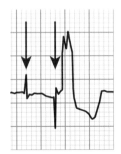

Fig. 10.12 Dual-chamber pacing. There are pacing spikes (arrows) before the P wave and the QRS complex, indicating pacing of both the atrium and ventricle. (Source: Urden, L., Stacy, K., Lough, M. (2002). Cardiac rhythm assessment and management. In: *Critical Care Nursing: Diagnosis and Management*, 4th ed. Mosby.)

MANAGEMENT

No management is necessary for normal pacemaker function, although concerns about pacemaker malfunction may warrant investigation (including pacemaker check and chest X-ray) and/or referral. Pacemaker malfunction can be diagnosed in some cases on an ECG, such as the absence of ventricular depolarisation after a pacing spike.

NORMAL ECG VARIANTS

No two ECGs are identical; for example, ECGs vary with body habitus, age and fitness. There are some features of ECGs that at first glance look abnormal and may lead you to think there is pathology present, when in fact some changes can be completely normal in some people.

It can be challenging to determine what is 'abnormal', particularly in children, athletes and pregnancy. Other findings not related to cardiac pathology can be observed in skeletal deformities (e.g. pectus excavatum), emphysema, dextrocardia, hyperventilation and ectopic heart beats.

ECGs IN ATHLETES

Since exercise has an effect on the heart, it makes sense that athletes can display some ECG changes. These changes typically become apparent in athletes who exercise to high intensity for an average of an hour a day or more.

The heart chambers enlarge (particularly with aerobic exercise) and hypertrophy to maintain cardiac output with a lower heart rate. ECG changes seen in athletes are listed in Box 10.3.

Box **10.3**   ECG changes in athletes

• Changes due to high vagal tone
  • Sinus bradycardia (Fig. 10.14)
  • Sinus arrhythmia
  • First-degree heart block
• Left ventricular hypertrophy
• Left or right atrial enlargement

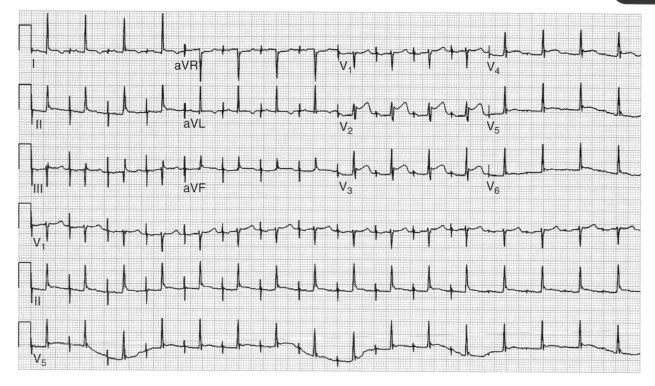

A

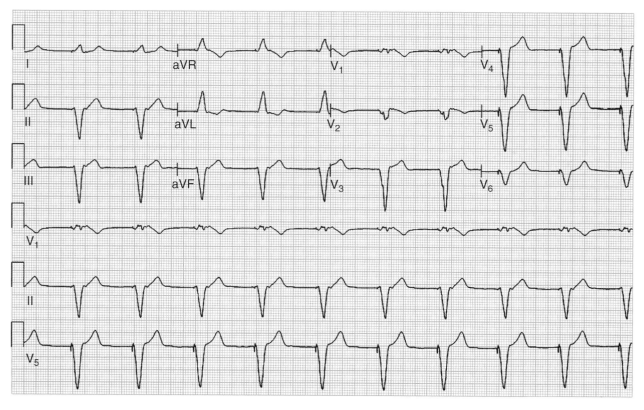

B

Fig. 10.13 ECGs of different types of pacing. (A) Single-chamber pacing – atrial (AAI). There are pacing spikes before every P wave. The ventricle activates normally through the AVN–His bundle and intraventricular conduction system, resulting in a narrow, normal-appearing QRS complex. (B) Single-chamber pacing – ventricular (VVI). There are pacing spikes before every QRS complex. Note that the QRS complex is wide because the ventricles are not depolarised with the His–Purkinje system. The left bundle branch block pattern is typically seen when pacing is from the right-ventricle apex.

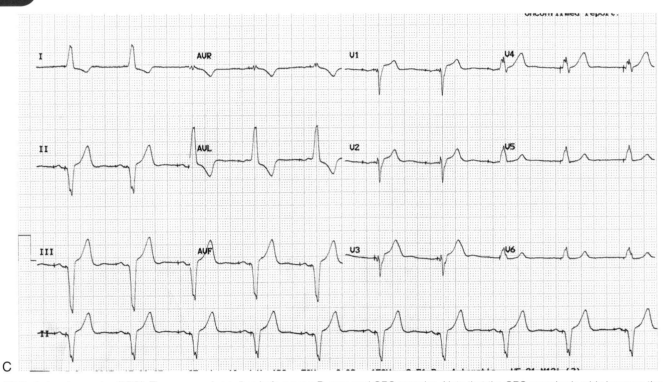

(C) Dual-chamber pacing (DDD). There are pacing spikes before every P wave and QRS complex. Note that the QRS complex is wide because the ventricles are not depolarised with the His–Purkinje system.

((A) Source: Olshansky, B., et al. (2016). Cardiac pacing and pacemaker rhythms. In: *Arrhythmia Essentials*, 2nd ed. Elsevier.

(B) Source: Olshansky, B., et al. (2016). Cardiac pacing and pacemaker rhythms. In: *Arrhythmia Essentials*, 2nd ed. Elsevier.)

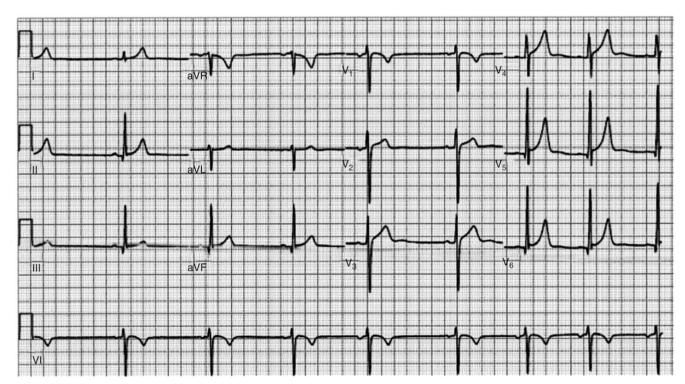

Fig. 10.14 ECG tracing from asymptomatic athlete. ECG shows sinus bradycardia with sinus arrhythmia, early repolarisation (benign ST segment elevation) and large precordial QRS complexes (associated with left ventricular hypertrophy). (Source: Zipes, D. P., Libby, P. (2018). Exercise and sports cardiology. In: *Braunwald's Heart Disease: A Textbook of Cardiovascular Medicine*, 11th ed. Elsevier.)

Box **10.4** ECG changes in pregnancy

- Increased sympathetic activity:
  - Sinus tachycardia
  - Increased frequency of atrial and ventricular ectopic beats
- Left-axis deviation – due to compensatory left ventricular dilatation and change in orientation of the heart in the chest
- Flattened or inverted T waves (Fig. 10.15)

Some of these ECG changes are seen in those with underlying cardiomyopathies. Given that cardio-myopathies increase the risk of sudden death, it is important to exclude these conditions if the above ECG findings are observed.

PREGNANCY

A number of changes occur to a woman's cardiovascular system when she is pregnant, and this leads to several ECG changes (Box 10.4). ECG changes usually manifest later in pregnancy.

PAEDIATRIC CASES

The normal resting heart depends on age. Children normally have higher heart rates than adults because of elevated sympathetic activity and smaller stroke volumes; for instance, a heart rate of 150 bpm is considered normal in newborn babies. In addition, they have a shorter PR interval as a result of faster AVN

conduction (Fig. 10.16). Heart rate gradually declines with age and reaches adult levels by approximately 15-years-old.

Furthermore, in early childhood, there is evidence of right ventricular dilatation due to in utero left-to-right shunting. This produces the following ECG changes:
- Right ventricular hypertrophy – prominent R wave in V_1, T-wave inversion V_1–V_3
- Right-axis deviation

Key Points

1. U wave: small waves occurring immediately following T wave. May indicate hypokalaemia
2. Delta wave: slurred upstroke appearance of QRS complex. Suggests pre-excitation, as seen in Wolff–Parkinson–White pattern
3. Wolff–Parkinson–White syndrome is diagnosed based on the presence of tachycardias in combination with pre-excitation:
   (a) Short PR interval (<120 ms; <3 small squares)
   (b) Wide QRS (>120 ms; >3 small squares)
   (c) Presence of delta waves
4. Osborn wave: elevated J-point. Suggests moderate to severe hypothermia
5. Pacemakers produce pacing spikes on the ECG. This can be atrial only, ventricular only or dual chamber. NBG pacemaker codes correspond to:
   (a) I: chamber paced
   (b) II: chamber sensed
   (c) III: response to sensing
   (d) IV: rate modulation

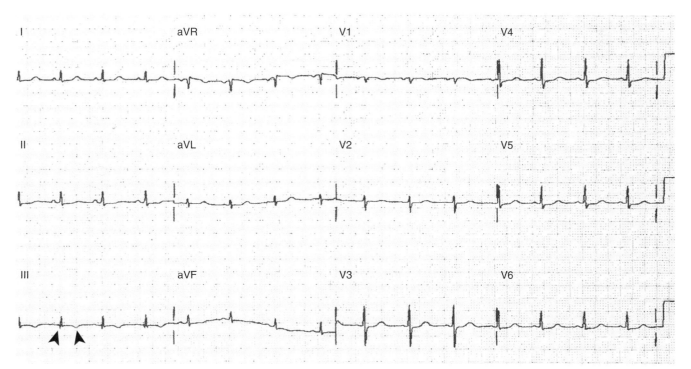

Fig. 10.15 Normal ECG changes in pregnancy. ECG taken in pregnancy showing normal changes: a small Q wave and an inverted T wave are seen in lead III (arrows). (Source: Saksena, S., et al. (2005). Arrhythmias during pregnancy. In: *Electrophysiological Disorders of the Heart*, 2nd ed. Churchill Livingstone.)

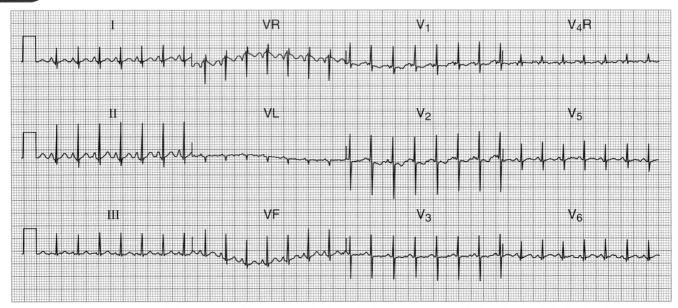

Fig. 10.16 Normal ECG of 1-month-old child. ECG of a 1-month-old child with normal findings for age, including heart rate of 170 bpm and dominant R waves in V$_1$. Lead V$_4$R (a position on the chest equivalent to V$_4$, but on the right side) has been recorded instead of V$_4$. (Source: Hampton, J., Adlam, D. (2019). The ECG in healthy people. In: *The ECG Made Practical*, 7th ed. Elsevier.)

FURTHER READING

Camm, A.J., Lüscher, T.F., Serruys, P.W., 2009. The ESC Textbook of Cardiovascular Medicine. Oxford University Press, Oxford.

Mareedu, R.K., et al., 2008. Classic EKG changes of hypothermia. Clin. Med. Res. 6 (3–4), 107–108.

Murphy, J.G., Lloyd, M.A., 2013. Mayo Clinic Cardiology: Concise Textbook. Oxford University Press, Oxford.

Osadchii, O.E., 2010. Mechanisms of hypokalemia-induced ventricular arrhythmogenicity. Fundam. Clin. Pharmacol. 24 (5), 547–559.

Viskin, S., Zelster, D., Antzelevitch, C., 2004. When U say 'U waves', what do U mean?. Pacing Clin. Electrophysiol. 27 (2), 145–147.

Cases

11

CASE 1 – QUESTIONS

A 72-year-old female patient on the cardiothoracic surgical ward reports palpitations and mild shortness of breath on exertion. She has a history of moderate to severe aortic stenosis, for which she is awaiting surgery, but no other significant medical history.

On examination, she has oxygen saturations of 94% on room air, respiratory rate 14 breaths/min, heart rate 144 bpm and blood pressure 107/76 mmHg. On auscultation of the chest, she has normal bilateral air entry, and an ejection systolic murmur can be heard loudest on the left side of the chest, radiating to the carotids.

A 12-lead ECG is performed.

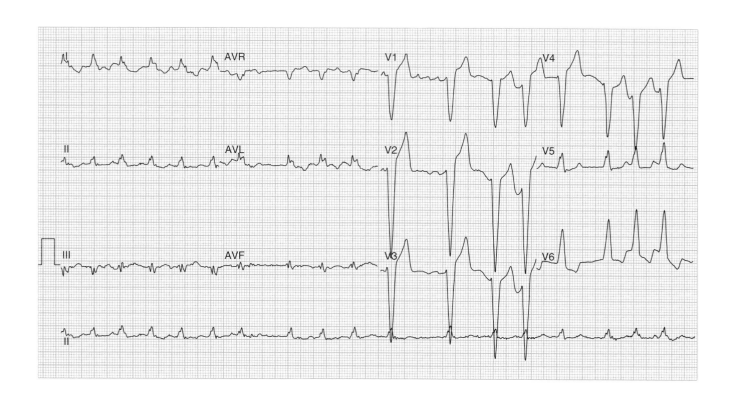

❓ QUESTIONS FOR CANDIDATE

1. **Which of the following may give rise to AF?**
   (a) Aortic stenosis
   (b) Chronic obstructive pulmonary disease (COPD)
   (c) Excessive alcohol consumption
   (d) Hypothyroidism
   (e) Sepsis
2. **Which of the following may be a consequence of AF?**
   (a) Bowel ischaemia
   (b) Deep-vein thrombosis
   (c) Heart failure
   (d) Intracranial haemorrhage
   (e) Myocardial infarction
3. **Which clinical scoring systems are important decision aids in the management of AF?**
   (a) $ABCD_2$ score
   (b) CHA_2DS_2-VASc score
   (c) GRACE score
   (d) HAS-BLED score
   (e) All of the above
   ❶ Note: Answers are on page 141.

CASE 2 – QUESTIONS

A 75-year-old male patient presents to the emergency department with shortness of breath on exertion and palpitations. He has a history of hypertension and type 2 diabetes mellitus, for which he takes ramipril and metformin, respectively. He is an ex-smoker with a 20-pack-year history.

On examination, he has saturations of 95% on room air, respiratory rate 17 breaths/min, heart rate 150 bpm and blood pressure 139/88 mmHg. On auscultation, he has normal breath sounds with good bilateral air entry. A pansystolic murmur can be heard across the precordium, loudest at the apex and radiating to the axilla.

A 12-lead ECG is performed as part of his diagnostic work-up.

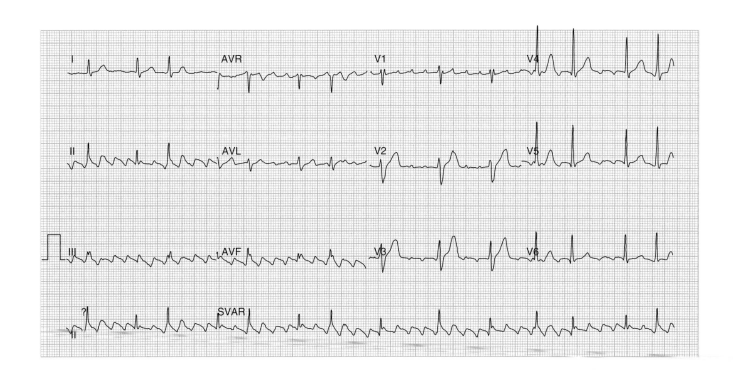

❓ QUESTIONS FOR CANDIDATE

1. What is the use of adenosine in atrial flutter?

(a) An adenosine bolus provides a rapid and effective method of terminating the arrhythmia.

(b) Adenosine can be used as a long-term method of rate control if DC cardioversion fails to terminate the arrhythmia.

(c) An adenosine bolus may block atrioventricular node (AVN) conduction to the ventricles, making flutter waves easier to visualise on ECG.

(d) Adenosine may reduce the atrial rate and therefore reduce the ventricular rate.

(e) Adenosine has no use in atrial flutter.

2. What is the most likely cause of the 2:1 and 3:1 conduction block in this patient?

(a) Myocardial ischaemia due to rapid activation of atria and ventricles

(b) Idiopathic fibrosis of the conduction system

(c) Excessive vagal tone due to elevated blood pressure

(d) Physiological effect of delayed conduction in the AVN

(e) Iatrogenic heart block as a result of ramipril therapy

3. Which of the following are risk factors for developing atrial flutter?

(a) Hypertension

(b) Diabetes mellitus

(c) Mitral regurgitation

(d) Male sex

(e) Younger age

❶ Note: Answers are on page 144.

CASE 3 – QUESTIONS

A 77-year-old female patient presents to the emergency department reporting dizziness, chest pain and fatigue. She has had previous short episodes of a similar nature but this is the first time she has experienced chest pain. Three months ago, she had a catheter ablation procedure for atrial fibrillation (AF). She has hypertension, for which she takes amlodipine, and has a history of ischaemic heart disease.

On examination, she has saturations of 97% on room air, respiratory rate 16 breaths/min, heart rate 150 bpm and blood pressure 110/79 mmHg. On auscultation, her breath sounds and heart sounds are normal.

An ECG is performed as part of her initial work-up.

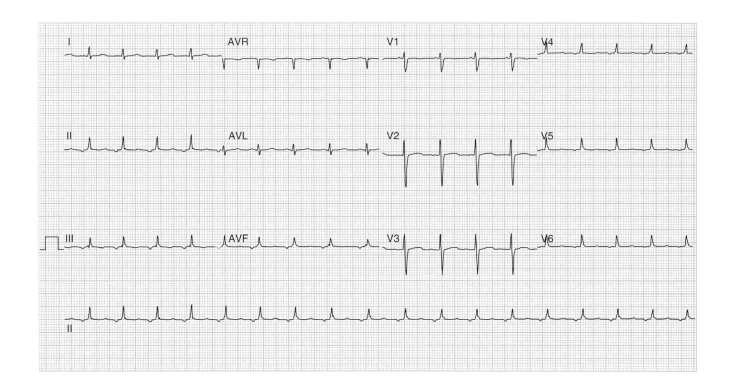

❓ QUESTIONS FOR CANDIDATE

1. **What mechanism gives rise to atrial tachycardia?**
   (a) Increased automaticity
   (b) Re-entry
   (c) Triggered activity
   (d) All of the above
   (e) None of the above

2. **Aside from atrial tachycardia, what other complications may arise from catheter ablation for AF?**
   (a) Aortic regurgitation
   (b) Cardiac tamponade
   (c) Femoral vein and arterial damage
   (d) Myocardial infarction
   (e) Stroke

3. **Where is the lesion (or lesions) giving rise to the atrial tachycardia most likely to be located?**
   (a) Adjacent to the atrioventricular node (AVN)
   (b) Anterior free wall of the right atrium

   (c) Left atrium
   (d) Right ventricular outflow tract
   (e) Sinoatrial node

   ❶ Note: Answers are on page 146.

CASE 4 – QUESTIONS

A 59-year-old male patient is brought to the emergency department with severe central crushing chest pain, nausea, increasing shortness of breath and dizziness for a duration of 3 day. He has a past medical history of hypertension and high cholesterol, for which he is taking ramipril and atorvastatin.

On examination, he has saturations of 95% on room air, respiratory rate 21 breaths/min, heart rate 60 bpm and blood pressure 99/65 mmHg. On auscultation, breath sounds are normal with good air entry bilaterally.

A paramedic hands you the patient's 12-lead ECG taken in the ambulance.

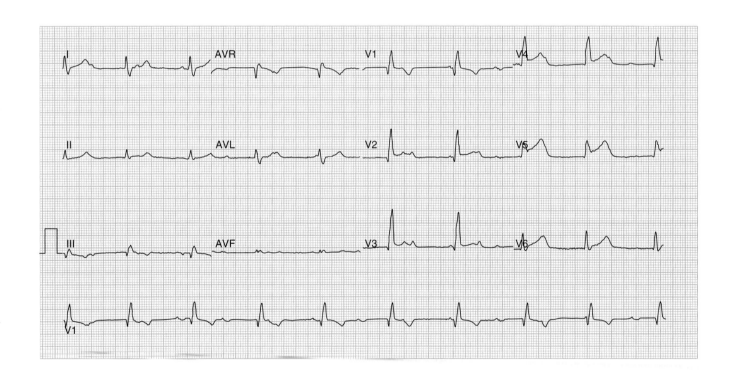

❓ QUESTIONS FOR CANDIDATE

1. **What coronary artery has been occluded in this patient?**
   (a) Left anterior descending (LAD) artery
   (b) Left circumflex (LCx) artery
   (c) Left main stem (LMS)
   (d) Posterior descending artery (PDA)
   (e) Right coronary artery (RCA)

Two days after admission, the patient begins to complain of chest pain and increasing shortness of breath at rest. His saturations read 83% on room air. On examination, he has fine crepitations in both lung bases and a harsh holosystolic murmur that is loudest over the tricuspid area of the heart. This murmur was not present on admission.

2. **Which complications of myocardial infarction (MI) may have occurred?**
   (a) Acute aortic regurgitation
   (b) Acute mitral regurgitation
   (c) Acute ventricular septal defect (VSD)
   (d) Dressler syndrome
   (e) Left ventricular aneurysm

3. **What ECG changes would you expect to see to indicate a full thickness infarction when following up with this patient 6 months later?**
   (a) Pathological Q waves
   (b) Peaked T waves
   (c) ST segment depression
   (d) ST segment elevation
   (e) None of the above

❶ Note: Answers are on page 148.

CASE 5 – QUESTIONS

An 81-year-old male patient is seen for a regular follow-up in the cardiology clinic. As part of his assessment, a 12-lead ECG is taken.

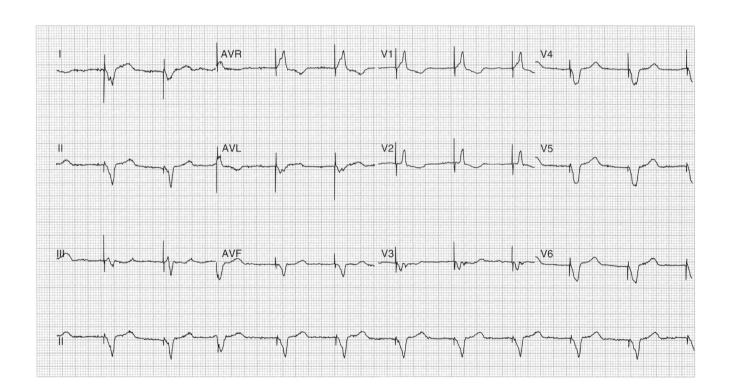

❓ QUESTIONS FOR CANDIDATE

1. **A different patient with a recent pacemaker insertion complains of pain overlying the site of the pacemaker. On examination, the area is red, swollen and warm to the touch. He is otherwise well with a temperature of 37.2°C. What complication of pacemaker insertion has occurred?**
   (a) Coronary sinus dissection
   (b) Device-related endocarditis
   (c) Pacemaker pocket haematoma
   (d) Pacemaker pocket infection
   (e) Pericardial effusion

2. **What pacing mode describes a pacemaker that generates impulses in the ventricles and stops when ventricular activity is detected?**
   (a) AAI
   (b) AVI
   (c) AVT
   (d) DDD
   (e) VVI

3. **In the clinic notes, the specialist nurse has written that this patient had a biventricular pacemaker. What is the most likely indication for this?**
   (a) Brugada syndrome
   (b) Complete heart block
   (c) Heart failure
   (d) Mobitz type II heart block
   (e) Wolff–Parkinson–White syndrome

❶ Note: Answers are on page 150.

CASE 6 – QUESTIONS

A 28-year-old male is brought into ED after being found unconscious in the water at a local swimming pool. He suffered no adverse effects as he was promptly rescued by the lifeguard, and regained consciousness in under a minute.

He has never lost consciousness while swimming before but described one previous episode of syncope while playing football. He also describes occasional dizziness and palpitations. His paternal uncle died suddenly aged 44. He is previously well with no past medical history of note and no current medication.

An ECG is performed as part of his diagnostic work-up.

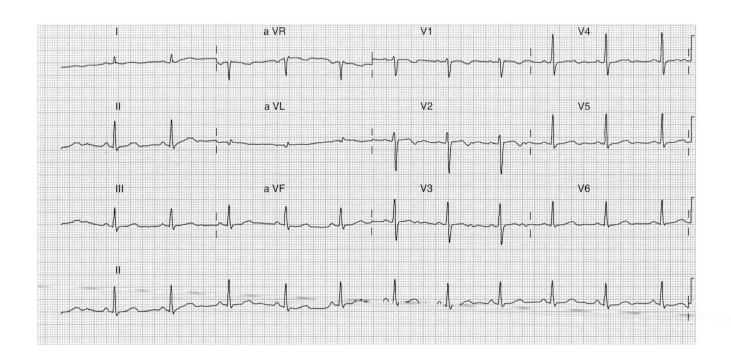

❓ QUESTIONS FOR CANDIDATE

1. **Which features of a clinical history support a diagnosis of syncope secondary to cardiac arrhythmia?**
   (a) Loss of consciousness after a prolonged period of standing up
   (b) Loss of consciousness when standing up from a sitting or lying position
   (c) Loss of consciousness associated with jerky movements
   (d) Loss of consciousness associated with a prolonged recovery period
   (e) Loss of consciousness without warning and with rapid recovery

2. **What ECG features would you expect to see before cardiac syncope in a patient with long QT syndrome?**
   (a) A narrow-complex tachycardia
   (b) A QT interval that progressively lengthens each beat until a beat is dropped
   (c) Ventricular fibrillation
   (d) A wide-complex tachycardia with many different-sized QRS complexes
   (e) A wide-complex tachycardia with identical QRS complexes

3. **Which of the following can prolong the QT interval?**
   (a) Erythromycin
   (b) Hypokalaemia
   (c) Hypocalcaemia
   (d) Quetiapine
   (e) Methotrexate

   ❶ Note: Answers are on page 152.

CASE 7 – QUESTIONS

A 35-year-old male patient presents to his general practitioner after a routine health check for private health insurance. He has been told that his ECG is abnormal and wishes to seek a second opinion. He has no significant past medical history and is not taking any regular medication. His clinical exam is normal.

A repeat ECG is performed.

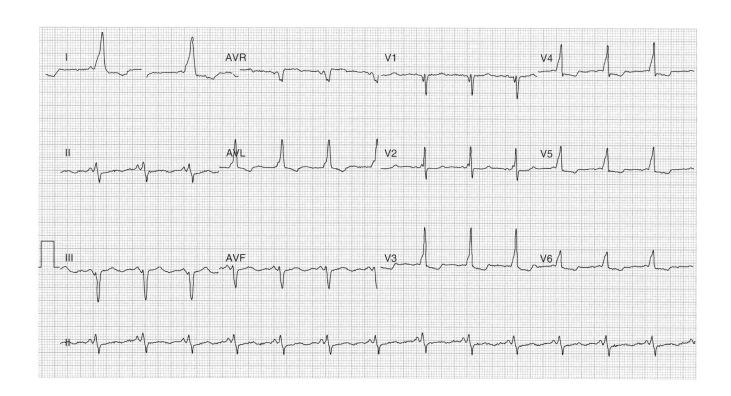

❓ QUESTIONS FOR CANDIDATE

1. **Which of the following are risk factors for the presence of pre-excitation on an ECG?**
   (a) Increasing age
   (b) Congenital cardiac abnormalities
   (c) Smoking
   (d) Diabetes mellitus
   (e) Family history of WPW syndrome

2. **What kind of arrhythmia is commonly associated with pre-excitation when the term WPW syndrome is used?**
   (a) Atrioventricular nodal re-entrant tachycardia (AVNRT)
   (b) Atrioventricular re-entrant tachycardia (AVRT)
   (c) Atrial tachycardia
   (d) Ventricular tachycardia
   (e) Torsades de pointes ventricular tachycardia

3. **Which of the following are thought to be the cause of sudden death in Wolff-Parkinson-White syndrome?**

(a) Atrial fibrillation
(b) Acute heart failure
(c) Stroke
(d) Complete heart block
(e) Myocardial infarction secondary to AVRT

❶ Note: Answers are on page 154.

CASE 8 – QUESTIONS

A 30-year-old female patient presents to the emergency department with palpitations associated with light-headedness and fatigue. She describes similar infrequent episodes that begin and terminate rapidly without warning. She has no significant past medical history.

On examination, her saturations are 96% on room air, respiratory rate 19 breaths/min with good bilateral air entry and clear lungs. Her heart rate is 165 bpm and is regular with a blood pressure of 134/83 mmHg. Heart sounds are normal.

An ECG is performed as part of her initial assessment.

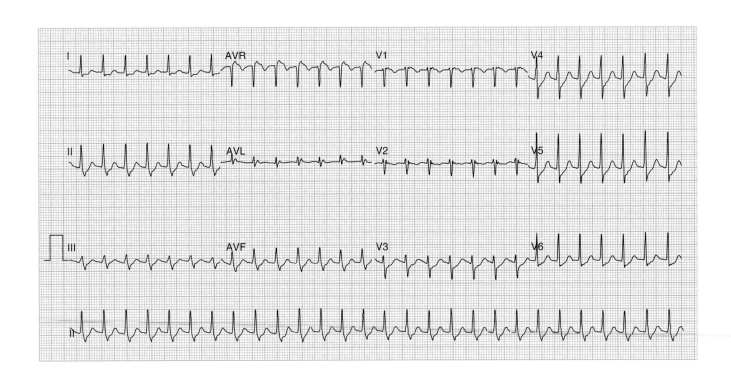

❓ QUESTIONS FOR CANDIDATE

1. What interventions could be attempted to terminate the arrhythmia before giving IV adenosine to this patient?

(a) Carotid sinus massage

(b) Head-up tilt test

(c) IV metoprolol infusion

(d) Synchronised DC cardioversion

(e) Valsalva manoeuvre

2. What symptoms may be experienced by a patient receiving an adenosine bolus?

(a) Chest tightness

(b) Flushing

(c) Hypertension

(d) Sense of impending doom

(e) Stroke

3. What is a possible cause of the negative deflection after the QRS complex in the inferior leads?

(a) Delayed depolarisation of the interventricular septum

(b) Delayed repolarisation of the atria

(c) Myocardial ischaemia due to the rapid heart rate

(d) Non-functional cardiac tissue creating an electrical window into the heart

(e) Retrograde 'p' wave

❶ Note: Answers are on page 156.

CASE 9 – QUESTIONS

A 67-year-old male presents to the emergency department with central chest pain and shortness of breath of 5 h duration. Shortly after admission, he complains of increasing shortness of breath, worsening pain and palpitations. He has a history of myocardial infarction, type 2 diabetes and hypercholesterolaemia.

On examination, his oxygen saturations are 91% on room air, respiratory rate 24 breaths/min, heart rate 190 bpm and blood pressure 105/69 mmHg. On auscultation, there is good air entry bilaterally with normal air entry with normal heart sounds.

A 12-lead ECG is performed as a matter of urgency.

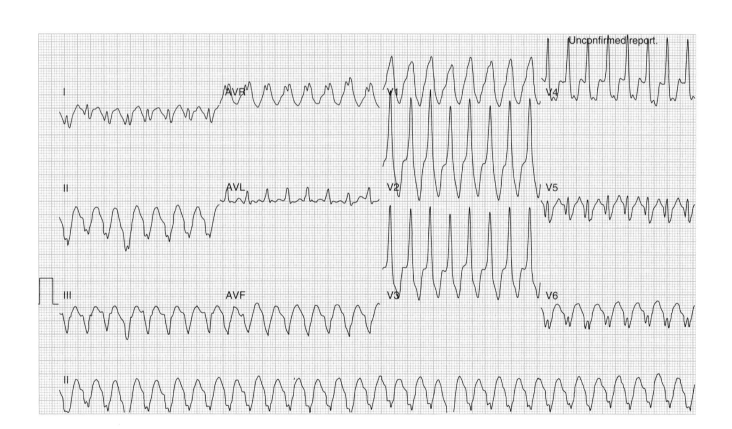

❓ QUESTIONS FOR CANDIDATE

1. **What features on examination would be indicative of cardiac arrest in this patient?**
   (a) Absent carotid pulse
   (b) Absent radial pulse
   (c) Apnoea
   (d) Blood pressure <90 mmHg systolic or <60 mmHg diastolic
   (e) Ventricular tachycardia on ECG lasting longer than 30 s

2. **Which rhythms can be treated by electrical defibrillation in cardiac arrest?**
   (a) Asystole
   (b) Pulseless electrical activity
   (c) Ventricular fibrillation
   (d) Ventricular tachycardia
   (e) All of the above

3. **What is the long-term management of patients at high risk of dangerous ventricular tachycardias?**
   (a) Discharge and monitor closely
   (b) Heart transplantation
   (c) Implantable cardiac defibrillator (ICD) insertion
   (d) Antiarrhythmic drug therapy – beta-blocker and/or amiodarone
   (e) Ventricular pacemaker insertion

   ❶ Note: Answers are on page 158.

CASE 10 – QUESTIONS

An 84-year-old male patient was admitted with dehydration and marked acute kidney injury to the Department of Medicine for the Elderly following a fall. He has a medical history of osteoarthritis, for which he takes regular naproxen, ischaemic heart disease and mild heart failure, for which he takes ramipril, bisoprolol, furosemide, digoxin and spironolactone.

Shortly after his admission, the patient complains of dizziness and breathlessness at rest. On examination, his saturations are 94% on room air, respiratory rate 24 breaths/min, heart rate 48 bpm and blood pressure 112/62 mmHg. Auscultation of the chest is normal.

A 12-lead ECG is performed.

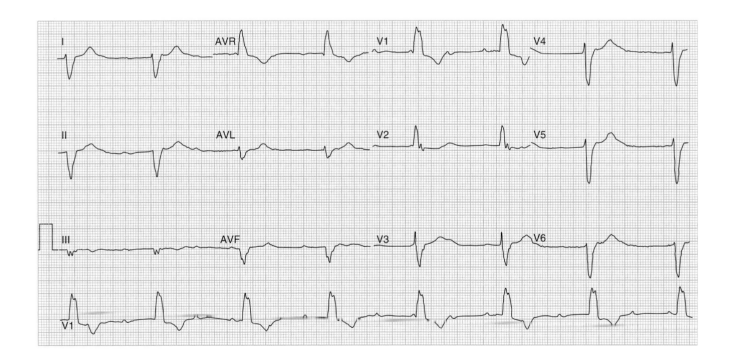

❓ QUESTIONS FOR CANDIDATE

1. **What are the likely contributing factors to the development of complete heart block in this patient?**
   (a) Acute kidney injury
   (b) Idiopathic fibrosis of the conduction system
   (c) Infiltrative heart disease such as sarcoidosis
   (d) Ischaemic heart disease
   (e) Medication-related heart block
2. **Which of the following medications may precipitate heart block?**
   (a) Amiodarone
   (b) Digoxin
   (c) Metoprolol
   (d) Spironolactone
   (e) Verapamil
3. **Which type(s) of heart block is/are associated with high risk of P wave asystole?**
   (a) First-degree heart block
   (b) Second-degree heart block (Mobitz type I)
   (c) Second-degree heart block (Mobitz type II)
   (d) Third-degree heart block (complete heart block)
   (e) None of the above

❶ Note: Answers are on page 160.

CASE 11 – QUESTIONS

A 62-year-old female patient attends the surgical day case service for an elective cholecystectomy. She is well with no current symptoms but has a past medical history of gallstones, type 2 diabetes mellitus and anterior myocardial infarction. She is currently taking aspirin, ramipril, bisoprolol and atorvastatin.

On examination, she has saturations of 96% on room air, respiratory rate 14 breaths/min, heart rate 72 bpm and blood pressure 136/86 mmHg. On auscultation, breath sounds are present and normal and heart sounds are normal.

A 12-lead ECG is performed as part of her preoperative assessment.

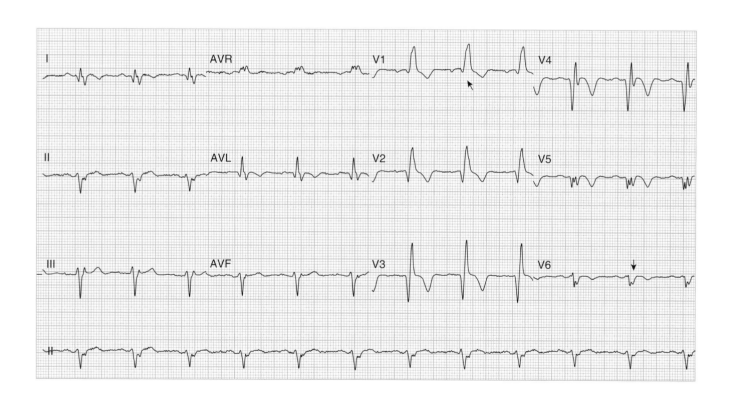

❓ QUESTIONS FOR CANDIDATE

1. **Which of the following aetiologies may give rise to bundle branch block?**
   - (a) Third-degree heart block
   - (b) Atrial fibrillation
   - (c) Hypertension
   - (d) Idiopathic fibrosis of the conduction system
   - (e) Myocardial infarction

2. **What pathological mechanism(s) may give rise to bifascicular block?**
   - (a) Impaired conduction in the left and right bundle branches
   - (b) Impaired conduction in the left bundle branch and the right anterior fascicle
   - (c) Impaired conduction in the left bundle branch and the right posterior fascicle
   - (d) Impaired conduction in the right bundle branch and the left anterior fascicle
   - (e) Impaired conduction in the right bundle branch and the left posterior fascicle

3. **The patient presents to the emergency department 6 months later with shortness of breath, light-headedness and chest pain. On examination, her heart rate is 32 bpm and blood pressure is 94/52 mmHg. What complication of bifascicular block is likely to have occurred?**
   - (a) Complete heart block
   - (b) Heart failure
   - (c) Pulmonary embolism
   - (d) Sick sinus syndrome
   - (e) Sinus bradycardia

   ❶ Note: Answers are on page 162.

CASE 12 – QUESTIONS

A 26-year-old female patient presents to the emergency department with shortness of breath, dizziness and palpitations of 5 h duration with mild central chest pain. She has no medical history of note but does describe previous episodes of palpitations and light-headedness. She is not taking any medication.

On examination, she has oxygen saturations of 98% on room air, respiratory rate 18 breaths/min, heart rate 174 bpm and blood pressure 118/78 mmHg. On auscultation, breath sounds are normal with equal air entry on both sides and heart sounds are normal.

An ECG is performed as part of her initial assessment.

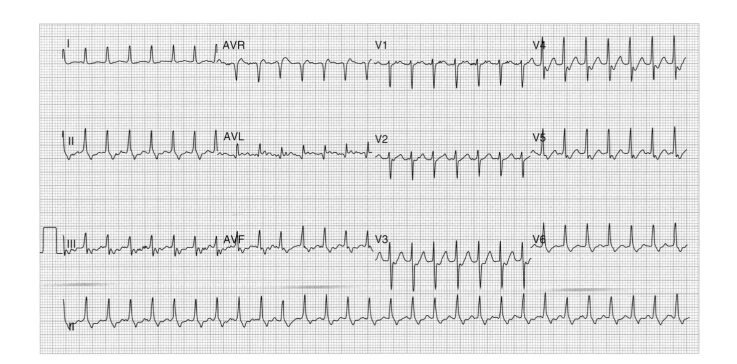

❓ QUESTIONS FOR CANDIDATE

1. Which cardiac condition is commonly associated with AVRT?
   (a) Arrhythmogenic right ventricular cardiomyopathy
   (b) Brugada syndrome
   (c) Heart failure
   (d) Pulmonary hypertension
   (e) Wolff–Parkinson–White syndrome

2. What is the mechanism underlying AVRT?
   (a) An atrial focus with rapid abnormal pacemaker activity
   (b) Re-entrant circuit in the right atrium
   (c) Re-entrant circuit around a slow pathway and a fast pathway located within or adjacent to the AVN
   (d) Re-entrant circuit from atria to ventricles via the AVN and back into atria via an accessory pathway
   (e) Re-entrant circuit in the left ventricle

3. What is the definitive long-term management of patients at risk of AVRT?
   (a) Ablation of the accessory pathway(s) to break the re-entrant circuit
   (b) Ablation of the AVN to break the re-entrant circuit
   (c) Dual-chamber pacemaker insertion
   (d) Implantable cardiac defibrillator (ICD) insertion
   (e) Long-term anticoagulation therapy

❶ Note: Answers are on page 164.

CASE 13 – QUESTIONS

A 90-year-old female patient presents to the cardiology clinic complaining of fatigue and poor exercise tolerance. She has a history of sick sinus syndrome, which was being monitored with cardiology outpatient appointment, but has noticed a significant decline in her exercise tolerance over the last few days. She also has a history of chronic obstructive pulmonary disease (COPD), aortic stenosis and rheumatoid arthritis.

On examination, her respiratory rate is 18 breaths/min, heart rate 42 bpm and blood pressure 126/88 mmHg. On auscultation, breath sounds are normal and lung bases are clear. A soft ejection systolic murmur can be heard on the right side of the sternum.

A 12-lead ECG is performed as part of her assessment.

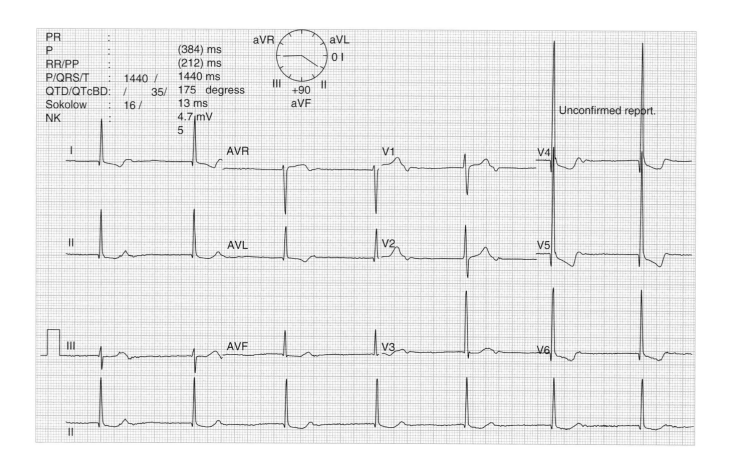

❓ QUESTIONS FOR CANDIDATE

1. Which of the following may give rise to sick sinus syndrome?

(a) Atropine
(b) Hypertension
(c) Idiopathic fibrosis of the sinoatrial node (SAN)
(d) Myocardial infarction
(e) Surgical damage to the SAN

2. Which of the following ECG patterns may feature in sick sinus syndrome?

(a) Alternating bradycardia and tachycardia
(b) Asystole
(c) Intermittently dropped sinus beats
(d) Sinus bradycardia
(e) All of the above

3. How should the junctional rhythm be managed?

(a) Anticoagulation with warfarin to prevent risk of thromboembolism
(b) Catheter ablation of the junctional rhythm focus
(c) No treatment is necessary as the rhythm is required to maintain cardiac output
(d) Suppression with amiodarone to reduce symptoms
(e) Vagal manoeuvres such as Valsalva to terminate the arrhythmia

❶ Note: Answers are on page 166.

CASE 14 – QUESTIONS

A 40-year-old female patient is referred to the cardiology clinic after presenting to her general practitioner with a history of recurrent 'attacks' of palpitations and mild shortness of breath. She has a history of gastro-oesophageal reflux disease but nothing else of note and has no family history of sudden death.

While in the waiting room for the cardiology clinic she reports palpitations and shortness of breath. On examination, she has oxygen saturations of 96% on room air, respiratory rate of 20 breaths/min, heart rate 168 bpm and blood pressure 116/84 mmHg.

A 12-lead ECG is immediately performed.

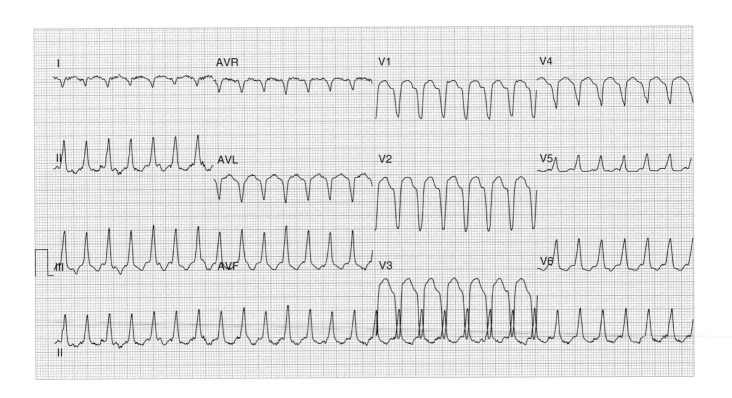

❓ QUESTIONS FOR CANDIDATE

1. What are the possible causes of VT in this patient?
(a) Brugada syndrome
(b) Arrhythmogenic Cardiomyopathy
(c) Idiopathic VT
(d) Ischaemic heart disease
(e) Long QT syndrome

2. Why does the blood pressure drop in VT?
(a) Decrease in myocardial contractility due to decreased ventricular filling
(b) Decrease in myocardial contractility due to depletion of calcium from the cardiomyocyte
(c) Decreased duration of systole causing a decrease in stroke volume
(d) Failure of excitation–contraction coupling
(e) Reflex vasodilation due to the excessively rapid heart rate

3. Which of the following clinical features suggest a good prognosis in VT?
(a) Family history of sudden death
(b) Reduced left ventricular systolic function
(c) The presence of known channelopathy
(d) The presence of structural heart disease
(e) VT with no known cause (idiopathic VT)

❶ Note: Answers are on page 168.

CASE 15 – QUESTIONS

A 31-year-old male presents to ED with palpitations and shortness of breath of 4 hours duration. He has had several similar episodes in the past but all had previously terminated by taking a deep breath. He was investigated previously for cardiac disease and was found to have left bundle branch block but no evidence of structural heart cardiac disease. He is otherwise well and takes no medication.

On examination, he has oxygen saturations of 99% on room air, respiratory rate 18 breaths/min, heart rate 190 bpm and blood pressure 134/88 mmHg. On auscultation, breath sounds are normal with equal bilateral air entry and heart sounds are normal.

A 12-lead ECG is performed as part of his diagnostic work-up.

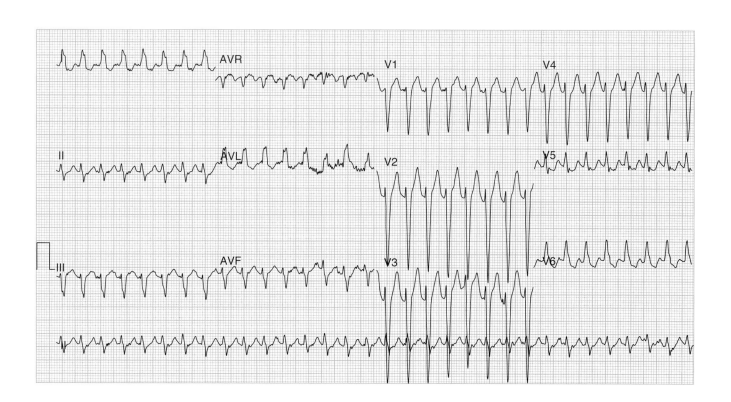

❓ QUESTIONS FOR CANDIDATE

1. Which clinical features may point to a diagnosis of SVT with aberrant conduction as opposed to VT?
(a) A history of left bundle branch block
(b) Age more than 35 years old
(c) Atrioventricular dissociation
(d) Extreme axis deviation
(e) QRS complex of greater than 160 ms in duration

2. The medical registrar attends to the patient rapidly and confirms that this patient has an atrioventricular nodal re-entrant tachycardia (AVNRT) with aberrant conduction. What first-line treatments could be attempted in this patient while in the emergency department?
(a) Adenosine bolus
(b) Catheter ablation
(c) Synchronised DC cardioversion
(d) Transcutaneous pacing
(e) Vagal manoeuvres

3. What symptoms may be associated with AVNRT?
(a) Chest pain
(b) Palpitations
(c) Polyuria
(d) Shortness of breath
(e) All of the above

❶ Note: Answers are on page 170.

CASE 16 – QUESTIONS

A 43-year-old female patient presents to the emergency department with sudden-onset shortness of breath, light-headedness, palpitations and chest pain. She reports several previous episodes of palpitations in the past but has never presented to a doctor for these. She takes the combined oral contraceptive pill but has no significant past medical history and takes no other regular medication.

On examination, she has a heart rate of 240 bpm, and her blood pressure is 122/72 mmHg. Oxygen saturations are 96% on air and her respiratory rate is 28 breaths/min. Her chest is clear to auscultation and heart sounds appear normal.

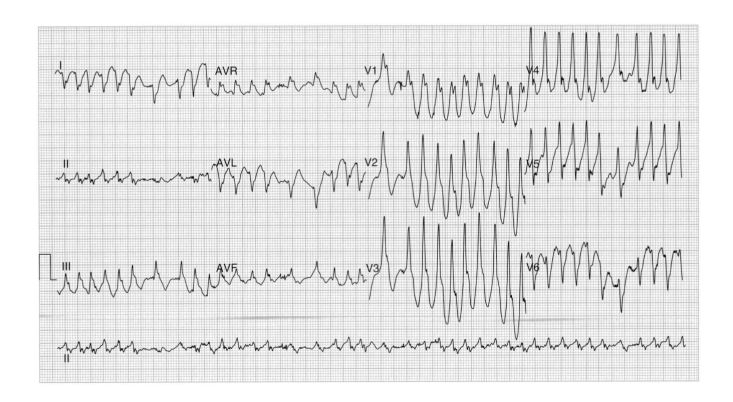

❓ QUESTIONS FOR CANDIDATE

1. What condition is characterised by the presence of an accessory pathway between the atria and the ventricles?
   (a) Arrhythmogenic right ventricular cardiomyopathy
   (b) Atrial flutter
   (c) Ebstein anomaly
   (d) Wolff–Parkinson–White syndrome
   (e) None of the above

2. Which antiarrhythmic drugs could be considered in pre-excited AF?
   (a) Adenosine
   (b) Amiodarone
   (c) Digoxin
   (d) Flecainide
   (e) Verapamil

3. What long-term management options should be considered for pre-excited AF?
   (a) Catheter ablation of accessory pathway
   (b) Insertion of an implantable cardiac defibrillator (ICD)
   (c) Oral adenosine
   (d) Oral anticoagulation
   (e) Oral flecainide

❶ Note: Answers are on page 172.

CASE 17 – QUESTIONS

You have been bleeped to review a 70-year-old man on the surgical ward who has developed new-onset shortness of breath. He is 5 days post-laparoscopic cholecystectomy and is currently being treated for pneumonia.

He has a past medical history of hypertension, diabetes mellitus, hypercholesterolaemia, gout and osteoarthritis of the spine. He smokes 10 cigarettes a day and drinks 20 units of alcohol per week.

On examination, he is apyrexic with a heart rate of 60 bpm, respiratory rate 20 breaths/min and blood pressure 165/80 mmHg and his JVP is elevated at 5 cm. Auscultation reveals normal heart sounds with no murmurs with bibasal crepitations at the lung bases.

An ECG is performed as part of his work-up.

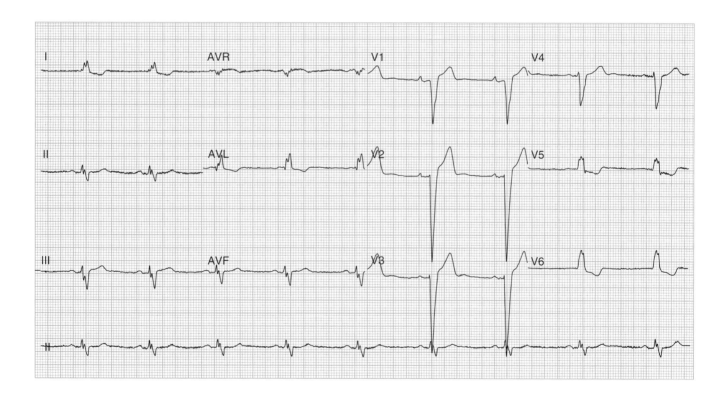

❓ QUESTIONS FOR CANDIDATE

1. **Which of the following conditions are associated with an LBBB?**
   (a) Aortic stenosis
   (b) Atrial septal defect
   (c) Cardiomyopathy
   (d) Hypokalaemia
   (e) Ischaemic heart disease

2. **Which of the following ECG changes can be produced by an LBBB?**
   (a) Left-axis deviation
   (b) Prolonged PR interval
   (c) Right-axis deviation
   (d) RSR′ pattern in V_1–V_3
   (e) Wide QRS complexes

3. **Which of the following are appropriate treatment options for this patient?**
   (a) ACE inhibitors
   (b) Adenosine
   (c) Calcium channel blockers
   (d) Biventricular pacing
   (e) Diuretics

❶ Note: Answers are on page 174.

CASE 18 – QUESTIONS

A 18-year-old female presents with shortness of breath and palpitations during physical activity. There is no chest pain.

Apart from experiencing severe and frequent chest infections each winter, there is no significant past medical history of note. There is a family history of 'heart problems'.

On examination, she is apyrexial with a heart rate of 86 bpm, respiratory rate 20 breaths/min and blood pressure 90/50 mmHg. There is an ejection systolic murmur on the second intercostal space at the left sternal edge with fixed splitting of S2. There is good bilateral air entry.

An ECG is performed as part of her work-up.

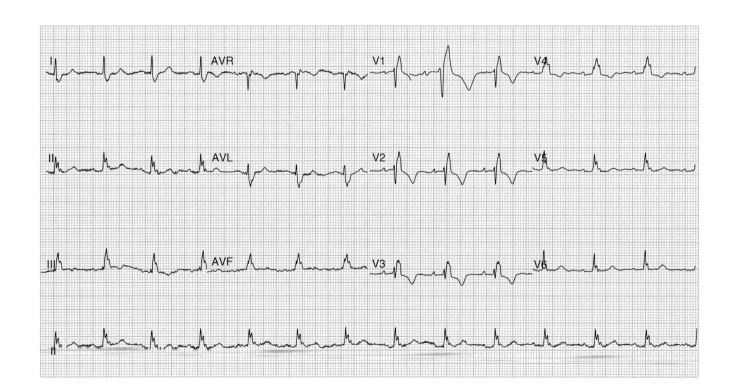

❓ QUESTIONS FOR CANDIDATE

1. Which of the following may produce an RBBB?
(a) Atrial septal defect
(b) Brugada syndrome
(c) Systemic hypertension
(d) Pulmonary embolism
(e) All of the above

2. Which of the following ECG changes can be produced by an RBBB?
(a) RSR′ pattern in V_1–V_3
(b) Right-axis deviation
(c) Widened QRS complex
(d) Left-axis deviation
(e) ST elevation in V_1–V_3

3. Which of the following statements is/are true with regard to RBBB?
(a) Bifascicular blocks involve the right bundle.
(b) Cardiac resynchronisation may be used in patients with heart failure and RBBB.
(c) RBBBs are always benign findings.
(d) RBBBs in young individuals are usually indicative of organic heart disease.
(e) Trifascicular blocks involve the right bundle.

❶ Note: Answers are on page 176.

CASE 19 – QUESTIONS

A 25-year-old man presents to the emergency department with chest pain worse on deep inspiration. He does not smoke and drinks a moderate amount and there is no significant past medical history.

On examination his blood pressure is 125/80 mmHg and oxygen saturations are 94% with a respiratory rate of 30 breaths/min. He is pyrexial with a temperature of 38.5°C. Heart sounds are normal and there are crackles at his right lung base.

An ECG is performed as part of his work-up.

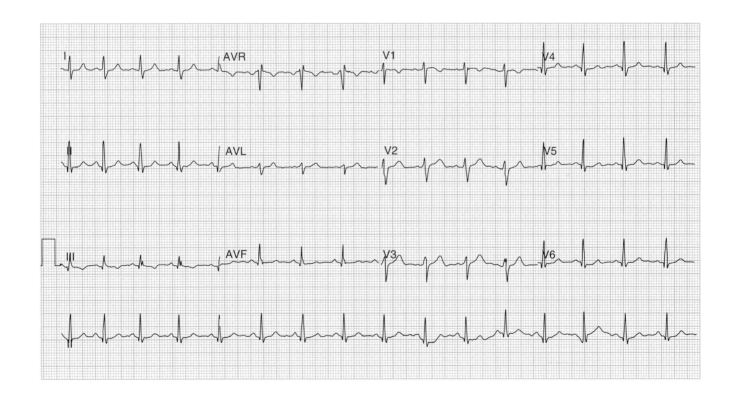

❓ QUESTIONS FOR CANDIDATE

1. **On a standard ECG trace what amount of time is represented by one small square?**
   - (a) 0.01 s
   - (b) 0.04 s
   - (c) 0.1 s
   - (d) 0.4 s
   - (e) 1 s

2. **What is the maximum normal duration for a QRS complex?**
   - (a) 50 ms
   - (b) 110 ms
   - (c) 150 ms
   - (d) 200 ms
   - (e) 1 s

3. **Which of the following can be a normal variant on an ECG?**
   - (a) No Q waves in any leads
   - (b) Prominent Q waves in aVR
   - (c) Prominent Q waves in lead III
   - (d) Prominent Q waves in V_1–V_3
   - (e) Small Q waves (<2 small squares) in V_4–V_6

❶ Note: Answers are on page 178.

CASE 20 – QUESTIONS

A 45-year-old man attends his pre-op review prior to a right hemicolectomy under the 2-week wait for right-sided colon carcinoma. He reports feeling generally well aside from feeling more tired than usual and weight loss.

On examination, he has oxygen saturations of 94% on room air, respiratory rate 14 breaths/min, heart rate 55 bpm and blood pressure 123/76 mmHg. Auscultation reveals normal heart and lung sounds.

An ECG is performed as part of his pre-op work-up.

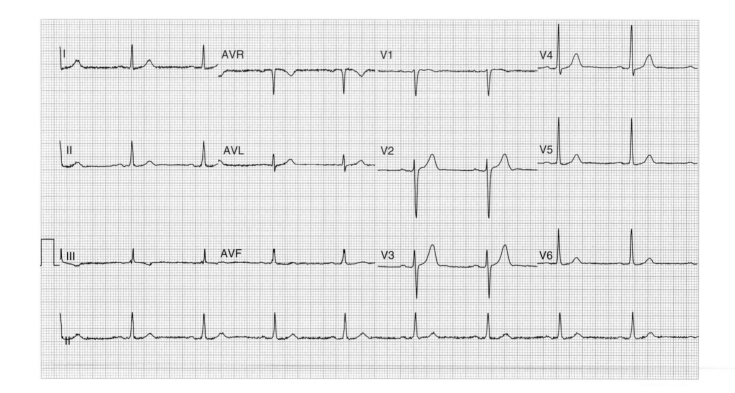

❓ QUESTIONS FOR CANDIDATE

1. Which of the following are possible causes of sinus bradycardia?

(a) Angiotensin-converting enzyme (ACE) inhibitors
(b) Beta-blockers
(c) Hyperthyroidism
(d) Hypoglycaemia
(e) Increased vagal tone

2. What symptoms is this patient likely to be experiencing because of the ECG changes seen?

(a) Chest pain
(b) None
(c) Orthopnoea
(d) Shortness of breath on exertion
(e) Syncope

3. Which of the following ECG changes can be caused by sinus bradycardia?

(a) Increased PR interval
(b) Increased QT interval
(c) Large Q waves in the inferior leads
(d) Presence of a delta wave
(e) Widened QRS complex

❶ Note: Answers are on page 180.

CASE 21 – QUESTIONS

You are the junior doctor covering the medical assessment unit and you are asked to review the admission ECG of a 78-year-old man admitted with confusion.

He has a past medical history of hypertension, type 2 diabetes, chronic obstructive pulmonary disease (COPD) and Parkinson disease. When you arrive, he is alert and comfortable but says he still has palpitations. He has no chest pain. His observations are: respiratory rate 20 breaths/min, oxygen saturations 98% on room air, heart rate 54 bpm, blood pressure 110/68 mmHg and temperature 36.5°C. Auscultation of the heart and chest is unremarkable.

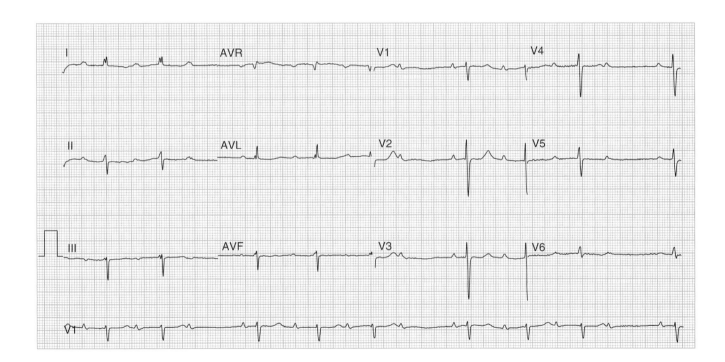

❓ QUESTIONS FOR CANDIDATE

1. What is the cause of this arrhythmia?
  (a) Accessory pathways between the atria and the ventricles
  (b) Electrolyte disturbances
  (c) AV node conduction disease
  (d) Malfunction of cells in the Purkinje fibres
  (e) Ventricular ischaemia

2. Which of the following would be appropriate acute investigations and management for this patient?
  (a) Administration of atropine
  (b) Administration of clopidogrel and aspirin
  (c) No management necessary
  (d) Percutaneous coronary intervention (PCI)
  (e) Thrombolysis using alteplase

3. Which of the following are potential complications arising from this heart block?
  (a) Asystole
  (b) Hypotension
  (c) Myocardial infarction (MI)
  (d) Progression to third-degree heart block
  (e) Syncope secondary to bradycardia
  ❶ Note: Answers are on page 181.

CASE 22 – QUESTIONS

You are a junior doctor working in a general practice surgery. A 57-year-old woman has booked an emergency appointment for the morning complaining of palpitations, shortness of breath and dizziness.

She has no significant past medical history and her only regular medication is simvastatin. Her heart rate is 75 bpm, blood pressure 123/82 mmHg, respiratory rate 18 breaths/min, oxygen saturation 98% on air and temperature 36.8°C. Auscultation of the heart and chest is unremarkable.

A 12-lead ECG is performed.

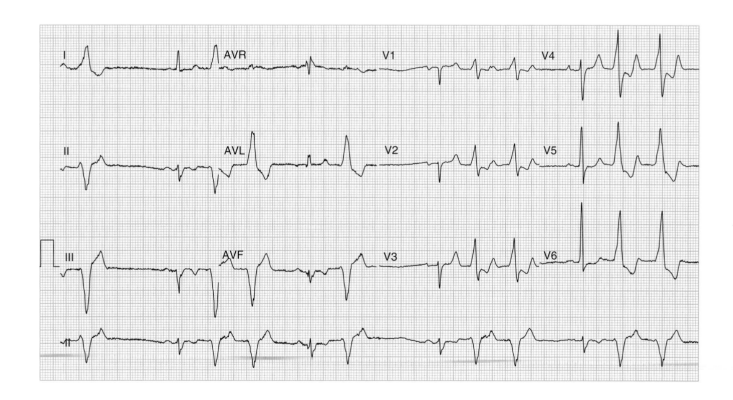

❓ QUESTIONS FOR CANDIDATE

1. What is the name for the condition where every third beat is a ventricular ectopic?

(a) Atrial bigeminy
(b) Atrial trigeminy
(c) Non-sustained ventricular tachycardia
(d) Ventricular bigeminy
(e) Ventricular trigeminy

2. In which of the following conditions may ventricular ectopic beats induce other arrhythmias?

(a) Aortic stenosis
(b) Atrial fibrillation
(c) Cor pulmonale
(d) Ischaemic heart disease
(e) Wolff–Parkinson–White

3. Which of the following would a patient with a long QTc be at risk of developing from frequent ventricular ectopics?

(a) Asystole

(b) Bundle branch block
(c) Pulseless electrical activity
(d) Torsades de pointes
(e) Ventricular fibrillation

❶ Note: Answers are on page 183.

CASE 23 – QUESTIONS

A 64-year-old man is brought into the emergency department by his daughter after he fell and sustained a head injury. The man does not remember what happened but his daughter says he suddenly collapsed and became unconscious while walking. He regained consciousness a few seconds later but sustained a head injury and has a visible scalp wound.

His observations are respiratory rate 22 breaths/min, oxygen saturations 98% on room air, heart rate 36 bpm, blood pressure 180/60 mmHg and temperature 36.3°C. The only examination finding is bradycardia.

An ECG is performed.

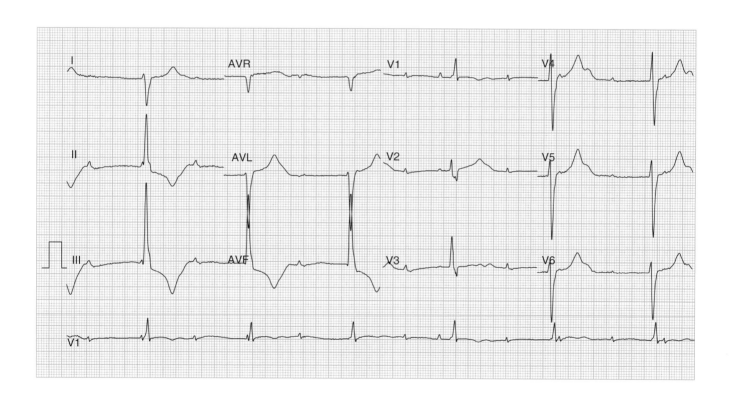

❓ QUESTIONS FOR CANDIDATE

1. Why are there still QRS complexes in complete heart block?

(a) Conduction through the atrioventricular (AV) node still occurs but is just delayed

(b) P waves are sporadically conducted through the AV node

(c) The AV node can generate an escape rhythm

(d) There are accessory pathways between the atria and the ventricles

(e) The ventricles can generate an escape rhythm

2. Which of the following are causes of complete heart block?

(a) Digoxin toxicity

(b) Hyperkalaemia

(c) Lev disease

(d) Inferior myocardial infarction

(e) Septal myocardial infarction

3. If complete heart block is symptomatic, what treatment may be required?

(a) Atropine

(b) No treatment required

(c) Permanent pacemaker insertion

(d) Regular outpatient follow-up with no acute treatment

(e) Transcutaneous pacing

❶ Note: Answers are on page 185.

CASE 24 – QUESTIONS

An 85-year-old woman is brought to the emergency department by ambulance after her neighbour became worried that she had not seen her for several days. When the ambulance crew arrived at the patient's home, they found the woman on the floor, apparently having fallen.

On arrival at the emergency department, the woman appeared very confused and unable to say when she fell. Her blood pressure is 110/75 mmHg, oxygen saturation is 93% on room air with a respiratory rate of 20 breaths/min. Her temperature is 34.0°C. From her medical records you notice that she takes warfarin for previous recurrent pulmonary emboli. Examination is unremarkable.

A 12-lead ECG is performed.

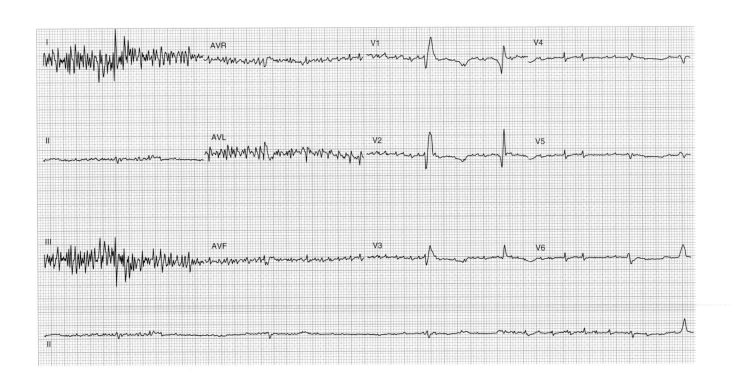

❓ QUESTIONS FOR CANDIDATE

1. **Which of the following are possible causes for an irregular baseline in this patient's ECG?**
   (a) Acute myocardial infarction (MI)
   (b) Confusion/agitation
   (c) Electrical interference from nearby equipment
   (d) Hypothermia
   (e) Rhabdomyolysis

2. **What immediate further investigations will this patient require?**
   (a) 24-h tape
   (b) Bloods, including creatinine kinase and urea and electrolytes (U&Es)
   (c) Computed tomography (CT) head
   (d) CT pulmonary angiogram
   (e) Echocardiogram

3. **What should be done before repeating this patient's ECG?**
   (a) Attempt to make her more comfortable and less agitated
   (b) Change the ECG machine as it is likely to be faulty
   (c) Give a beta-blocker to slow the heart rate
   (d) Slowly warm her up
   (e) Turn off any nearby machinery/equipment

❶ Note: Answers are on page 187.

CASE 25 – QUESTIONS

You are the junior doctor working in ED. A 58-year-old man presents with a fall.

As you are taking a history, he mentions that he thinks he has previously been diagnosed with a 'funny rhythm' and is taking pills for this, although he cannot remember what they are called. He has no other past medical history or regular medications.

His observations are respiratory rate 22 breaths/min, oxygen saturations 96% on room air, heart rate 35 bpm, blood pressure 140/80 mmHg and temperature 37.0°C. On examination he has a right-sided facial droop with slight slurring of speech. Power is 5/5 bilaterally.

You record an ECG as part of your work-up.

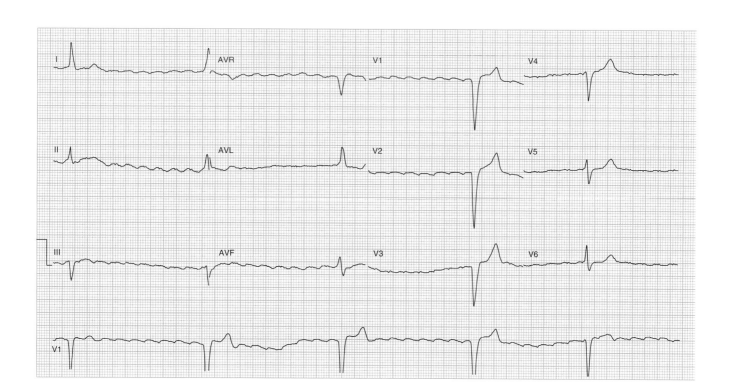

❓ QUESTIONS FOR CANDIDATE

1. Why are the QRS complexes wide?
  (a) He also has complete heart block
  (b) He has been successfully rhythm-controlled
  (c) He has had electrophysiological ablation
  (d) The atrial flutter is paroxysmal
  (e) The man was wrong about his previous diagnosis

2. Based on this ECG, which of the following drugs is this patient most likely to be taking?
  (a) Amiodarone
  (b) Amlodipine
  (c) Digoxin
  (d) Pravastatin
  (e) Ramipril

3. If he is not already on an equivalent medication, which of the following medications would it be most appropriate to start this patient on?
  (a) Amiodarone
  (b) Apixaban
  (c) Aspirin
  (d) Clopidogrel
  (e) Low-molecular-weight heparin

❶ Note: Answers are on page 189.

CASE 26 – QUESTIONS

A 65-year-old man presents to the emergency department with severe abdominal pain. He has a past medical history of depression and diverticulosis.

His observations are respiratory rate 30 breaths/min, oxygen saturations 95% on 4 L oxygen, heart rate 50 bpm, blood pressure 82/64 mmHg and temperature 37.2°C. On examination, his abdomen is rigid with rebound tenderness and guarding. The surgical team organised computed tomography (CT) which showed a perforated sigmoid diverticulum. They plan to take him to theatre for an emergency laparotomy.

After initial stabilisation with fluid resuscitation, the anaesthetist is called to review the patient before theatre and requests an ECG. As the junior doctor on the emergency department, the nurse asks you to review the ECG.

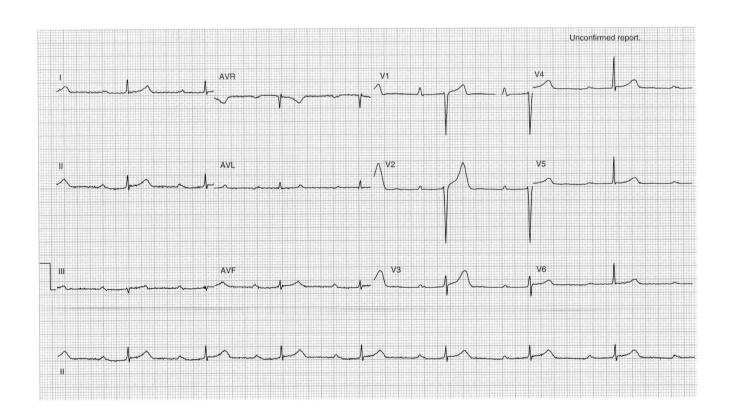

❓ QUESTIONS FOR CANDIDATE

1. What is the normal PR interval?
(a) 0.10–0.15 s
(b) 0.12–0.20 s
(c) 0.15–0.25 s
(d) 0.20–0.30 s
(e) 0.30–0.38 s

2. Which of the following can cause first-degree heart block?
(a) Athletic training
(b) Digoxin
(c) Electrolyte disturbances
(d) Pericarditis
(e) Posterior myocardial infarction (MI)

3. Assuming this patient has no underlying heart disease, what treatment is indicated?
(a) Atropine
(b) Dual-chamber pacemaker
(c) Catheter ablation
(d) No treatment
(e) Ventricular pacemaker

❶ Note: Answers are on page 191.

CASE 27 – QUESTIONS

A 42-year-old woman presents to the emergency department with worsening confusion and lethargy. She has a 7-day history of vomiting and diarrhoea and has not been able to tolerate much oral intake over the past few days. She has no significant past medical history.

Her observations are heart rate 60 bpm, blood pressure 98/70 mmHg, respiratory rate 26 breaths/min, oxygen saturation 96% on room air and she is apyrexial. Her examination is largely normal aside from some mild abdominal pain and power 4/5 in her lower limbs. She also appears clinically dehydrated.

A 12-lead ECG is recorded.

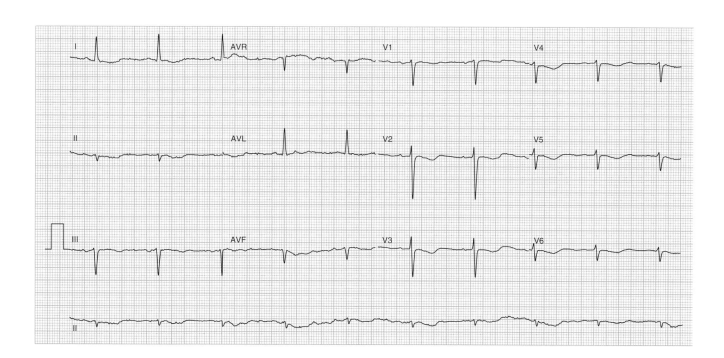

❓ QUESTIONS FOR CANDIDATE

1. **Which of the following would be appropriate in the initial management of this patient?**
   (a) Bloods, including U&Es and magnesium
   (b) Give calcium gluconate 10%
   (c) Give intravenous (IV) insulin and dextrose 20%
   (d) IV fluids, including potassium chloride
   (e) IV magnesium replacement

2. **Which of the following are complications of hypokalaemia?**
   (a) Left bundle branch block
   (b) Supraventricular tachycardia
   (c) Torsades de pointes
   (d) Ventricular fibrillation
   (e) Ventricular tachycardia

3. **Which of the following are risk factors for hypokalaemia?**
   (a) Burns
   (b) Diarrhoea
   (c) Hypomagnesaemia
   (d) Increased sweating
   (e) Vitamin D deficiency

❶ Note: Answers are on page 193.

CASE 28 – QUESTIONS

A 65-year-old man is seen in the cardiology outpatient clinic following pacemaker insertion for severe symptomatic bradycardia.

His only past medical history is prostate cancer, for which he is currently under surveillance. He is feeling well and has had no symptoms.

His observations are respiratory rate 22 breaths/min, oxygen saturation 97% on room air, heart rate 60 bpm, blood pressure 110/68 mmHg and temperature 37.0°C. Examination shows a device implanted below his left clavicle with a well-healed wound.

A routine ECG is recorded.

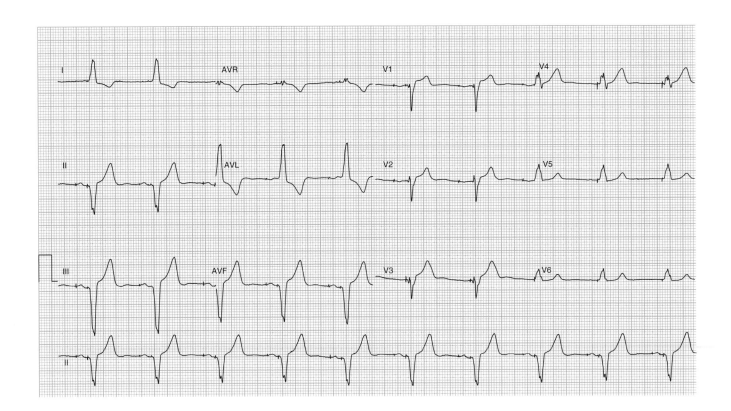

❓ QUESTIONS FOR CANDIDATE

1. Which chamber(s) are being paced?
  (a) Both ventricles only
  (b) Left ventricle and one atrium
  (c) Left ventricle only
  (d) Right ventricle and one atrium
  (e) Right ventricle only

2. Which of the following is/are an indication for this type of pacemaker?
  (a) Atrial flutter
  (b) Complete heart block
  (c) Ischaemic heart disease
  (d) Sick sinus syndrome
  (e) Wolff–Parkinson–White

3. Which of the following investigations should be routinely performed following pacemaker insertion?
  (a) 24-h tape
  (b) Bloods, including C-reactive protein (CRP)
  (c) Chest X-ray
  (d) Computed tomography (CT) chest
  (e) Device check

❶ Note: Answers are on page 195.

CASE 29 – QUESTIONS

A 67-year-old man presents to the emergency department with a several-day history of crushing central chest pain. He initially ignored it but has presented because the pain did not go away. The pain came on while he was climbing the stairs and since it started it has got gradually worse. He has a background of type 2 diabetes and stable angina but previously his angina has always been relieved by rest, which this pain has not.

His observations are: blood pressure 135/70 mmHg, heart rate 90 bpm, respiratory rate 25 breaths/min, oxygen saturation 93% on room air and temperature 36.5°C. On examination he is clammy to touch and has mild bibasal crackles on auscultation.

A 12-lead ECG is recorded in view of his chest pain.

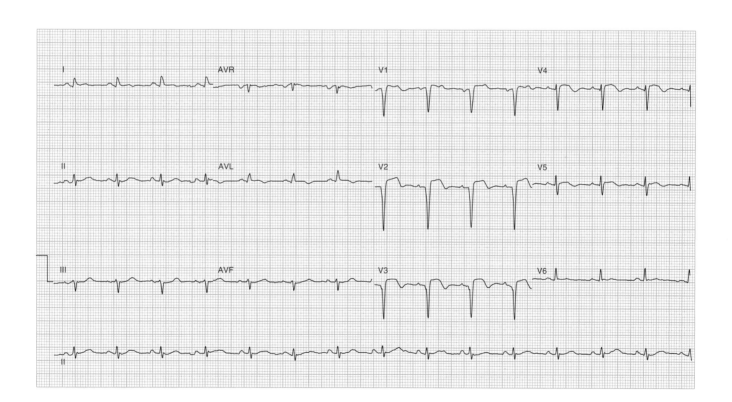

❓ QUESTIONS FOR CANDIDATE

1. **What size of Q waves are the minimum to be considered significant?**
   (a) 1 mm
   (b) 2 mm
   (c) 3 mm
   (d) 4 mm
   (e) 5 mm
2. **Which of the following can cause significant Q waves?**
   (a) Acute ischaemia
   (b) Cardiomyopathy
   (c) Lead misplacement
   (d) Previous infarction
   (e) Rotation of the heart
3. **Which of the following are risk factors for this patient's presentation?**
   (a) Diabetes mellitus
   (b) Hypertension
   (c) Hypercholesterolaemia
   (d) Family history of ischaemic heart disease
   (e) Pulmonary artery hypertension

❶ Note: Answers are on page 197.

CASE 30 – QUESTIONS

A 50-year-old man presents to the emergency department with sudden-onset shortness of breath, dizziness and light-headedness. The symptoms came on at rest around 1 h ago and he called an ambulance immediately. The ambulance crew report that on arrival his heart rate was 30 bpm. His observations now show respiratory rate 26 breaths/min, oxygen saturations 95% on room air, heart rate 38 bpm, blood pressure 90/68 mmHg and temperature 36.8°C. He has no significant past medical history, and examination is unremarkable aside from severe bradycardia.

A 12-lead ECG is recorded.

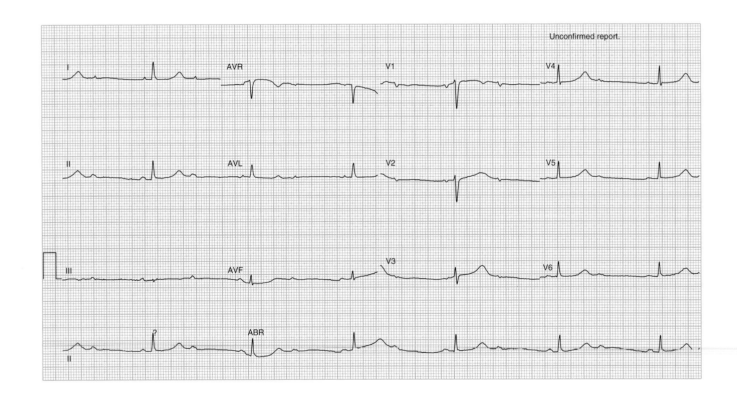

❓ QUESTIONS FOR CANDIDATE

1. **Which of the following may be the site of the lesion in 2:1 heart block?**
   (a) Atrioventricular (AV) node
   (b) Bundle of His
   (c) Purkinje fibres
   (d) Sinoatrial node
   (e) Ventricular myocardium

2. **Which of the following treatment options may be appropriate in an asymptomatic patient with 2:1 heart block?**
   (a) Daily beta-blockers
   (b) DC cardioversion
   (c) Cardiac catheter ablation
   (d) No treatment may be necessary
   (e) Permanent pacemaker insertion

3. **Which of the following would be the appropriate treatment for this patient?**
   (a) Amiodarone infusion
   (b) Isoprenaline infusion
   (c) No treatment is necessary
   (d) Permanent pacemaker insertion
   (e) Transcutaneous pacing before urgent permanent pacemaker insertion

❶ Note: Answers are on page 199.

CASE 31 – QUESTIONS

A 64-year-old woman presents to the emergency department with a 2-day history of vomiting and diarrhoea. She reports being sick several times and having multiple episodes of watery stool with abdominal pain.

Her past medical history includes chronic kidney disease stage 4 and a recent diagnosis of atrial fibrillation for which she has been started on digoxin 125 mcg OD. Her observations show respiratory rate 22 breaths/min, oxygen saturations 95% on room air, heart rate 70 bpm, blood pressure 108/82 mmHg and temperature 36.2°C. On examination, her abdomen is diffusely tender with no guarding or rigidity.

Her ECG is shown below.

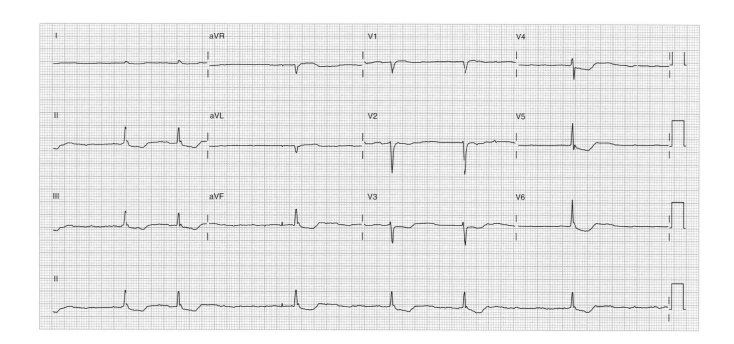

❓ QUESTIONS FOR CANDIDATE

1. What is the mechanism of action of digoxin?
(a) Activation of Na^+/K^+-ATPase
(b) Activation of voltage-gated potassium channels
(c) Activation of voltage-gated sodium channels
(d) Inhibition of Na^+/K^+-ATPase
(e) Inhibition of voltage-gated calcium channels

2. Which of these can be caused by digoxin toxicity?
(a) Complete heart block
(b) Hyperkalaemia
(c) Hypokalaemia
(d) Ventricular fibrillation
(e) Xanthopsia

3. Which of the following are appropriate in the management of digoxin toxicity?
(a) Administration of digoxin-specific antibody
(b) Discontinue digoxin
(c) Immediate transcutaneous pacing
(d) Intravenous calcium if hyperkalaemia is present
(e) Intravenous fluid resuscitation if hypotension is present

❶ Note: Answers are on page 201.

CASE 32 – QUESTIONS

You are the junior doctor on call covering the surgical wards. You are asked to review a 42-year-old woman on the orthopaedic ward, 1-week post-knee replacement, who reported sudden-onset shortness of breath and chest pain.

There is no past medical history of note. She is on the oral contraceptive pill for occasional menorrhagia.

On examination, she is apyrexial with a heart rate of 110 bpm, respiratory rate of 30 breaths/min and blood pressure 130/80 mmHg. Heart sounds are normal and there is good bilateral air entry.

An ECG is performed as part of her work-up.

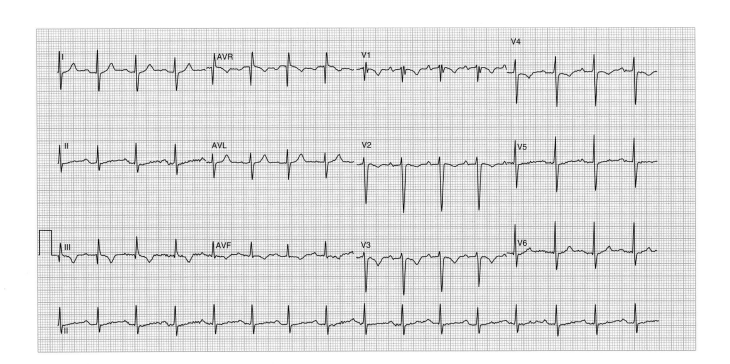

？ QUESTIONS FOR CANDIDATE

1. Which of the following is/are a risk factor(s) for developing pulmonary embolism?

(a) Diabetes mellitus

(b) Malignancy

(c) Oral contraceptive pills

(d) Polycythaemia

(e) Previous myocardial infarction

2. Which of the following ECG changes can be produced by a pulmonary embolism?

(a) Deep S wave in lead I

(b) P mitrale

(c) Peaked T wave

(d) Sinus tachycardia

(e) T-wave inversion in V_1–V_4

3. Which of the following is/are true with regard to the management of pulmonary embolism?

(a) CTPA is the gold-standard diagnostic tool for pulmonary embolism

(b) D-dimer should be used to diagnose pulmonary embolism

(c) Echocardiography may be used if pulmonary embolism is suspected

(d) Thrombolytic therapy is only indicated in patients with acute pulmonary embolism with low bleeding risk who are haemodynamically stable

(e) Wells score can be used as a probability scoring tool for diagnosing pulmonary embolism

❶ Note: Answers are on page 203.

CASE 33 – QUESTIONS

A 68-year-old woman presents to the emergency department with a 2-month history of worsening exertional breathlessness and a purulent cough. She has also noticed a recent increase in the size of her ankles.

Her past medical history includes hypertension, type 2 diabetes mellitus and ischaemic heart disease.

On examination, she is apyrexial with a heart rate 85 bpm, respiratory rate 25 breaths/min and blood pressure 160/90 mmHg. A pansystolic murmur is noted in the fifth intercostal space in the mid-clavicular line. There is good bilateral air entry.

An ECG is performed as part of her work-up.

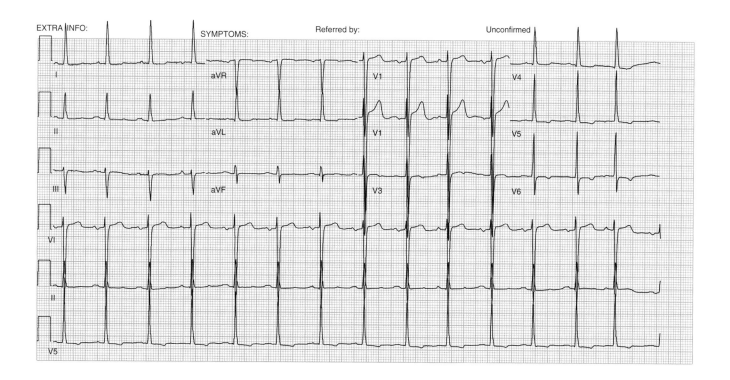

❓ QUESTIONS FOR CANDIDATE

1. **Which two of the following are the LEAST likely to be an aetiology of left ventricular hypertrophy?**
   (a) Aortic regurgitation
   (b) Aortic stenosis
   (c) Hypertension
   (d) Mitral regurgitation
   (e) Mitral stenosis

2. **Which of the following ECG changes can be produced by left ventricular hypertrophy?**
   (a) Dominant R wave in V_1
   (b) Increased R-wave amplitude in V_6
   (c) Left-axis deviation
   (d) Prolonged PR interval
   (e) ST elevation in lateral leads

3. **Which of the following statements is/are true regarding left ventricular hypertrophy?**
   (a) A total sum of 22 mm from R-wave amplitude in aVL plus S-wave amplitude in V_3 indicates left ventricular hypertrophy
   (b) Large ventricular amplitude is a normal finding in patients older than 45 years
   (c) Left ventricular hypertrophy is diagnosed if the sum of R-wave height in V_1 plus S-wave depth in V_5–V_6 is greater than 35 mm
   (d) Left ventricular hypertrophy may be a sign of left ventricular failure
   (e) Left-sided heart failure can cause portal hypertension and peripheral oedema

❶ Note: Answers are on page 205.

CASE 34 – QUESTIONS

A 65-year-old gentleman presents to ED with a 24-hour history of severe central chest pain radiating to the neck, shortness of breath and dizziness. He denies any cough, haemoptysis and loss of consciousness.

He has a past medical history of hypertension, diabetes mellitus, hypercholesterolaemia and chronic obstructive pulmonary disease (COPD). He smokes 20 cigarettes a day and drinks 10 units of alcohol per week.

On examination, he is apyrexial with a heart rate 70 bpm, respiratory rate 25 breaths/min and blood pressure 150/90 mmHg. Auscultation reveals normal heart sounds with no murmurs, and good bilateral air entry with no added sounds.

An ECG is performed as part of his work-up.

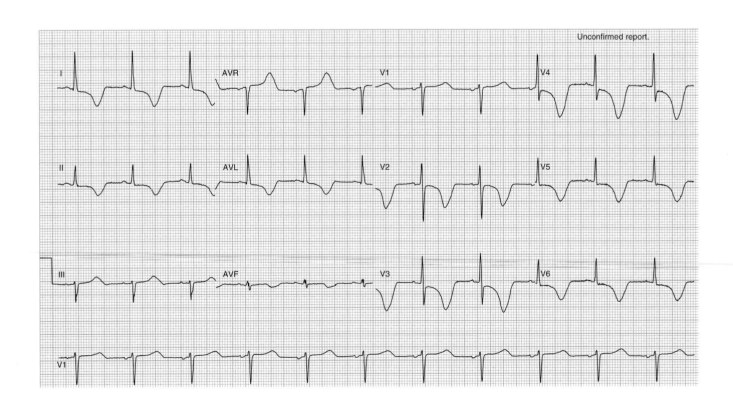

❓ QUESTIONS FOR CANDIDATE

1. **Which of the following ECG changes can be produced by an NSTEMI?**
   (a) Hyperacute T waves
   (b) P-wave flattening
   (c) Prolonged PR interval
   (d) ST depression
   (e) T-wave inversion
2. **Which of the following treatments should be routinely offered in the acute management of NSTEMIs?**
   (a) Antiplatelet therapy
   (b) Aspirin
   (c) Coronary angiography
   (d) Spironolactone
   (e) Statin
3. **Which of the following would most likely describe the underlying pathology?**
   (a) Reversible cardiac ischaemia
   (b) Subendocardial infarct due to atherosclerosis
   (c) Subendocardial infarct due to vasospasm
   (d) Transmural infarct due to atherosclerosis
   (e) Transmural infarct due to vasospasm
   ❶ Note: Answers are on page 207.

CASE 35 – QUESTIONS

A 40-year-old man presents to the emergency department with a 3-day history of chest pain that is relieved by leaning forward. He is slightly short of breath and has complained of a recent cough alongside feeling cold and feverish. He denies any palpitations and dizziness.

His past medical history includes asthma and a 'funny heart rhythm', although he has not needed medication for this. There is no family history of any heart condition. He smokes 10 cigarettes a day and drinks 10 units of alcohol per week.

On examination, he has a temperature of 38.9°C, heart rate 80 bpm, respiratory rate 20 breaths/min and blood pressure 130/80 mmHg. Auscultation reveals normal heart sounds with no murmurs, and there is good bilateral air entry.

An ECG is performed as part of his work-up.

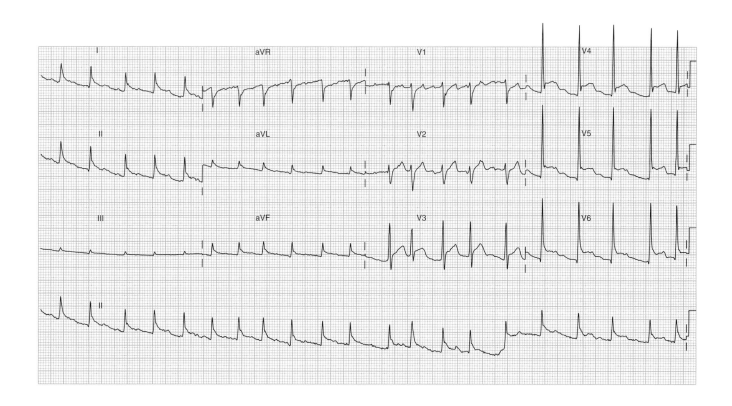

❓ QUESTIONS FOR CANDIDATE

1. **Which of the following may produce pericarditis?**
   (a) Cardiac surgery
   (b) Myocardial infarction
   (c) Rheumatic heart disease
   (d) Viral respiratory tract infection
   (e) All of the above
2. **Which of the following ECG changes can be produced by acute pericarditis?**
   (a) PR depression
   (b) Sinus tachycardia
   (c) Slurred upstroke in the QRS complex
   (d) ST depression
   (e) T-wave inversion
3. **Which of the following are effective in the management of pericarditis?**
   (a) Anticoagulants
   (b) Beta-blockers
   (c) NSAIDs
   (d) Pericardiocentesis
   (e) Thiazide diuretics

❶ Note: Answers are on page 209.

CASE 36 – QUESTIONS

A 64-year-old man presents to the emergency department with severe central crushing chest pain and difficulty in breathing.

He has a 40-pack year smoking history but there is no significant past medical history.

On examination, he has saturations of 91% on air, respiratory rate 16 breaths/min, heart rate 80 bpm, blood pressure 120/80 mmHg and is afebrile. Auscultation reveals normal heart sounds with no murmurs, and good bilateral air entry with no added sounds.

An ECG is performed as part of his work-up.

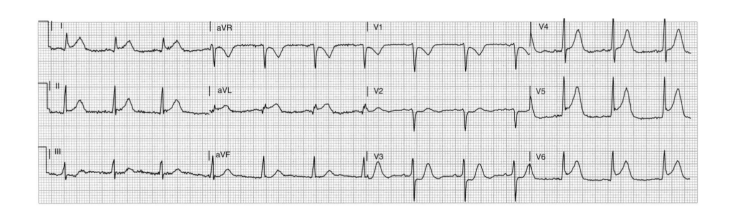

❓ QUESTIONS FOR CANDIDATE

1. Which of the following is/are a risk factor(s) for developing myocardial infarction?

(a) Diabetes mellitus

(b) Male sex

(c) Smoking

(d) Use of angiotensin-converting enzyme (ACE) inhibitors

(e) Use of combined oral contraceptive pill

2. What of the following best describes the classic characteristics of chest pain due to myocardial ischaemia?

(a) Burning, diffuse bilateral chest pain

(b) Central crushing chest pain radiating to the left shoulder

(c) Sharp, well-localised left chest pain with overlying tenderness

(d) Sharp, well-localised right chest pain worse on inspiration

(e) Tearing chest pain radiating to the back

3. What is the most likely coronary artery to have been affected in this patient?

(a) Left anterior descending artery

(b) Left circumflex artery

(c) Posterior descending artery

(d) Right coronary artery

(e) Right marginal artery

❶ Note: Answers are on page 211.

CASE 37 – QUESTIONS

A 40-year-old man presents to the emergency department with central crushing chest pain. He was playing football when he developed sudden crushing pain in his central chest radiating to his jaw. He had no past medical history of note. He is a non-smoker and non-drinker.

On examination, he is tachycardic with a heart rate of 110 bpm. His pulse is regular and his oxygen saturation is 92% on air. Respiratory rate is 18 breaths/min. Blood pressure was 160/80 mmHg. Auscultation reveals normal heart sounds with no murmurs, and good bilateral air entry with no added sounds.

An ECG is performed as part of his work-up.

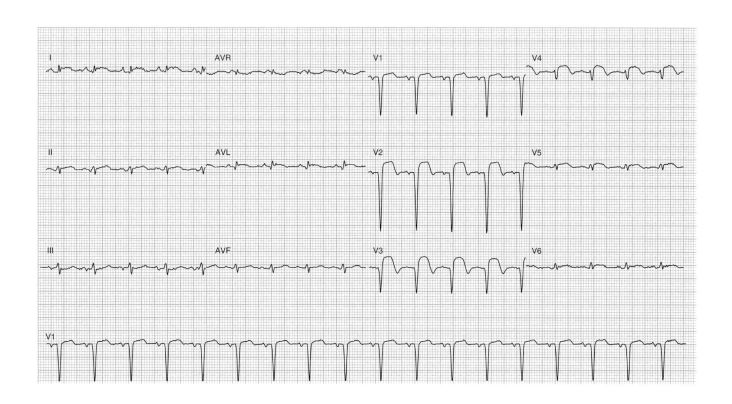

❓ QUESTIONS FOR CANDIDATE

1. Which of the following would most likely describe the underlying pathology?

(a) Reversible cardiac ischaemia
(b) Subendocardial infarct due to atherosclerosis
(c) Subendocardial infarct due to vasospasm
(d) Transmural infarct due to atherosclerosis and plaque rupture
(e) Transmural infarct due to vasospasm

2. Which of the following can lead to myocardial ischaemia?

(a) Atherosclerosis
(b) Anaemia
(c) Cocaine use
(d) Infective endocarditis
(e) All of the above

3. Which of the following is/are a diagnostic ECG finding(s) for a STEMI?

(a) >1 mm ST elevation in two or more limb leads
(b) >1 mm ST elevation in two or more precordial leads (V_1–V_6)
(c) New left bundle branch block
(d) New right bundle branch block
(e) T-wave inversion

❶ Note: Answers are on page 214.

CASE 38 – QUESTIONS

A 50-year-old man presents to the emergency department after developing severe central chest pain and dizziness. He has a past medical history of gastro-oesophageal reflux disease, hiatus hernia and obesity. He is on glyceryl trinitrate spray as required, omeprazole, ramipril and simvastatin.

On examination, his heart rate is 70 bpm. He is tachypnoeic with a respiratory rate of 25 breaths/min with an oxygen saturation of 95% on 4 L oxygen. His blood pressure is 155/95 mmHg. Auscultation reveals normal heart sounds with no murmurs, and reduced air entry with some minimal wheeze.

An ECG is performed as part of his work-up.

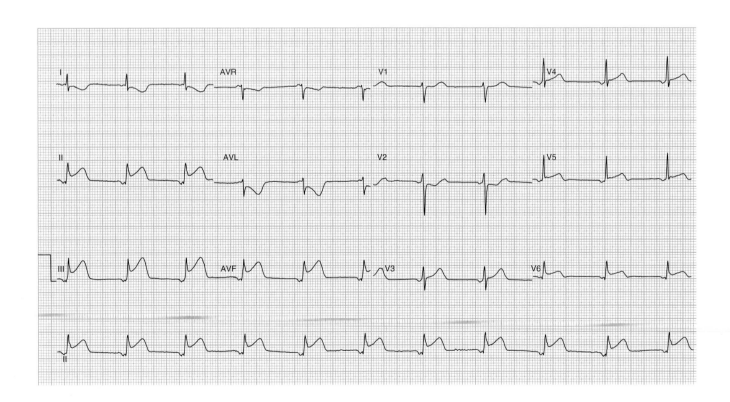

❓ QUESTIONS FOR CANDIDATE

1. **What is the most appropriate cardiac biomarker for investigating myocardial infarction?**
   (a) Aspartate aminotransferase
   (b) Creatine kinase
   (c) Lactate dehydrogenase
   (d) Myoglobin
   (e) Troponin I and T

2. **What is the most appropriate immediate treatment for this patient?**
   (a) Aspirin 300 mg and primary percutaneous coronary intervention (PCI)
   (b) Aspirin, clopidogrel, fondaparinux, beta-blocker and pain relief
   (c) Coronary artery bypass graft (CABG)
   (d) Heart transplant
   (e) High-flow oxygen and intravenous (IV) atropine

3. **A few days following admission, the patient complained of acute shortness of breath. A new pansystolic murmur and bibasal lung crackles can be heard on auscultation. Which of the following is the most likely complication that the patient has developed?**
   (a) Complete heart block
   (b) Heart failure
   (c) Papillary muscle rupture
   (d) Pericarditis
   (e) Ventricular aneurysm
   ❶ Note: Answers are on page 216.

CASE 39 – QUESTIONS

A 30-year-old man with a history of acute lymphoblastic leukaemia (ALL) treated with marrow transplant and chemotherapy 18 years ago presented to the emergency department with acute-onset chest pain and shortness of breath that started 4 h prior to arrival. He rated the pain as 10/10. His father had a history of coronary artery disease in his late 40s. The patient is currently in remission from ALL and he has no other medical conditions.

On examination, his heart rate is 90 bpm and his respiratory rate is 25 breaths/min. His blood pressure is 130/80 mmHg. He is saturating at 95% on 8 L oxygen. Auscultation reveals normal heart sounds with no murmurs, and good bilateral air entry with no added sounds.

An ECG is performed as part of his work-up.

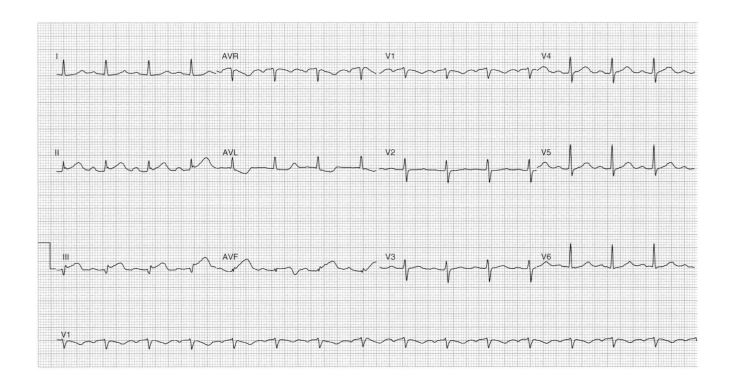

❓ QUESTIONS FOR CANDIDATE

1. **What drugs should be offered for the following 12 months, assuming no contraindications?**
   (a) Aspirin, clopidogrel, spironolactone, statin, beta-blocker, angiontensin-converting enzyme (ACE) inhibitor
   (b) Aspirin, clopidogrel, statin, beta-blocker, ACE inhibitor
   (c) Aspirin, statin, ACE inhibitor
   (d) Aspirin, statin, beta-blocker
   (e) Aspirin, statin, beta-blocker, ACE inhibitor

2. **The following medications are matched to drug classes. Which of the following is/are correct?**
   (a) Abciximab – cyclooxygenase inhibitor
   (b) Bivalirudin – direct thrombin inhibitor
   (c) Clopidogrel – phosphodiesterase inhibitor
   (d) Prasugrel – non-thienopyridine adenosine diphosphate (ADP) platelet receptor inhibitor
   (e) Ticagrelor – thienopyridine ADP platelet receptor inhibitor

3. **Which of the following statement(s) regarding reperfusion strategy after myocardial infarction is/are false?**
   (a) Coronary artery bypass can be considered as a reperfusion strategy when PCI fails
   (b) Patients presenting within 12 h of symptom onset of STEMI should be considered for a reperfusion strategy, unless they have severe comorbidities
   (c) Primary PCI is preferred for reperfusion therapy over fibrinolytic therapy in patients with STEMI if it can be performed within 4 h of first medical contact
   (d) The ideal reperfusion therapy for STEMIs is acute PCI
   (e) Thrombolysis using alteplase may be considered as a reperfusion strategy after myocardial infarction

❶ Note: Answers are on page 218.

CASE 40 – QUESTIONS

An 85-year-old woman with a background history of hypertension, type 2 diabetes mellitus, hypercholesterolaemia, peripheral vascular disease, angina and congestive cardiac failure was admitted to the acute medical unit for treatment of pneumonia. She was treated with intravenous (IV) co-amoxiclav. She developed a sudden-onset 6-h history of sudden central chest pain radiating to the left arm. She also complained of worsening shortness of breath and syncope.

On examination, her heart rate is 54 bpm. She looks pale and clammy. She is tachypnoeic at a respiratory rate of 30 breaths/min and is agitated. Her blood pressure is 120/60 mmHg. She is saturating at 88% on high-flow oxygen. Auscultation reveals systolic murmur, and reduced air entry bibasally with some crackles.

An ECG is performed as part of her work-up.

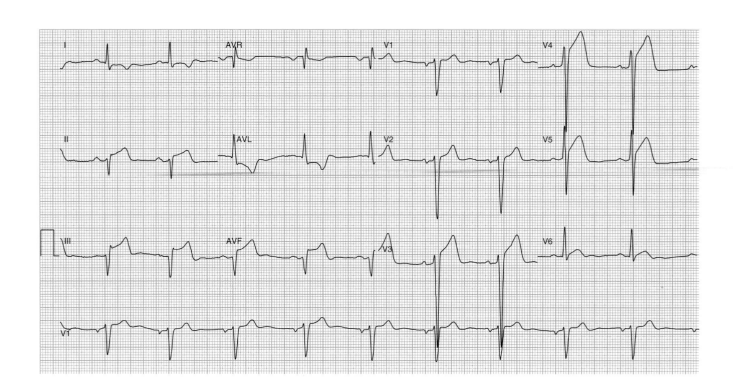

❓ QUESTIONS FOR CANDIDATE

1. **A few days after presenting to the emergency department, the patient developed a drop in blood pressure, raised jugular venous pressure and muffled heart sounds. Which of the following best describes the complication that she has developed?**
   (a) Arrhythmia
   (b) Left-to-right shunting due to ventricular septal defect
   (c) Pericarditis
   (d) Pulmonary oedema due to mitral regurgitation
   (e) Tamponade due to ventricular rupture

2. **Following successful treatment, the patient returns 8 weeks later complaining of a fever and a sharp, well-localised chest pain that is relieved by leaning forwards. What complication has this patient developed?**
   (a) Arrhythmia
   (b) Dressler syndrome
   (c) Heart failure
   (d) New myocardial infarction
   (e) Reflux oesophagitis

3. **Twelve months later, the patient returns for a routine check-up at her general practice. What is the most likely finding on the ECG?**
   (a) Delta waves
   (b) PR prolongation
   (c) Q waves
   (d) ST elevation
   (e) ST depression

❶ Note: Answers are on page 220.

ECG Annotation Key
Blue = P wave
Green = QRS complex
Yellow = T wave
Purple = Interval
Bright red = Abnormal morphology/feature

CASE 1 – ANSWERS

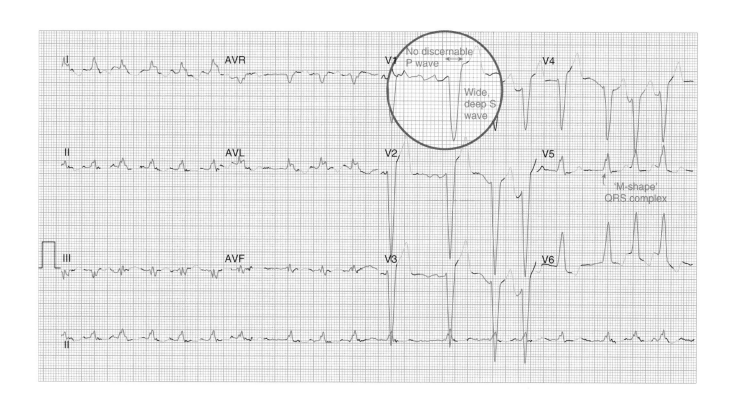

Present Your Findings

BASIC DETAILS

This is an anonymised ECG of unknown date and time.

I would like to ensure that this is calibrated to the usual 25 mm/s paper speed and 1 mV/cm gain.

KEY FEATURES

The major abnormalities in this ECG are an irregularly irregular rhythm, absent P waves and wide QRS complexes.

HEART RATE AND RHYTHM

The heart rate is approximately 144 bpm with an irregularly irregular rhythm.

CARDIAC AXIS

The cardiac axis is normal (between –30° and +90°).

PR AND QT INTERVAL

There is no identifiable PR interval. The QT interval is normal (320 ms).

WAVE MORPHOLOGY

There are no visible P waves. The QRS complexes are wide (120 ms), predominantly negative in V_1 and predominantly positive in V_6. ST segment and T waves are normal in morphology.

In Summary

This ECG is consistent with atrial fibrillation (AF), given the irregular rhythm and absent P waves. There is also evidence of left bundle branch block (LBBB).

This ECG should be compared to a previous ECG if available to confirm that the LBBB is long-standing (as new-onset LBBB may indicate a myocardial infarction) and to look for previous evidence of AF. As this is an irregular wide-complex tachycardia, urgent referral to cardiology may be warranted for further advice.

Further investigations should aim to investigate a precipitant for the AF, particularly if this is new-onset. Urea and electrolytes, bone profile and magnesium should be measured for electrolyte disturbances, thyroid-stimulating hormone should be assessed to exclude hyperthyroidism and sepsis or infection should be considered as an underlying cause.

If this episode of AF is of less than 48 h duration, pharmacological cardioversion could be considered with amiodarone. However, if the patient has been symptomatic for longer than 48 h, rate control with a beta-blocker followed by anticoagulation is necessary.

★ ANSWERS FOR CANDIDATES

1. Which of the following may give rise to atrial fibrillation?

The correct answers are: (a) aortic stenosis; (b) COPD; (c) excessive alcohol consumption; (d) hypothyroidism; and (e) sepsis

A wide range of underlying medical conditions can lead to atrial fibrillation. The mechanisms by which AF arises include acute or chronic changes to atrial chamber dimensions (such as in pulmonary embolism and heart failure, respectively), and stimulation of atrial tissue, as in hyperthyroidism and caffeine consumption.

(a) **Aortic stenosis – correct: valvular heart disease of all types can cause AF. In mitral regurgitation, this is due to enlargement of the left atrium, while in aortic stenosis, the mechanism is unclear.**

(b) **COPD – correct: COPD and other chronic lung diseases contribute to the occurrence of AF, which may be in part due to altered haemodynamics of the heart (such as increased right-sided pressures in severe COPD and cor pulmonale) and may also relate to CO_2 retention.**

(c) **Excessive alcohol consumption – correct: consumption of alcohol is known to increase the risk of AF, with increasing alcohol consumption conferring increased risk. Stimulants such as caffeine also increase the risk of developing AF.**

(d) **Hypothyroidism – correct: while hyperthyroidism is a well-known cause of AF, hypothyroidism may also be a risk factor for AF. The association of subclinical hypothyroidism and AF is multifactorial due to its indirect effect on myocardial function and coexisting risk of coronary artery disease. Patients with AF without a known cause should have their thyroid function investigated, particularly in younger patients.**

(e) **Sepsis – correct: critical illness such as sepsis is a common trigger for AF, particularly in elderly patients. This is often associated with poorer outcomes in very unwell patients.**

¹²₃ Key Points

A wide range of risk factors exist for AF, including:
- Ischaemic heart disease
- Valvular heart disease
- Acute lung disease, e.g. pulmonary embolism
- Chronic lung disease, e.g. COPD
- Diabetes mellitus
- Thyroid disease
- Acute infection
- Acid–base disruption
- Electrolyte disturbances
- Alcohol
- Stimulant drugs (e.g. caffeine, recreational drugs)

2. Which of the following may be a consequence of AF?

The correct answers are: (a) bowel ischaemia; (c) heart failure; and (e) myocardial infarction

The major complications of AF are due to systemic thromboembolism. This is caused by stagnation of blood in the atria, permitting formation of clots which can dislodge and enter the systemic circulation. AF also increases the oxygen consumption of the heart, which may predispose to myocardial ischaemia and failure.

(a) **Bowel ischaemia – correct: AF leads to stagnation of blood in the atria and subsequent thrombosis. Disrupted thrombi enter the peripheral circulation, where they commonly travel to the brain, causing ischaemic stroke. However, thromboembolism may also cause thromboembolism in the mesenteric vasculature, causing ischaemic bowel.**

(b) Deep-vein thrombosis – incorrect: AF causes thrombosis in the arterial circulation only, normally as a result of clot formation in the left atrium, not venous thrombosis.

(c) **Heart failure – correct: the combination of increased oxygen demand, poor filling and rapid heart rate can predispose patients with AF to heart failure. In permanent AF (AF that does not respond to cardioversion), rate control management aims to prevent the development of heart failure.**

(d) Intracranial haemorrhage – incorrect: strokes caused by AF are ischaemic in origin due to thromboembolism. However, intracranial haemorrhage is an important complication of anticoagulation, which forms the mainstay of long-term management for persistent or permanent AF.

(e) **Myocardial infarction – correct: AF increases the myocardial oxygen demand in the heart, which may lead to myocardial ischaemia, particularly in the context of coronary artery disease. A rapid ventricular response (so-called 'fast AF') may reduce the cardiac output (as a result of decreased diastolic filling) and further increase the risk of myocardial infarction. In addition, peripheral emboli can cause coronary ischaemia and infarction.**

Key Points

AF causes the formation of clots in the atria that may enter the arterial circulation, causing thromboembolism, especially stroke. AF also increases myocardial oxygen demand and reduces diastolic filling time, which may contribute to myocardial ischaemia, myocardial infarction or heart failure.

3. Which clinical scoring systems are important decision aids in the management of AF?

The correct answers are (b) CHA_2DS_2-VASc score; and (d) HAS-BLED score.

Scoring systems are used to aid in clinical decision making and have proved highly important in balancing the benefits of anticoagulation in AF against the risk of morbidity and mortality associated with bleeding.

(a) $ABCD_2$ score – incorrect: the $ABCD_2$ score is a clinical score used in patients with a recent transient ischaemic attack to identify the risk of a subsequent stroke.

(b) **CHA_2DS_2-VASc score – correct: this score is used to evaluate the risk of stroke in patients with AF. Usually, a CHA_2DS_2-VASc score of ≥ 2 warrants anticoagulation, such as with warfarin or direct oral anticoagulants.**

(c) GRACE score – incorrect: this score is used to estimate the prognosis of patients with acute coronary syndrome and is not used in AF.

(d) **HAS-BLED score – correct: the HAS-BLED score is used to evaluate the risk of bleeding in patients with AF on anticoagulation. It scores patients based on: *hypertension, abnormal liver function, abnormal renal function, history of stroke, bleeding tendency, labile international normalised ratio, elderly age and drugs/alcohol.***

(e) All of the above – incorrect: $ABCD_2$ and GRACE scores are not normally used in the management of AF.

Key Points

Scoring systems are frequently used to evaluate risk in patients with AF. The CHA_2DS_2-VASc score is used at the point of diagnosis to establish the risk of stroke and make decisions regarding anticoagulation. In contrast, the HAS-BLED score is used to identify patients at risk of major bleeding, with high-risk patients requiring additional risk factor management and close monitoring.

CASE 2 – ANSWERS

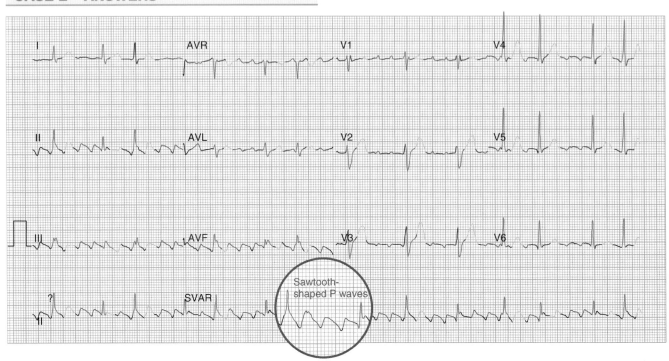

Sawtooth-shaped P waves

Present Your Findings

BASIC DETAILS
This is an anonymised ECG of unknown date and time.
I would like to ensure that this is calibrated to the usual 25 mm/s paper speed and 1 mV/cm gain.

KEY FEATURES
There is a sawtooth baseline pattern, most visible in leads III and V$_1$.

HEART RATE AND RHYTHM
The heart rate is approximately 84 bpm with an irregularly irregular rhythm.

CARDIAC AXIS
The cardiac axis is normal (between –30° and +90°).

PR AND QT INTERVAL
There is no clearly identifiable PR interval. The QT interval is normal (360 ms).

WAVE MORPHOLOGY
There is a sawtooth baseline with evident flutter waves. There is variable conduction of flutter waves into the ventricles, ranging from 2:1 to 3:1. The QRS complexes are narrow. ST segment and T waves are normal in morphology.

In Summary

This ECG is strongly suggestive of atrial flutter with variable 2:1 to 3:1 conduction block. All patients should initially be started on an anticoagulant if there are no contraindications.
Options for the atrial flutter itself include:
1) Rhythm control: To try and restore a normal rhythm with a synchronised DC cardioversion. This should be performed if there are any signs of haemodynamic compromise thought to be secondary to atrial flutter or if the patient is very symptomatic with a clear onset of symptoms <48 hours if the patient is not anticoagulated. Further

considerations to reduce the risk of atrial flutter recurrence is to refer for catheter ablation which is effective in treating this rhythm.
2) Rate control: We would recommend in the majority of cases initially adopting a rate control strategy, whilst further evaluation is being performed, This would be initially with beta-blockers +/- digoxin if this is ineffective.
Bloods tests (including thyroid function tests, urea & electrolytes (U&E), bone profile, magnesium, and full blood count (FBC)) and an echocardiogram (particularly given the findings of a murmur suggestive of mitral regurgitation) should be arranged.

★ ANSWERS FOR CANDIDATES

1. What is the use of adenosine in atrial flutter?
The correct answer is: (c) an adenosine bolus may block AVN conduction to the ventricles, making flutter waves easier to visualise on ECG.

Adenosine blocks conduction of depolarisation impulses through the AVN. This will not terminate atrial flutter, which propagates through the atria alone, but will cause a brief ventricular pause that makes flutter waves much easier to see. Although adenosine in this case is not necessary as the flutter waves are clearly visible on the ECG, in other cases, particularly when 2:1 or 1:1 flutter is present, adenosine can be useful in making the diagnosis.

(a) An adenosine bolus provides a rapid and effective method of terminating the arrhythmia – incorrect: adenosine acts predominantly at the AVN and blocking conduction through the AVN. Atrial flutter is a self-sustaining atrial arrhythmia: blocking the AVN will prevent conduction of flutter waves to the ventricles but will not terminate the arrhythmia.

(b) Adenosine can be used as a long-term method of rate control if DC cardioversion fails to terminate the arrhythmia – incorrect: adenosine cannot be used as long-term management of atrial flutter. Instead, long-term rate control may be used in the form of beta-blockers or calcium channel blockers, usually in conjunction with an antiarrhythmic drug.

(c) **An adenosine bolus may block AVN conduction to the ventricles, making flutter waves easier to visualise on ECG – correct: often flutter waves can be difficult to distinguish on ECG, making a definitive diagnosis difficult. If atrioventricular nodal re-entrant tachycardia (AVNRT) or atrial flutter is suspected, an adenosine bolus may terminate the AVNRT or be diagnostic for atrial flutter by slowing down the overall ventricular rate, and revealing the sawtooth baseline.**

(d) Adenosine may reduce the atrial rate and therefore reduce the ventricular rate – incorrect: adenosine has no effect on the atrial rate in atrial flutter. Some antiarrhythmic drugs may reduce atrial rate, but there is a risk that this will allow the AVN to conduct at a 1:1 rate, paradoxically increasing the ventricular rate.

(e) Adenosine has no use in atrial flutter – incorrect: adenosine is useful as a diagnostic aid in atrial flutter, though it has no use in terminating the arrhythmia.

> **1₂₃ Key Points**
>
> Adenosine may be used to aid diagnosis in atrial flutter: a bolus dose briefly blocks AVN conduction and will reveal flutter waves in atrial flutter. However, it will not terminate atrial flutter.

2. What is the most likely cause of the 2:1 and 3:1 conduction block in this patient?

The correct answer is: (d) physiological effect of delayed conduction in the AVN.

Variable AV conduction in atrial flutter is not a pathological effect but rather a physiological role of the AVN, which acts to prevent rapid atrial rates from being conducted into the ventricles. Indeed, the existence of pathways that bypass the AVN (such as in Wolff–Parkinson–White) bypass this protective mechanism and can be very dangerous.

(a) Myocardial ischaemia due to rapid activation of atria and ventricles – incorrect: while myocardial ischaemia may be present, this is unlikely to significantly impact AVN conduction without evidence on ECG.

(b) Idiopathic fibrosis of the conduction system – incorrect: idiopathic fibrosis of the conduction disease is possible and increases with age. However, there is no evidence in this ECG to suggest that it is present. Evidence of heart block on a baseline ECG without atrial flutter may support this diagnosis.

(c) Excessive vagal tone due to elevated blood pressure – incorrect: vagal tone sufficient to induce conduction block is unlikely in a patient of this age; young patients and very athletic individuals may be more prone to this type of conduction block.

(d) **Physiological effect of delayed conduction in the AVN – correct: under normal physiological circumstances, the AVN slows conduction from atria into ventricles, generating the PR interval. This role has the added advantage of causing physiological conduction block (which may be 2:1, 3:1, etc.) at high atrial rates, preventing excessively rapid rates from being conducted into the ventricles.**

(e) Iatrogenic heart block as a result of ramipril therapy – incorrect: ramipril does not have an effect on the AVN. Other antihypertensive medication, such as calcium channel blockade, however, may contribute to AV block in these circumstances.

> **1₂₃ Key Points**
>
> The AVN causes physiological conduction block at high atrial rates, which prevents rapid atrial rates (e.g. atrial fibrillation, atrial flutter) from being conducted into the ventricles and causing haemodynamic compromise.

3. Which of the following are risk factors for developing atrial flutter?

The correct answers are: (a) hypertension; (b) diabetes mellitus; (c) mitral regurgitation; and (d) male sex.

Atrial flutter shares similar pathophysiology to atrial fibrillation and therefore has a lot of overlap in terms of its risk factors and aetiology.

(a) **Hypertension – correct: hypertension promotes structural changes to the left side of the heart, which may increase the risk of both atrial fibrillation and flutter.**

(b) **Diabetes mellitus – correct: atrial flutter is more common in patients with diabetes than in the general population.**

(c) **Mitral regurgitation – correct: dilatation of the atria due to valvular disease is a frequent cause of atrial flutter.**

(d) **Male sex – correct: men are approximately 2.5 times more likely to suffer from atrial flutter than women.**

(e) Younger age – incorrect: increasing age is one of the most important risk factors for atrial flutter. Flutter is over 100 times more common in patients >80 years old than in those <50 years old.

> **1₂₃ Key Points**
>
> Risk factors for atrial flutter are similar to risk factors for atrial fibrillation and include:
> * Age
> * Male sex
> * Hypertension
> * Diabetes mellitus
> * Valvular disease
> * Acute or chronic lung disease
> * Thyroid disease
> * Stimulant drugs

CASE 3 – ANSWERS

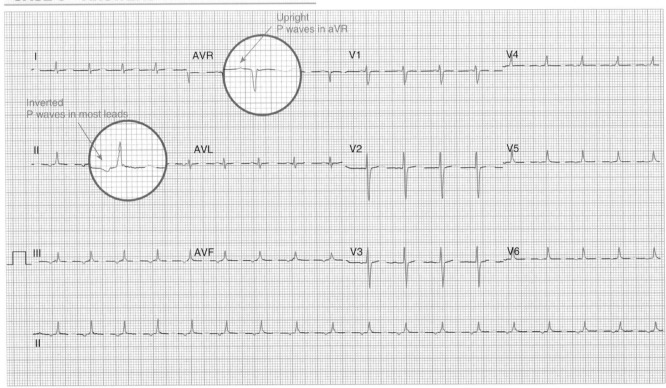

Upright P waves in aVR

Inverted P waves in most leads

Present Your Findings

BASIC DETAILS

This is an anonymised ECG of unknown date and time.

I would like to ensure that this is calibrated to the usual 25 mm/s paper speed and 1 mV/cm gain.

KEY FEATURES

This is a rapid, narrow-complex tachycardia. P waves appear to be inverted in leads II, III, aVF and V_4–V_6 while upright in lead aVR.

HEART RATE AND RHYTHM

The heart rate is approximately 108 bpm with a regular rhythm.

CARDIAC AXIS

The cardiac axis is normal (between −30° and +90°).

PR AND QT INTERVAL

The PR interval is normal (200 ms), and the QT interval is normal (360 ms).

WAVE MORPHOLOGY

The P waves are inverted leads II, III, aVF and V_4–V_6 (i.e. there is an abnormal P wave axis).

The QRS complexes are narrow (<120 ms). ST segment and T waves are normal in morphology.

In Summary

Abnormal P waves in a regular, narrow-complex tachycardia are suggestive of atrial tachycardia, particularly in a patient who has recently undergone catheter ablation, of which atrial tachycardia is a well-recognised complication.

Alongside medical history, baseline blood tests including electrolytes (U&E, calcium, magnesium) and thyroid function should be obtained. If the patient is taking digoxin or theophylline, plasma levels should be assessed to rule out toxicity. First line management is to control the heart rate with beta-blockers or if contraindicated a Calcium channel blocker. Further considerations once rate control and reversible causes excluded would be to consider restoring sinus rhythm with a synchronised DC cardioversion and ensuring the patient is anticoagulated.

⭐ **ANSWERS FOR CANDIDATES**

1. What mechanism gives rise to atrial tachycardia?

The correct answer is: (d) all of the above.

The term 'atrial tachycardia' is a descriptive term ascribed to any atrial abnormality that gives rise to tachycardia. As such, any mechanism of arrhythmogenesis may give rise to atrial tachycardia.

(a) **Increased automaticity – correct: this mechanism is common among patients with catecholamine** excess or excessive alcohol consumption. It tends to resolve when the cause is treated appropriately.

(b) **Re-entry – correct: small re-entry circuits can be generated by scar tissue in patients who have undergone atrial ablation procedures. This mechanism is also a feature in patients with structural changes to the atrium. This is different to the re-entry circuits in the AVN/ septum, as they are occurring in the atria themselves, thus still triggering a P wave.**

(c) **Triggered activity – correct: this mechanism may be associated with cardiomyopathies and digoxin toxicity.**

(d) **All of the above – correct: all three mechanisms may contribute to the occurrence of atrial tachycardia under differing circumstances.**

(e) None of the above – incorrect: all of these mechanisms can cause atrial tachycardia.

 Key Points

Atrial tachycardia can arise due to any of the three major mechanisms of arrhythmogenesis, and the aetiology will have an impact on the management and outcome.

---

2. Aside from atrial tachycardia, what other complications may arise from catheter ablation for AF?

The correct answers are: (b) cardiac tamponade; (c) femoral vein and arterial damage; and (e) stroke.

Cardiac catheter ablation is, relatively speaking, a very safe procedure with a low complication rate. However, as with any medical procedure, complications do occur and can range from mild to life-threatening.

(a) Aortic regurgitation – incorrect: for atrial ablation, access to the right atrium is usually achieved via the femoral vein and inferior vena cava, while the left atrium is accessed by inserting the catheter through the interatrial septum from the right atrium. Since there is no access via the aorta, aortic regurgitation is rare. However, aortic regurgitation can occur in left-ventricle ablations, where the ventricle is accessed via the aorta.

(b) **Cardiac tamponade – correct: perforation of the myocardium and bleeding into the pericardial space are rare but potentially fatal complications of catheter ablation.**

(c) **Femoral vein and arterial damage – correct: Although access for these procedures is via the femoral vein, it is possible to puncture** the artery, resulting in complications such as arterial pseudoaneurysms and arterial-venous fistulae.

(d) Myocardial infarction – incorrect: myocardial infarction can theoretically occur as a result of catheter ablation due to embolic events, but it is extremely unlikely. However, myocardial infarction is a recognised complication of angiography due to the placement of the catheter in the coronary arteries.

(e) **Stroke – correct: both stroke and transient ischaemic attacks are recognised complications of AF ablation, and patients must be appropriately anticoagulated before treatment.**

 Key Points

Catheter ablation for AF is associated with a number of complications that differ from those associated with catheterisation of the coronary arteries.

---

3. Where is the lesion (or lesions) giving rise to the atrial tachycardia most likely to be located?

The correct answer is: (c) left atrium.

The left atrium is the commonest location for an atrial tachycardia following catheter ablation for AF.

(a) Adjacent to the AVN – incorrect: this location is a possible target for ablation of AV nodal re-entrant tachycardia but not for ablation for AF.

(b) Anterior free wall of the right atrium – incorrect: the anterior free wall of the right atrium may be ablated in cases of atypical atrial flutter but is not routinely ablated for AF.

(c) **Left atrium – correct: the left atrium is the most common site for catheter ablation for AF, which normally involves electrically isolating the pulmonary veins as they enter the left atrium.**

(d) Right ventricular outflow tract – incorrect: this would give rise to a ventricular, rather than atrial, tachycardia.

(e) Sinoatrial node – incorrect: a tachycardia arising from the sinoatrial node is by definition a sinus tachycardia.

 Key Points

As with ventricular axis, the axis of P waves in atrial tachycardia can be useful to identify the location of the lesion. This can be useful to identify the cause or inform further management.

CASE 4 – ANSWERS

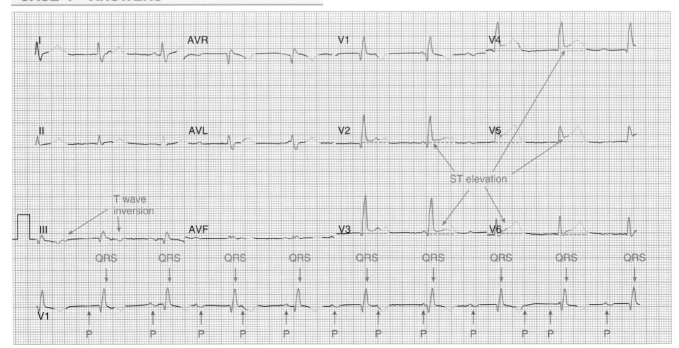

Present Your Findings

BASIC DETAILS

This is an anonymised ECG of unknown date and time.

I would like to ensure that this is calibrated to the usual 25 mm/s paper speed and 1 mV/cm gain.

KEY FEATURES

There is dissociation between P waves and QRS complexes. There is ST elevation in leads V_2–V_6 with no reciprocal ST depression in the inferior leads.

HEART RATE AND RHYTHM

The patient has a ventricular rate of 60 bpm with regular rhythm.

The atrial rate is approximately 78 bpm, so this is not a sinus rhythm.

CARDIAC AXIS

The cardiac axis is normal (between –30° and +90°).

PR AND QT INTERVAL

There is complete dissociation of the P wave and QRS complexes with no regular PR interval.

The QT interval is normal (400 ms).

WAVE MORPHOLOGY

The P waves are of normal morphology, though not related to the QRS.

The QRS complexes are borderline prolonged (120 ms). There is ST segment elevation in leads V_4–V_6.

In Summary

This ECG has evidence of regional ST elevation consistent with an ST elevation myocardial infarction (STEMI) in the anterolateral territory. There is also evidence of atrioventricular dissociation with a ventricular escape rhythm which is suspicious for complete heart block, which may be secondary to the STEMI.

This patient should be treated immediately with aspirin and clopidogrel and referred to the cardiac catheter laboratory without delay for primary percutaneous coronary intervention (PCI). Cardiac troponin should be measured urgently, but this should not delay PCI.

★ ANSWERS FOR CANDIDATES

1. What coronary artery has been occluded in this patient?

The correct answer is: (a) Left Anterior Descending Artery.

ST elevation in the anterior leads is indicative of a blockage to the left anterior descending artery, although localisation of the exact site of the infarct does not always correlate with ECG changes. Complete heart block is usually more common in inferior MI (occurring in around 7% of cases) but can complicate infarction of any part of the heart.

(a) **LAD artery – correct: LAD occlusion causes ST elevation in the anterior leads, namely V_1–V_4.**

(b) LCx artery – incorrect: LCx occlusion, or occlusion of marginal branches associated with LCx, causes ST elevation in the lateral leads (V_4–V_6). There is often ST elevation in the so-called 'high-lateral' leads, leads I and aVL, in large lateral infarcts.

(c) LMS – incorrect: LMS occlusion leads to very widespread ischaemia, which generally presents as ST elevation in most or all of the chest leads.

(d) PDA – incorrect: PDA occlusion leading to a posterior MI can be easy to miss, presenting as reciprocal ST depression in the anterior leads V_1–V_3. Often this ST depression is considerably more marked than in simple myocardial ischaemia and, if the ECG is viewed upside down, closely resembles ST elevation that would be expected in other territories.

(e) RCA – incorrect: RCA occlusion leads to ST elevation in the inferior leads, II, III and aVF.

 Key Points

Generally the location of the infarct can be approximated by the affected leads in STEMI, although this assessment is not always accurate.

---

2. Which complications of MI may have occurred?

The correct answers are: (b) acute mitral regurgitation; and (c) acute VSD.

Complications of MI follow a defined time course, which results from the process of inflammation, healing and remodelling of the injured myocardium. Sudden haemodynamic compromise associated with new heart sounds is usually indicative of a mechanical complication such as VSD formation or papillary muscle rupture.

(a) Acute aortic regurgitation – incorrect: aortic regurgitation does not tend to occur after an acute MI. Patients with aortic regurgitation usually have a diastolic murmur in the tricuspid area.

(b) **Acute mitral regurgitation – correct: this is a possible diagnosis in this patient. Mitral regurgitation due to rupture of left ventricular papillary muscle may occur up to a week after MI and presents with acute left heart failure with a pansystolic murmur. An echocardiogram is appropriate to confirm the diagnosis.**

(c) **Acute VSD – correct: this is a possible diagnosis in this patient. Rupture of the interventricular septum may be asymptomatic if small or may cause pulmonary oedema and heart failure if large. An echocardiogram is appropriate to confirm diagnosis.**

(d) Dressler syndrome – incorrect: Dressler syndrome is characterised by recurrent pericarditis with pleuritic chest pain, occurring weeks to months after MI.

(e) Left ventricular aneurysm – incorrect: ventricular aneurysms tend to occur days to weeks after the acute MI. They may be asymptomatic or present with heart failure. Classically they are associated with prolonged ST segment elevation on ECG.

Key Points

MI is associated with a number of complications, which may be arrhythmic (such as complete heart block), mechanical (such as mitral regurgitation or VSD) or another pathology, such as pericarditis.

---

3. What ECG changes would you expect to see to indicate a full thickness infarction when following up this patient 6 months later?

The correct answer is: (a) pathological Q waves.

As with complications of MI, the ECG changes associated with MI follow a well-defined time course that may support diagnosis. Pathological Q waves are the most enduring changes on ECG, and usually occur when there has been a delay in reperfusing the cardiac muscle and indicates a full thickness infarction. However, with the widespread access to centres offering primary PCI, this finding is now fortunately less common.

(a) **Pathological Q waves – correct: pathological Q waves occur in the context of an old full thickness STEMI and, once present, do not tend to resolve.**

(b) Peaked T waves – incorrect: in MI, peaked T waves are considered a 'hyperacute' ECG change, and usually resolve very quickly, often before the patient presents to the medical team.

(c) ST segment depression – incorrect: ST segment depression is a feature of acute myocardial ischaemia and is unlikely in the context of a routine follow-up.

(d) ST segment elevation – incorrect: ST segment elevation is an acute sign of MI and usually resolves hours to days after the MI.

(e) None of the above – incorrect: pathological Q waves may be expected on this patient's ECG.

Key Points

MI is associated with a number of ECG changes that evolve over the course of the patient's presentation, management and follow-up. Serial ECGs may give an idea of the stage that a patient is in post-MI.

CASE 5 – ANSWERS

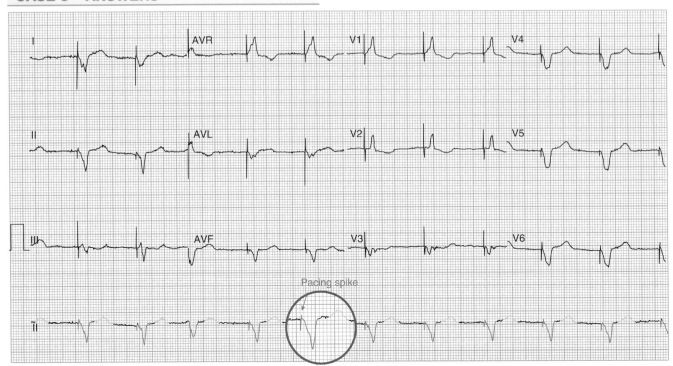

Pacing spike

 Present Your Findings

BASIC DETAILS

This is an anonymised ECG of unknown date and time.
I would like to ensure that this is calibrated to the usual 25 mm/s paper speed and 1 mV/cm gain.

KEY FEATURES

There are pacing spikes before the QRS complex in all leads. The QRS complex is wide and cardiac axis is extreme axis deviation.

HEART RATE AND RHYTHM

The heart rate is 60 bpm and the rhythm is regular. There are no appreciable P waves, excluding sinus rhythm.

CARDIAC AXIS

There is extreme axis deviation (between +180° and −90°).

PR AND QT INTERVAL

There is no appreciable PR interval. The QT interval is normal (440 ms).

WAVE MORPHOLOGY

There are no visible P waves. The QRS complex is preceded by a pacing spike and there is QRS prolongation (>160 ms). There is T-wave inversion in leads V_1–V_3.

 In Summary

This ECG shows prominent pacing spikes before the QRS complex with no appreciable P waves and therefore likely atrial fibrillation and demonstrates marked derangement of the QRS complex morphology and axis. These findings are characteristic of a ventricular paced rhythm. Pacing spikes are not always visible on ECG and such findings in the absence of obvious pathology may point towards a paced rhythm.

The morphology of the QRS would also give information about the site of ventricular pacing; a positive R in V_1 suggests left ventricular pacing (in this case biventricular pacing) and a negative S in V_1 right ventricular only pacing.

A thorough history of symptoms should be taken for this patient to ensure there are no new findings, and this ECG should be compared to a previous paced ECG to ensure there are no new morphological changes that could indicate new pathology.

★ **ANSWERS FOR CANDIDATES**

1. **A different patient with a recent pacemaker insertion complains of pain overlying the site of the pacemaker. On examination, the area is red, swollen and warm to the touch. He is otherwise well with a temperature of 37.2°C. What complication of pacemaker insertion has occurred?**

The correct answer is: (d) pacemaker pocket infection.

As with any invasive medical procedure, pacemaker insertion is associated with complications which may range from very mild to severe and life-threatening. Infection is a worrisome complication that may require replacement of the pacemaker and may lead to device-related endocarditis.

(a) Pericardial effusion – incorrect: while this is a recognised complication of pacemaker insertion, this may be asymptomatic or present with pericarditis. There would not be localised redness or swelling.

(b) Device-related endocarditis – incorrect: the patient is not systemically unwell and does not have a fever, suggesting that this diagnosis is unlikely.

(c) Pacemaker pocket haematoma – incorrect: while the swelling may be consistent with haematoma, the redness and pain suggest alternative pathology.

(d) **Pacemaker pocket infection – correct: the erythema, swelling and pain are suggestive of a local infection.**

(e) Coronary sinus dissection – incorrect: this is a rare but serious complication of pacemaker lead insertion, which is usually detected intra-operatively or may present with pericardial effusion or tamponade.

$1_2{}_3$ Key Points

Pacemaker insertion is associated with a number of complications, as with any surgical procedure. Serious and potentially life-threatening complications include coronary sinus dissection and endocarditis, while complications such as perioperative pain and haematoma are fairly common.

2. **What pacing mode describes a pacemaker that generates impulses in the ventricles and stops when ventricular activity is detected?**

The correct answer is: (e) VVI.

Pacemaker modes are named by the NGB code, which is composed of three to five letters. The first letter describes the chamber that is paced (atrial or ventricular or dual); the second letter describes the chamber that is sensed (atrial or ventricular or dual); and the third letter describes how the pacemaker responds to sensed activity (inhibit or …).

(a) AAI – incorrect: this pacing mode would inhibit atrial activity in response to endogenous atrial activity – this type of pacing is often used in sick sinus syndrome.

(b) AVI – incorrect: this pacing mode would inhibit atrial activity in response to ventricular activity. This pacing mode is not routinely used.

(c) AVT – incorrect: this pacemaker mode triggers the atria in response to ventricular activation. This pacing mode is not routinely used.

(d) DDD – incorrect: this would a pacemaker that senses and responds to leads in both the atria and ventricles. This is the most commonly used pacing mode and can be used in the treatment of atrioventricular conduction block and atrial fibrillation.

(e) **VVI – correct: this type of pacemaker is often used for atrial fibrillation or flutter with concomitant heart block or symptomatic bradycardia.**

$1_2{}_3$ Key Points

Pacemaker codes give useful information about the function of the pacemaker and the possible reasons for its insertion.

3. **In the clinic notes, the specialist nurse has written that this patient had a biventricular pacemaker. What is the most likely indication for this?**

The correct answer is: (c) heart failure.

In most circumstances, pacing in just one ventricle is sufficient to cause contraction of both ventricles. Biventricular pacing is most commonly used when there is dyssynchrony between contraction of the left and right ventricle, which can lead to a reduced cardiac output. This often occurs in the setting of heart failure.

(a) Brugada syndrome – incorrect: Brugada syndrome is not normally paced but may be managed by insertion of an implantable cardiac defibrillator.

(b) Complete heart block – incorrect: single-chamber pacing or dual atrial and ventricular pacing is usually appropriate for complete heart block.

(c) **Heart failure – correct: biventricular pacing in heart failure is known as cardiac resynchronisation therapy and is used in heart failure with bundle branch block to increase cardiac output by synchronising ventricular contraction.**

(d) Mobitz type II heart block – incorrect: this may sometimes be paced, particularly if associated with bradycardia or periods of asystole. However, biventricular pacing is not usually used for this.

(e) Wolff–Parkinson–White syndrome – Wolff–Parkinson–White syndrome is not normally managed by pacing.

$1_2{}_3$ Key Points

Biventricular pacing or cardiac resynchronisation therapy is used in heart failure with bundle branch block (usually LBBB) to increase cardiac output. It works by synchronising ventricular contraction, which improves stroke volume.

CASE 6 – ANSWERS

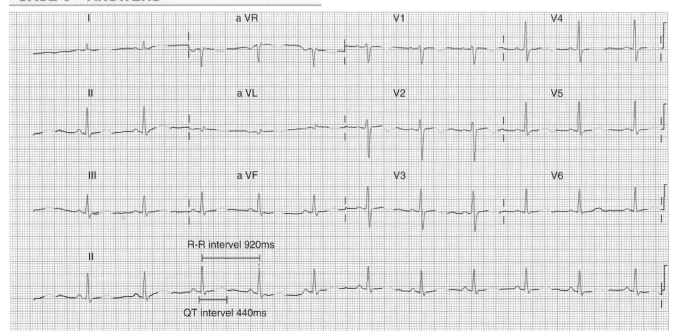

R-R interval 920ms

QT interval 440ms

Present Your Findings

BASIC DETAILS

This is an anonymised ECG of unknown date and time.

I would like to ensure that this is calibrated to the usual 25 mm/s paper speed and 1 mV/cm gain.

KEY FEATURES

The QT interval is prolonged (440 ms) with a corrected QT interval of 452 ms.

HEART RATE AND RHYTHM

The heart rate is 66 bpm with a sinus rhythm.

CARDIAC AXIS

The cardiac axis is normal (between –30° and +90°).

PR AND QRS INTERVAL

The PR interval is normal (120 ms). The QT interval is prolonged (440 ms) with a corrected QT interval of 452 ms.

$$QTc = \frac{440}{\sqrt[3]{0.92}} = 452ms$$

WAVE MORPHOLOGY

The P waves are normal in morphology. The QRS complexes are narrow with no evidence of ventricular hypertrophy. The ST segment and T waves are normal.

In Summary

This ECG demonstrates a long QT interval. In a young man with no other medical history, no current medication and a family history of sudden death, this is suspicious for a congenital long QT syndrome.

A thorough history of acquired causes of prolonged QT interval (particularly an in-depth medication history) should be taken, and any QT-prolonging medications should be stopped if safe to do so. Blood tests, including urea and electrolytes, calcium and magnesium, should be performed to rule out electrolyte abnormalities.

Following an episode of syncope, we would recommend a period of cardiac monitor on a cardiac ward, with initiation of beta-blockers. Information regarding avoiding QT prolonging drugs, avoidance of high intensity sports and swimming should be given.

★ ANSWERS FOR CANDIDATES

1 Which features of a clinical history support a diagnosis of syncope secondary to cardiac arrhythmia?

The correct answer is: (e) loss of consciousness without warning and with rapid recovery.

Syncope can be a challenging symptom to diagnose, given its varied presentation and often limited history. Often a collateral history from a relative or bystander is important to support the diagnosis.

(a) Loss of consciousness after a prolonged period of standing up – incorrect: this is a common cause of syncope and is usually related to orthostatic intolerance or vasovagal syncope.

(b) Loss of consciousness when standing up from a sitting or lying position – incorrect: this is characteristic of orthostatic intolerance, which is particularly prevalent in the elderly, and is due to poor or delayed activation of the baroreceptor reflex in response to standing.

(c) Loss of consciousness associated with jerky movements – incorrect: this presentation is most characteristic of a seizure, although myoclonic jerks may also occur after cardiogenic syncope. As a result, other diagnostic features such as recovery from the event should be considered.

(d) Loss of consciousness associated with a prolonged recovery period – incorrect: a prolonged recovery period after loss of consciousness is more suggestive of a seizure, especially if associated with disorientation or confusion.

(e) Loss of consciousness without warning and with rapid recovery – correct: rapid recovery is frequent with arrhythmic causes of loss of consciousness, normally without confusion. There may be no warning, or symptoms such as palpitations or shortness of breath may precede the episode.

Key Points

There are many different causes of transient loss of consciousness, some of which are benign (such as vasovagal syncope), while others need further investigation (such as seizures or cardiogenic causes).

Based on history alone, cardiac symptoms, rapid onset and rapid recovery are suggestive of cardiac causes while unusual movements and prolonged recovery are suggestive of neurological causes.

2. What ECG features would you expect to see before cardiac syncope in a patient with long QT syndrome?

The correct answer is: **(d) a wide-complex tachycardia with many different-sized QRS complexes;**

Syncope in long QT syndrome is most often caused by torsades de pointes ventricular tachycardia, which arises due to a cardiac impulse during repolarisation of ventricular tissue.

(a) A narrow-complex tachycardia – incorrect: this is suggestive of a supraventricular tachycardia, which is not normally a cause of syncope in long QT syndrome.

(b) A QT interval that progressively lengthens each beat until a beat is dropped – incorrect: this pattern of progressive lengthening followed by a dropped beat is known as the Wenckebach phenomenon and is seen in Mobitz type I heart block or, more rarely, in sinus node dysfunction.

(c) Ventricular fibrillation – incorrect: ventricular fibrillation is not normally associated with transient loss of consciousness and would only be seen in a patient in cardiac arrest.

(d) A wide-complex tachycardia with many different-sized QRS complexes – correct: this is the torsades de pointes ventricular tachycardia associated with prolonged QT interval.

(e) A wide-complex tachycardia with identical QRS complexes – incorrect: this describes a monomorphic ventricular tachycardia and his type of VT is more common in patients with myocardial scar, such as from a previous MI.

Key Points

Long QT syndrome is associated with ventricular arrhythmias, usually polymorphic ventricular tachycardia. It is classically associated with the torsades de pointes pattern of ventricular tachycardia on ECG, which occurs as a result of abnormal repolarisation of cardiac myocytes.

3. Which of the following can prolong the QT interval?

The correct answers are: **(a) erythromycin; (b) hypokalaemia; (c) hypocalcaemia; and (d) quetiapine.**

QT interval can be prolonged by medications or electrolyte abnormalities. This may not be problematic in healthy individuals, but in patients who have pre-existing long QT syndrome or those with multiple QT-prolonging factors, care should be taken to avoid triggering ventricular tachycardia.

(a) Erythromycin – correct: macrolide antibiotics such as erythromycin and clarithromycin may prolong the QT interval and should be avoided in long QT syndrome.

(b) Hypokalaemia – correct: hypokalaemia hyperpolarises the membranes of cardiac cells and therefore causes a longer duration of repolarisation. Drugs that may cause hypokalaemia, such as diuretics, should be used with caution in long QT syndrome.

(c) Hypocalcaemia – correct: low extracellular calcium increases the duration of the plateau phase of the cardiac action potential, increasing the QT interval duration.

(d) Quetiapine – correct: many antipsychotics and antidepressants may cause prolongation of the QT interval. Patients should have a baseline ECG to exclude the presence of long QT syndrome before starting on antipsychotic medication.

(e) Methotrexate – incorrect: methotrexate does not increase the QT interval.

Key Points

A number of medications and electrolyte disturbances can have a detrimental effect on the QT interval. Patients receiving QT-prolonging drugs should have a baseline ECG to exclude the presence of long QT syndrome. Treatment of electrolyte abnormalities may normalise the QT interval and is especially important in patients with congenital long QT syndrome.

CASE 7 – ANSWERS

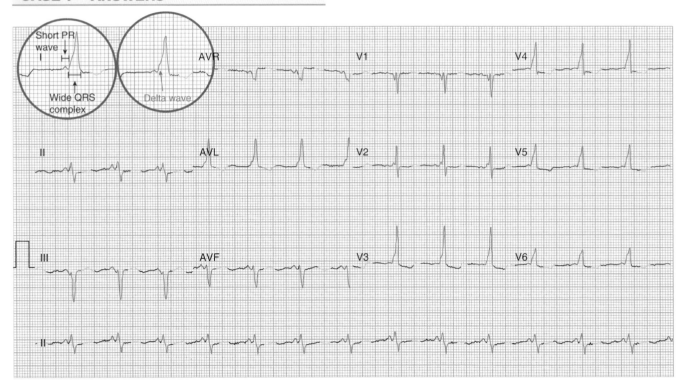

Present Your Findings

BASIC DETAILS

This is an anonymised ECG of unknown date and time.

I would like to ensure that this is calibrated to the usual 25 mm/s paper speed and 1 mV/cm gain.

KEY FEATURES

There is a slurred upstroke of the QRS complex, consistent with a delta wave and a short PR interval.

HEART RATE AND RHYTHM

The heart rate is 80 bpm and is in regular sinus rhythm.

CARDIAC AXIS

There is left-axis deviation (cardiac axis is between –30° and –90°).

PR AND QT INTERVAL

The PR interval is short (80 ms) and the QT interval is normal (400 ms).

WAVE MORPHOLOGY

P wave and T wave are normal in morphology. There is a slurred upstroke to the QRS complex suggestive of a delta wave.

In Summary

This ECG demonstrates a patient in sinus rhythm with a short PR interval and a delta wave. This is strongly suggestive of ventricular pre-excitation.

No acute treatment is necessary but this patient should be referred to a cardiologist (electrophysiologist) for risk stratification and, if necessary, further monitoring.

★ ANSWERS FOR CANDIDATES

1. Which of the following are risk factors for the presence of pre-excitation on an ECG?

The correct answers are: (b) congenital cardiac abnormalities; and (e) family history of WPW syndrome.

WPW syndrome occurs because of an anatomical accessory pathway in the heart. As a result, the risk of developing WPW syndrome is determined by developmental or genetic factors.

(a) Increasing age – incorrect; WPW syndrome can manifest at any age. However, increasing age is associated with an increased risk of sudden death in WPW.

(b) **Congenital cardiac abnormalities – correct: a number of congenital cardiac abnormalities are associated with WPW, of which the most noticeable is Ebstein anomaly (inferior displacement of the tricuspid valve into the right ventricle). The prevalence of WPW among people with Ebstein anomaly is around 20%.**

(c) Smoking – incorrect: smoking does not increase the likelihood of WPW syndrome.

(d) Diabetes mellitus – incorrect: diabetes does not increase the risk of developing WPW syndrome.

(e) **Family history of WPW syndrome – correct: familial WPW syndrome can occur, although rare, and accounts for around 3% of WPW in people with accessory pathways.**

Key Points

Risk factors for WPW syndrome include the development of congenital cardiac abnormalities, in particular Ebstein's anomaly, and the presence of a family history of WPW syndrome.

---

2. What kind of arrhythmia is commonly associated with pre-excitation when the term WPW syndrome is used?

The correct answer is: (b) AVRT.

Atrial extrasystoles may trigger a re-entrant tachycardia due to depolarisation passing through the atrioventricular node (AVN), into the ventricles, and then back into the atria via the accessory pathway.

(a) AVNRT – incorrect: AVNRT is caused by the existence of re-entrant pathway within the AVN and is not related to WPW syndrome.

(b) **AVRT – correct: this normally occurs due to conduction of the wave of depolarisation in the normal direction through the AVN and then back into atria via the accessory pathway (orthodromic conduction). Rarely, depolarisation may pass from atria to ventricles via the accessory pathway and then backwards through the AVN (antidromic conduction).**

(c) Atrial tachycardia – incorrect: atrial tachycardia is not commonly associated with WPW syndrome.

(d) Ventricular tachycardia – incorrect: rapid ventricular rates in WPW syndrome are more frequently caused by AVRT arrhythmias or conduction of atrial fibrillation via the accessory pathway.

(e) Torsades de pointes ventricular tachycardia – incorrect: torsades de pointes is characteristically associated with prolongation of the QT interval, and is not normally associated with WPW syndrome.

Key Points

In WPW syndrome, atrial extrasystoles may trigger an AVRT that may be conducted normally through the AVN or backwards through the AVN (orthodromic or antidromic AVRT, respectively). This tachycardia may be terminated by vagal manoeuvres, by rate-controlling drugs such as beta-blockers or by a bolus of adenosine.

---

3. Which of the following are thought to be the cause of sudden death in Wolff-Parkinson-White syndrome?

The correct answer is: (a) atrial fibrillation.

Sudden cardiac death in WPW syndrome is most commonly caused by rapid conduction of very rapid atrial rates into the ventricles via the accessory pathway, such as atrial flutter or fibrillation.

(a) **Atrial fibrillation – correct: normally the AVN prevents atrial fibrillation from being conducted into the ventricles by only allowing a small number of atrial impulses to pass through into the ventricles. However, the accessory pathway may lack this protection and permit very rapid ventricular rates that rapidly degenerate into ventricular fibrillation.**

(b) Acute heart failure – incorrect: WPW syndrome does not tend to cause acute heart failure.

(c) Stroke – incorrect: stroke may occur secondary to atrial fibrillation in WPW syndrome, but the primary concern with atrial fibrillation and WPW syndrome is rapid ventricular conduction.

(d) Complete heart block – incorrect: it is rare for complete heart block and WPW syndrome to occur together, and this does not tend to cause sudden death.

(e) Myocardial infarction secondary to AVRT – incorrect: AVRT episodes can cause ischaemia but tend to be relatively well tolerated and rarely lead to myocardial infarction of sufficient severity to cause sudden death.

Key Points

The accessory pathway in WPW can allow rapid conduction of atrial impulses, which can then degenerate into ventricular fibrillation.

CASE 8 – ANSWERS

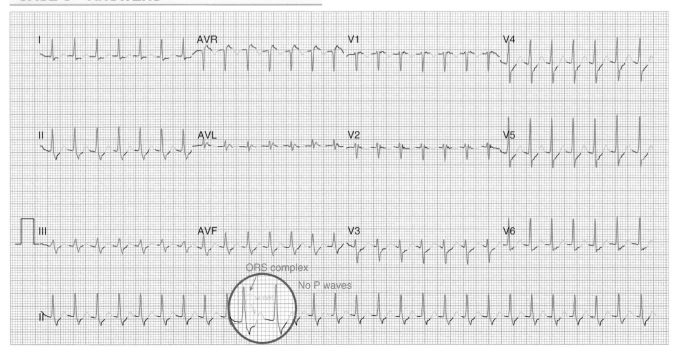

QRS complex

No P waves

 Present Your Findings

BASIC DETAILS
This is an anonymised ECG of unknown date and time.
I would like to ensure that this is calibrated to the usual 25 mm/s paper speed and 1 mV/cm gain.

KEY FEATURES
There is a narrow-complex tachycardia that is not preceded by P waves.

HEART RATE AND RHYTHM
The patient is tachycardic with a heart rate of 168 bpm.

CARDIAC AXIS
The cardiac axis is normal (between –30° and +90°).

PR AND QT INTERVAL
There is no visible PR interval. QT interval is normal for rate (240 ms).

WAVE MORPHOLOGY
There are some P waves visible after the QRS complex buried in the ST segment. The QRS complex is narrow. T waves are normal.

 In Summary

This ECG demonstrates a rapid narrow-complex tachycardia without preceding P waves (although with some P waves visible after the QRS complex), suggestive of an atrioventricular nodal re-entrant tachycardia (AVNRT) or an atrioventricular re-entrant tachycardia (AVRT).

Investigations should include urea and electrolytes, bone profile (checking calcium level), magnesium level and thyroid function tests.

As the patient is stable, an intravenous (IV) adenosine bolus is appropriate to attempt to terminate the arrhythmia. This patient can be discharged once the acute episode is terminated and should be followed up with a referral to cardiology for definitive management.

★ **ANSWERS FOR CANDIDATES**

1. What interventions could be attempted to terminate the arrhythmia before giving IV adenosine in this patient?
The correct answers are: (a) carotid sinus massage; and (e) Valsalva manoeuvre.

Interventions that slow conduction of depolarisation through the atrioventricular node (AVN) are appropriate to attempt to terminate the arrhythmia. Vagal manoeuvres can be attempted first to avoid the need for pharmacological intervention.

(a) **Carotid sinus massage – correct: massaging the neck at the level of the carotid bifurcation (approximately the level of the superior border of the thyroid cartilage) for 5 s activates carotid baroreceptors and causes reflex vagal activation, slowing heart rate and conduction through the AVN. This may terminate an AVNRT or AVRT. This should be avoided if there is a history of carotid disease.**

(b) Head-up tilt test – incorrect: the head-up tilt test is a test of orthostatic tolerance and works by progressively increasing sympathetic outflow by activating the sympathetic arm of the baroreceptor reflex. As such, it will not help to terminate an AVNRT or AVRT.

(c) IV metoprolol infusion – incorrect: IV beta-blockers or calcium channel blockers may be used in the management of AVNRT that is refractory to adenosine, but they are not first line.

(d) Synchronised DC cardioversion – incorrect: in a stable patient, cardioversion is not necessary, and manoeuvres or adenosine should be first line. If the patient shows signs of haemodynamic instability, such as a severely low blood pressure, cardioversion is appropriate.

(e) Valsalva manoeuvre – correct: forced expiration against a closed glottis transiently raises intrathoracic pressure and causes reflex vagal activation. There is also brief vagal activation after releasing the pressure by breathing out. Both of these events may terminate an AVNRT or AVRT.

 Key Points

Vagal manoeuvres are suitable to attempt to terminate AVNRT or AVRT arrhythmias before pharmacological interventions are attempted in stable patients. If the patient is haemodynamically unstable, DC cardioversion should be a priority.

2. What symptoms may be experienced by a patient receiving an adenosine bolus?

The correct answers are: (a) chest tightness; (b) flushing; and (d) sense of impending doom.

Adenosine causes a brief period of sinus arrest, which may manifest with transient symptoms. However, due to its very short duration of effect, it does not tend to cause longer-term effects.

(a) **Chest tightness – correct: chest tightness, discomfort or pain is common following adenosine administration.**

(b) **Flushing – correct: the vasodilatory properties of adenosine can commonly lead to flushing and occasionally headaches.**

(c) Hypertension – incorrect: in addition to its cardiac effects, adenosine also has vasodilatory effects, which are most marked in the coronary circulation. It can cause hypotension on bolus infusion but does not normally cause hypertension.

(d) **Sense of impending doom – correct: classically described as a 'sense of impending doom', this feeling tends to occur as a result of the sinus arrest caused by adenosine.**

(e) Stroke – incorrect: adenosine use is not linked with strokes.

 Key Points

Adenosine causes a range of cardiac and non-cardiac adverse effects, but these are almost always transient.

3. What is a possible cause of the negative deflection after the QRS complex in the inferior leads?

The correct answer is: (e) Retrograde 'p' wave.

In AVNRT arrhythmias, depolarisation cycles around the AVN and depolarises the ventricles anterogradely and the atria retrogradely. This causes a normal QRS and a negative P wave which is usually either concealed within the QRS complex or appears as a negative deflection just after the QRS or within the T wave.

(a) Delayed depolarisation of the interventricular septum – incorrect: in the absence of conduction system pathology, depolarisation of the septum proceeds as normal in AVNRT.

(b) Delayed repolarisation of the atria – incorrect: repolarisation of the atria is not normally visible on the ECG and does not tend to be delayed by AVNRT.

(c) Myocardial ischaemia due to the rapid heart rate – incorrect: myocardial ischaemia may occur because of prolonged tachycardia, but this will cause depression of the entire ST segment. It does not tend to cause isolated negative deflections after the QRS complex. Furthermore, this tends to be a global effect and is seen across most leads rather than in one territorial region.

(d) Non-functional cardiac tissue creating an electrical window into the heart – incorrect: this type of pathology is a feature of ST elevation myocardial infarction, leading to the formation of pathological Q waves on ECG. It is not a feature of AVNRT.

(e) **Retrograde 'p' wave – correct: retrograde conduction through the atria occurs due to cyclic activation of the AVN. This causes an inverted P wave that may either be concealed in the QRS complex or, as in this case, manifest as a negative deflection after the QRS complex.**

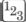 **Key Points**

AVNRT leads to anterograde conduction through the His–Purkinje system and ventricles and retrograde conduction through the atria.

CASE 9 – ANSWERS

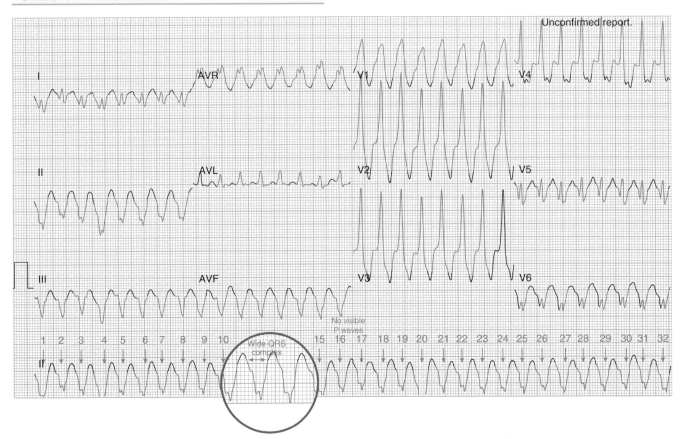

Unconfirmed report.

No visible P waves

Wide QRS complex

Present Your Findings

BASIC DETAILS

This is an anonymised ECG of unknown date and time.

I would like to ensure that this is calibrated to the usual 25 mm/s paper speed and 1 mV/cm gain.

KEY FEATURES

There is a regular, rapid wide-complex tachycardia.

HEART RATE AND RHYTHM

The patient is tachycardic with a heart rate of 192 bpm.

CARDIAC AXIS

There is left-axis deviation (cardiac axis is between –30° and –90°).

PR AND QT INTERVAL

There is no visible PR interval. QT interval is normal for rate (approximately 240 ms).

WAVE MORPHOLOGY

There is no visible P wave. QRS complex is wide (approximately 160 ms) and the complexes are monomorphic. T-wave morphology is difficult to determine.

In Summary

This ECG demonstrates a very rapid monomorphic ventricular tachycardia. In view of the patient's medical history, this is likely to be due to his previous myocardial infarction.

This presentation is a medical emergency and a periarrest call or equivalent is likely to be appropriate. Resuscitation equipment should be readily available as this patient is at risk of deteriorating into cardiac arrest. The patient is likely to require DC cardioversion with sedation, and urgent senior input is necessary.

Once the patient is stabilised, urgent investigations should be sought, including blood tests for electrolytes (including potassium, calcium and magnesium) and thyroid function tests. A repeat ECG should be performed when the patient is back in sinus rhythm, and an urgent echocardiogram performed to look for regional wall motion abnormalities.

★ ANSWERS FOR CANDIDATES

1. What features on examination would be indicative of cardiac arrest in this patient?

The correct answers are: (a) absent carotid pulse; and (c) apnoea.

In any clinical setting, the absence of carotid pulse and apnoea is diagnostic for cardiac arrest and warrants immediate life support. Ventricular tachycardia with a palpable pulse and retained breathing is a medical emergency but is not considered cardiac arrest.

(a) **Absent carotid pulse** – correct: ventricular tachycardia associated with absent carotid pulse (pulseless ventricular tachycardia) is one of the four cardiac rhythms associated with cardiac arrest.

(b) Absent radial pulse – incorrect: radial pulse can be unreliable and can be lost in patients with a blood pressure of less than 70–80 mmHg. In addition, cardiac patients may have coexisting vascular disease causing poor radial flow or may have had their radial artery removed for use as a coronary bypass graft.

(c) **Apnoea – correct: absence of breath sounds and chest movement is strongly indicative of cardiac arrest. Occasionally, patients in cardiac arrest may appear to take shallow, gasping breaths. This is known as agonal breathing and is a feature of cardiac arrest. If in doubt, treat as cardiac arrest.**

(d) Blood pressure <90 mmHg systolic or <60 mmHg diastolic – incorrect: this is suggestive of shock but does not itself indicate cardiac arrest.

(e) Ventricular tachycardia on ECG lasting longer than 30 s – incorrect: this is known as sustained ventricular tachycardia and is more likely to be associated with symptoms than short episodes of ventricular tachycardia. However, episodes longer than 30 s are not necessarily associated with cardiac arrest.

1₂₃ Key Points

An absence of breathing activity and/or a palpable carotid pulse is indicative of cardiac arrest. Theses should be managed in accordance with life support guidelines.

2. Which rhythms can be treated by electrical defibrillation in cardiac arrest?

The correct answers are: (c) ventricular fibrillation; and (d) ventricular tachycardia.

Defibrillation works by triggering depolarisation of the entire myocardium, terminating any cardiac rhythm and allowing the underlying spontaneous rhythm of the heart to take over.

(a) Asystole – incorrect: in asystole, there is an absence of spontaneous depolarisation of the heart; defibrillation therefore has no effect. Instead, asystolic cardiac arrest is treated with intravenous adrenaline between cycles of cardiopulmonary resuscitation.

(b) Pulseless electrical activity – incorrect: pulseless electrical activity is cardiac arrest with an underlying heart rhythm that would normally be associated with a pulse. Defibrillation only corrects abnormal heart rhythms but will not correct other abnormalities, such as loss of contractile function that may cause pulseless electrical activity.

(c) **Ventricular fibrillation – correct: as with ventricular tachycardia, ventricular fibrillation may respond to electrical cardioversion with progressively greater-energy shocks.**

(d) **Ventricular tachycardia – correct: pulseless ventricular tachycardia can potentially be cardioverted back into sinus rhythm by electrical defibrillation. The first shock is usually 150 J or greater, with higher energy for subsequent shocks.**

(e) All of the above – incorrect: asystole and pulseless electrical activity cannot be treated with defibrillation and are instead treated with cardiopulmonary resuscitation, intravenous adrenaline and treatment of reversible causes of cardiac arrest if present.

1₂₃ Key Points

Rhythms with underlying spontaneous cardiac activity and functional excitation–contraction coupling can be treated by electrical defibrillation. These rhythms (ventricular fibrillation and pulseless ventricular tachycardia) account for around 20% of all cardiac arrests.

3. What is the long-term management of patients at high risk of dangerous ventricular tachycardias?

The correct answer is: (c) ICD insertion; (d) Antiarrhythmic drug therapy – beta-blocker and/or amiodarone

Ventricular tachycardia can be managed long-term with anti-arrhythmic medication including beta-blocker therapy, amiodarone and catheter ablation or by ICD insertion. ICD insertion is indicated in patients at high risk of life-threatening VT.

(a) Discharge and monitor closely – incorrect: patients with ventricular tachycardia are at risk of sudden cardiac arrest and death. Treatment to reduce the risk of life-threatening ventricular tachycardias is usually necessary.

(b) Heart transplantation – incorrect: the main indication for heart transplantation is heart failure. While frequent ventricular arrhythmias can sometimes be an indication for transplantation, this is a rare occurrence.

(c) **ICD insertion – correct: ICDs are highly effective at terminating ventricular arrhythmias and should be considered first line in high-risk patients. However, they are not usually implanted in patients with a life expectancy of less than 1 year or in patients with continuous ventricular arrhythmias (who may anticipate numerous shocks from the ICD).**

(d) **Antiarrhythmic drug therapy – beta-blocker and/or amiodarone – incorrect: it is important to establish these patients on antiarrhythmic therapy. Although ICDs are effective in treating VT, they do not stop VT from being initiated which, if recurrent, could result in shocks from the ICD.**

(e) Ventricular pacemaker insertion – incorrect: pacemakers are predominantly used for treatment of bradycardias and are not used for ventricular tachycardia. However, some ICDs use a method called 'antitachycardia pacing' to terminate ventricular arrhythmias by briefly pacing the heart at a faster rate than the tachycardia.

1₂₃ Key Points

Patients at high risk of malignant ventricular tachycardias (recurrent sustained ventricular tachycardia) should be considered for ICD implantation, which is highly effective at preventing sudden cardiac death.

CASE 10 – ANSWERS

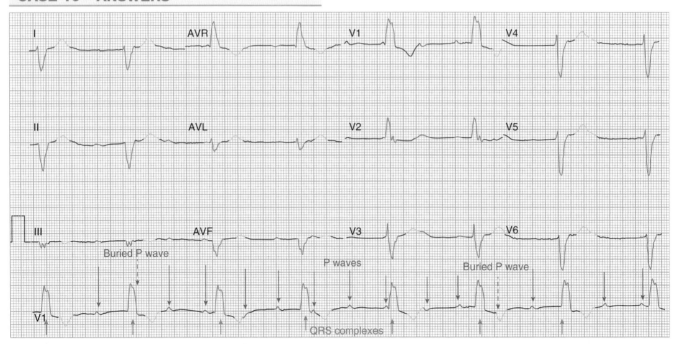

Present Your Findings

BASIC DETAILS
This is an anonymised ECG of unknown date and time.
  I would like to ensure that this is calibrated to the usual 25 mm/s paper speed and 1 mV/cm gain.

KEY FEATURES
There is complete dissociation of atrial and ventricular activity with an atrial rate of 100 bpm and a ventricular rate of 48 bpm.

HEART RATE AND RHYTHM
The patient is bradycardic with a heart rate of 48 bpm. There is dissociation of atrial and ventricular activity with an atrial rate of approximately 100 bpm.

CARDIAC AXIS
There is extreme axis deviation (between +180° and –90°).

PR AND QT INTERVAL
There is complete dissociation of the P waves and QRS complexes. The QT interval is 480 ms.

WAVE MORPHOLOGY
P waves are normal in morphology. QRS complex is wide (approximately 140 ms). There is T-wave inversion in leads III and V$_1$.

In Summary

The atrioventricular dissociation and bradycardia in this ECG are supportive of complete heart block. The wide QRS complexes and extreme axis deviation are suggestive of a ventricular escape rhythm.
  The patient should be treated as a medical emergency with an ABCDE approach. Early investigations should include full blood count, electrolytes (including calcium, magnesium and urea and electrolytes). Medications that may be causing or contributing to the heart block should be assessed and stopped if appropriate.
  This patient requires urgent cardiology review and they may require transcutaneous or transvenous pacing.

★ ANSWERS FOR CANDIDATES

1. What are the likely causes of the acute complete heart block in this patient?
The correct answer is: (b) Idiopathic fibrosis of the conduction system; and (e) medication-related heart block.

There are many potential causes of complete heart block, including drug toxicity, ischaemia and conduction system disease. Identification of reversible causes such as drug toxicity should be an important part of the history and investigation of patients with heart block.

(a) Acute kidney injury – incorrect: acute kidney injury may contribute to the occurrence of heart block, particularly in patients taking antiarrhythmic medication, but it is not a direct cause of heart block.

(b) **Idiopathic fibrosis of the conduction system – correct: fibrosis of the conduction system is a variation of normal ageing. It is a contributing feature and commonest cause of heart block in this age group.**

(c) Infiltrative heart disease such as sarcoidosis – incorrect: rarely, infiltrative diseases such as amyloidosis and sarcoidosis may cause damage or destruction of the conduction system, causing complete heart block. However, there are no signs or symptoms in this case to support this diagnosis.

(d) Ischaemic heart disease – incorrect: ischaemia is an important cause of heart block, which may occur as an acute complication of myocardial infarction, particularly if the right coronary artery is occluded. However, the lack of chest pain and acute onset of symptoms do not support ischaemic heart block in this patient.

(e) **Medication-related heart block – correct: this is an important cause of heart block and is a result of atrioventricular node (AVN)-blocking drugs, including beta-blockers, calcium channel blockers and digoxin. It is more likely to occur in the setting of renal failure (due to reduced clearance of drugs) and is especially likely when AVN-blocking drugs are combined, as in this patient. Although this may have precipitated heart block in this patient, he will have significant underlying conduction disease and therefore should be considered for a permanent pacemaker.**

123 Key Points

Toxicity from AVN-blocking medications, particularly in the context of renal disease, is an important cause and precipitant of complete heart block and should be considered in patients presenting with new-onset bradycardia. Withdrawal of offending medications is an important feature of the management of heart block initially.

2. **Which of the following medications may give rise to heart block?**
The correct answers are: (a) amiodarone; (b) digoxin; (c) metoprolol; and (e) verapamil.

Vaughan–Williams class II (beta-blockers) or Vaughan–Williams class IV (calcium channel blockers) drugs slow conduction through the AVN and therefore may predispose to heart block. Amiodarone and digoxin may also lead to the development of heart block.

(a) **Amiodarone – correct: amiodarone has a wide range of effects on the cardiac action potential and has similar effects to both beta-blockers and calcium channel blockers on the sinoatrial node (SAN) and AVN. As a result, amiodarone may cause or predispose to heart block.**

(b) **Digoxin – correct: cardiac glycosides, such as digoxin, are positive inotropes by inhibiting Na^+/K^+-ATPase activity but also have a poorly understood effect on SAN and AVN function by increasing parasympathetic stimulation of the heart. This leads to decreased conduction through the AVN and may contribute to heart block.**

(c) **Metoprolol – correct: β_1-adrenergic receptors in the heart lead to increased conduction velocity, particularly at the AVN. Blockade of this receptor with beta-blockers will therefore slow conduction rate through the AVN and can predispose to heart block. Glucagon can be used as an antidote for beta-blocker toxicity.**

(d) Spironolactone – incorrect: spironolactone is an aldosterone antagonist used in heart failure. Its primary effect is potassium-sparing diuresis by preventing potassium excretion in the distal convoluting tubule of the kidney. While spironolactone does have cardiac effects, these predominantly relate to cardiac remodelling and do not affect AVN conduction.

(e) **Verapamil – correct: non-dihydropyridine calcium channel blockers (verapamil and diltiazem) delay conduction through the AVN by reducing calcium channel currents. This can lead to heart block at high doses or in patients with pre-existing conduction system disease. Calcium can be used as an antidote for calcium channel blocker toxicity.**

123 Key Points

Drugs that delay conduction of depolarisation impulses through the AVN can lead to the occurrence of heart block. Combinations of these drugs, which are frequently used in heart disease, carry an increased risk of heart block.

3. **Which type(s) of heart block is/are associated with high risk of P wave asystole?**

The correct answers are: (c) second-degree heart block (Mobitz type II); and (d) third-degree heart block (complete heart block).

High-grade heart block is associated with a risk of progressively declining ventricular rate with associated worsening of symptoms and an increased risk of P wave asystole. These patients should be managed even if asymptomatic.

(a) First-degree heart block – incorrect: first-degree heart block is rarely associated with progression to more severe heart block in the acute setting and does not predispose to asystole.

(b) Second-degree heart block (Mobitz type I) – incorrect: Mobitz type I heart block (Wenckebach phenomenon), where there is progressive prolongation of the PR interval until a beat is dropped, does not frequently cause symptoms, and is usually managed satisfactorily by removal of AVN-blocking medications. It does not predispose to asystole.

(c) **Second-degree heart block (Mobitz type II) – correct: Mobitz type II heart block is** characterised by a regular PR interval but intermittent failure of conduction from atria to ventricles. It is at high risk of progression to complete heart block and asystole.

(d) **Third-degree heart block (complete heart block) – correct: complete heart block is associated with a high risk of asystole, especially in patients with a wide QRS complex. It indicates extensive damage to the conduction system.**

(e) None of the above – incorrect: sudden death is an infrequent but important presentation associated with second-degree (Mobitz II) or complete heart block.

¹²₃ Key Points

First-degree or second-degree Mobitz type I heart block is relatively benign and can be treated on a symptomatic basis. However, higher-grade heart block carries a risk of progression to complete heart block and P wave asystolic cardiac arrest. Therefore, they should be treated, usually with pacemaker insertion, to mitigate this risk.

CASE 11 – ANSWERS

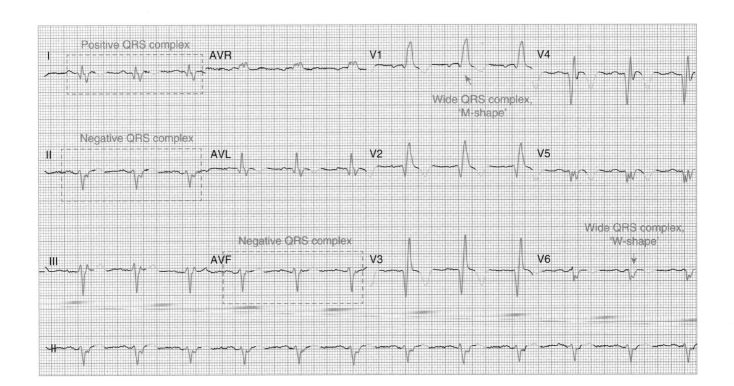

Present Your Findings

BASIC DETAILS
This is an anonymised ECG of unknown date and time.
I would like to ensure that this is calibrated to the usual 25 mm/s paper speed and 1 mV/cm gain.

KEY FEATURES
There is left-axis deviation with concomitant right bundle branch block.

HEART RATE AND RHYTHM
The patient is in sinus rhythm with a heart rate of 72 bpm.

CARDIAC AXIS
There is left-axis deviation (cardiac axis is between –30° and –90°).

PR AND QT INTERVAL
The PR interval is approaching the upper limit of normal duration (200 ms). The QT interval is 400 ms.

WAVE MORPHOLOGY
P wave is normal in morphology. The QRS complexes are wide (approximately 160 ms) with an RSR' pattern in V_1 and a prominent S wave in leads I, V_5 and V_6. T waves are inverted in leads I and V_1–V_6.

In Summary
This ECG is suggestive of right bundle branch block with left-axis deviation. This is consistent with bifascicular block. This pattern suggests right bundle branch block with left anterior fascicular block, which is the most common bifascicular block pattern.

No specific acute treatment is necessary for this patient, although comparison with a previous ECG is appropriate to assess if the block is of new onset. If symptomatic (e.g. syncope), referral to a cardiologist for consideration of further management may be appropriate.

★ ANSWERS FOR CANDIDATES

1. Which of the following aetiologies may give rise to bundle branch block?
The correct answers are: (c) hypertension; (d) idiopathic fibrosis of the conduction system; and (e) myocardial infarction.

Bundle branch block arises due to the same mechanism that causes heart block: functional or structural damage to the cardiac conduction system. As a result, the aetiologies for bundle branch block are similar to those of heart block.

(a) Atrial fibrillation – incorrect: atrial fibrillation is not considered a cause of bundle branch block. However, bundle branch block and atrial fibrillation may coexist, especially in heart failure, which tends to lead to a poorer prognosis than either condition alone.

(b) Complete heart block – incorrect: complete heart block does not cause bundle branch block.

Complete heart block may, however, be a consequence of some forms of bundle branch block, such as bifascicular block.

(c) **Hypertension – correct: hypertension is a frequent cause of right, left and bifascicular bundle branch block. This occurs to hypertrophic and fibrotic changes in the heart's structure and function.**

(d) **Idiopathic fibrosis of the conduction system – correct: just as in heart block, idiopathic fibrosis of the conduction system at the level of the bundle branches can give rise to bundle branch block.**

(e) **Myocardial infarction – correct: damage to the bundle branches of the conduction system is a common occurrence after myocardial infarction, affecting over 10% of patients with acute myocardial infarction.**

Key Points
Bundle branch block and heart block share a common pathological mechanism and, therefore, common underlying aetiologies. These include:
- Hypertension
- Ischaemic heart disease
- Idiopathic fibrosis
- Myocarditis and cardiomyopathies
- Hyperkalaemia

2. What pathological mechanism(s) may give rise to bifascicular block?
The correct answers are: (d) impaired conduction in the right bundle branch and the left anterior fascicle; and (e) impaired conduction in the right bundle branch and the left posterior fascicle.

Bifascicular block occurs as a result of damage to the cardiac conduction system resulting in impaired conduction through the right bundle branch and one of the two fascicles of the left bundle branch.

(a) Impaired conduction in the left and right bundle branches – incorrect: impaired conduction in the right bundle branch and both fascicles of the left bundle branch will lead to complete heart block, as the depolarisation impulse cannot be conducted into the ventricles.

(b) Impaired conduction in the left bundle branch and the right anterior fascicle – incorrect: the left bundle branch divides into left anterior and left posterior fascicles, while the right fascicle does not divide. As such the 'right anterior fascicle' does not exist.

(c) Impaired conduction in the left bundle branch and the right posterior fascicle – incorrect: as in (b), the right fascicle is a single entity and the 'right posterior fascicle' does not exist.

(d) **Impaired conduction in the right bundle branch and the left anterior fascicle – correct:**

this pattern is a common cause of bifascicular block, and causes a right bundle branch morphology on ECG with left-axis deviation.

(e) Impaired conduction in the right bundle branch and the left posterior fascicle – correct: this is a rarer cause of bifascicular block, which leads to right bundle branch morphology with right-axis deviation.

¹₂₃ Key Points

Bifascicular block is caused by right bundle branch block and one of left anterior fascicular block or left posterior fascicular block, which manifest on ECG as right bundle branch block with left-axis deviation or right-axis deviation, respectively.

3. **The patient presents to the emergency department 6 months later with shortness of breath, lightheadedness and chest pain. On examination, her heart rate is 32 bpm and blood pressure is 94/52 mmHg. What complication of bifascicular block is likely to have occurred?**

The correct answer is: (a) complete heart block.

Bifascicular block may be asymptomatic, present with syncope or, in exceptional circumstances, may lead to sudden cardiac death. The development of additional symptoms, such as bradycardia and frequent light-headedness or recurrent syncope, generally represents a progression to heart block.

(a) **Complete heart block – correct: blocked conduction in the right bundle branch and one of the two fascicles of the left bundle branch leaves only one functional route to conduct** depolarisation from the atria to ventricles. If this route is compromised due to drugs that slow cardiac conduction, ischaemia or fibrosis, this will lead to complete heart block.

(b) Heart failure – incorrect: acute heart failure is not a common complication of bifascicular block and usually presents with profound dyspnoea, tachycardia and peripheral oedema.

(c) Pulmonary embolism – incorrect: pulmonary embolism is not normally a feature of bifascicular block and presents with tachycardia as well as dyspnoea.

(d) Sick sinus syndrome – incorrect: sick sinus syndrome may occur in conjunction with bundle branch block as a result of widespread fibrosis of the conduction system. However, it is not a complication of bifascicular block.

(e) Sinus bradycardia – incorrect: sinus bradycardia is not a feature or complication of heart block, although it may coexist if there is widespread fibrosis of the whole cardiac conduction syndrome. This is unlikely to be the case in this patient.

¹₂₃ Key Points

Bifascicular block predisposes to the development of complete heart block. Under some circumstances, such as persistent syncope, it may be appropriate to treat bifascicular block with permanent pacemaker insertion in anticipation of complete heart block.

CASE 12 – ANSWERS

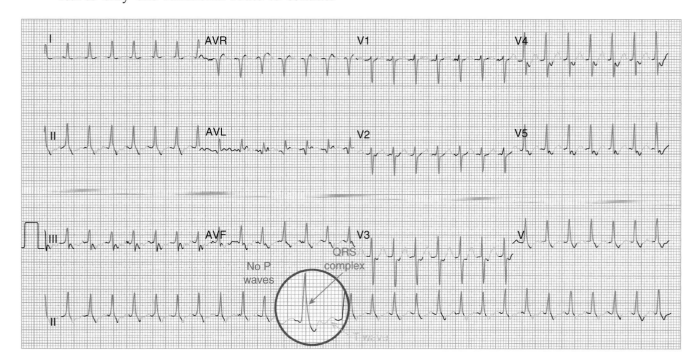

Present Your Findings

BASIC DETAILS
This is an anonymised ECG of unknown date and time.
I would like to ensure that this is calibrated to the usual 25 mm/s paper speed and 1 mV/cm gain.

KEY FEATURES
There is a rapid narrow-complex tachycardia without appreciable P waves.

HEART RATE AND RHYTHM
The heart rate is approximately 174 bpm and is regular.

CARDIAC AXIS
The cardiac axis is normal (between −30° and +90°).

PR AND QT INTERVAL
There is no appreciable PR interval. The QT interval is approximately 240 ms.

WAVE MORPHOLOGY
There are no visible P waves. The QRS complex is narrow, and T wave is normal in morphology. There is a negative deflection after the QRS complex in the inferior leads (II, III, aVF) and in V_4–V_6.

In Summary

This ECG shows a regular narrow-complex tachycardia of over 170 bpm, which in a young patient with no significant medical history is most likely to represent an atrioventricular re-entrant tachycardia (AVRT) or an atrioventricular nodal re-entrant tachycardia (AVNRT).

In the acute phase, attempts can be made to terminate the arrhythmia by prolonging atrioventricular node (AVN) conduction, either by vagal manoeuvres such as Valsalva or by giving an intravenous (IV) bolus of adenosine.

If the patient is clinically unstable (with hypotension or evidence of syncopal symptoms), a periarrest call is appropriate for urgent support.

Once the patient is back in sinus rhythm, a baseline 12-lead ECG may help in making a diagnosis.

★ ANSWERS FOR CANDIDATES

1. Which cardiac condition is commonly associated with AVRT?

The correct answer is: (e) Wolff–Parkinson–White syndrome.

AVRT occurs due to the existence of an accessory pathway that allows depolarisation to cycle between atria and ventricles. This accessory pathway also allows pre-excitation of the ventricles, which usually appears as a delta wave on ECG. The existence of pre-excitation on ECG and symptoms of tachyarrhythmias are together known as the Wolff–Parkinson–White syndrome.

(a) Arrhythmogenic right ventricular cardiomyopathy – incorrect: this condition is an inherited disease of the myocardial tissue which is commonly associated with ventricular arrhythmias and sudden death.

(b) Brugada syndrome – incorrect: Brugada syndrome is an inherited channelopathy of sodium ion channels which predisposes to ventricular tachyarrhythmias and sudden death.

(c) Heart failure – incorrect: heart failure predisposes to both atrial and ventricular arrhythmias due to several mechanisms, including structural and functional changes to the heart. However, no abnormal connection between the atria and ventricles forms in heart failure.

(d) Pulmonary hypertension – incorrect: pulmonary hypertension increases the afterload on the right side of the heart and induces right ventricular hypertrophy. It also causes right atrial dilatation and predisposes to atrial fibrillation and flutter. However, there is no abnormal anatomical communication between atria and ventricles, so AVRT cannot occur.

(e) **Wolff–Parkinson–White syndrome – correct: Wolff–Parkinson–White syndrome is the most common cause of AVRT. Other pre-excitation syndromes exist that can cause AVRT, such as the Lown–Ganong–Levine syndrome (short PR interval and absent delta waves), but these are much rarer.**

 Key Points

AVRT requires the existence of a congenital anatomical communication between the atria and ventricles in addition to the AVN. This is most commonly seen in Wolff–Parkinson–White syndrome and other pre-excitation syndromes.

2. What is the mechanism underlying AVRT?

The correct answer is: (d) Re-entrant circuit from atria to ventricles via the AVN and back into atria via an accessory pathway.

AVRT is usually caused by a re-entrant circuit of depolarisation that passes from atria to ventricles via the AVN, and then returns from the atria back into the ventricles via the accessory pathway (orthodromic AVRT). As ventricular activation is via the normal His-Purkinje system, the QRS complex is narrow. Conversely, in around 5% of cases, this circuit is reversed, with depolarisation travelling into the ventricles via the accessory pathway and conducting retrogradely through the AVN back into the atria (antidromic AVRT); since ventricular activation is NOT via the His-Purkinje system, the QRS would be wide.

(a) An atrial focus with rapid abnormal pacemaker activity – incorrect: this mechanism is one of several that can give rise to atrial tachycardia.

(b) Re-entrant circuit in the right atrium – incorrect: this is a common mechanism that underlies atrial flutter. This circuit may be clockwise or, more commonly, anticlockwise.

(c) Re-entrant circuit around a slow pathway and a fast pathway located within or adjacent to the AVN – incorrect: this is the mechanism that gives rise to AVNRT.

(d) **Re-entrant circuit from atria to ventricles via the AVN and back into atria via an accessory pathway – correct: AVRT requires the existence of an accessory pathway to propagate. The ECG features of AVRT, including the direction** of the cardiac axis and the breadth of the QRS complex, depend on the location of this pathway and the direction of conduction through it.

(e) Re-entrant circuit in the left ventricle – incorrect: this arrhythmia arises in the ventricles and is therefore a ventricular arrhythmia (ventricular tachycardia).

1₂₃ Key Points

The maintenance of an AVRT depends on the function of the accessory pathway between atria and ventricles. Blocking the accessory pathway will always terminate the arrhythmia. Conversely, tachyarrhythmias that do not terminate when the accessory pathway is blocked are not AVRTs.

3. What is the definitive long-term management of patients at risk of AVRT?

The correct answer is: (a) ablation of the accessory pathway(s) to break the re-entrant circuit.

Long-term management of AVRT focuses on prevention by blocking the accessory pathway and preventing the re-entrant circuit forming. This is most commonly managed by catheter ablation, as this one-off and low-risk procedure is usually curative. It may also be achieved pharmacologically with beta-blockers, calcium channel blockers or Vaughan–Williams type 1 antiarrhythmics.

(a) **Ablation of the accessory pathway(s) to break the re-entrant circuit – correct: this is a relatively safe procedure and generally proves curative by ablating the accessory pathway.**

(b) Ablation of the AVN to break the re-entrant circuit – incorrect: ablation of the AV node is sometimes performed in patients with pacemakers and atrial fibrillation to disconnect the atria from the ventricles to help with symptoms associated with AF and rapid ventricular rates not controlled with medication.

(c) Dual-chamber pacemaker insertion – incorrect: dual-chamber pacing has no role in the long-term management of AVRT-related syndromes. However, in the acute setting, rapid pacing of the atria may help to terminate the AVRT if pharmacological interventions such as adenosine are ineffective.

(d) ICD insertion – incorrect: an ICD is not usually required in pre-excitation syndromes or AVRT; dangerous tachyarrhythmias or pre-excited atrial fibrillation are better managed with accessory pathway ablation.

(e) Long-term anticoagulation therapy – incorrect: anticoagulation is not necessary for the management of AVRT as this arrhythmia does not tend to predispose to clot formation. However, anticoagulation should be considered if comorbid atrial fibrillation is present.

1₂₃ Key Points

The definitive long-term management of AVRT is to break the atrioventricular accessory pathway to prevent the arrhythmia from occurring. This is usually achieved with a catheter ablation procedure that has a high success rate and a low rate of complications.

CASE 13 – ANSWERS

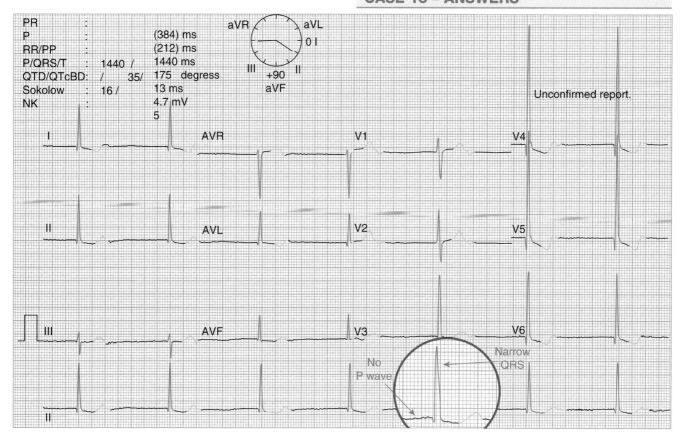

Present Your Findings

BASIC DETAILS
This is an anonymised ECG of unknown date and time.

I would like to ensure that this is calibrated to the usual 25 mm/s paper speed and 1 mV/cm gain.

KEY FEATURES
There is bradycardia with narrow QRS complexes, and no appreciable P waves. There is also downsloping ST depression in the lateral leads with tall QRS complexes in V_4–V_6.

HEART RATE AND RHYTHM
The heart rate is 42 bpm and regular.

CARDIAC AXIS
The cardiac axis is normal (between –30° and +90°).

PR AND QT INTERVAL
There is no appreciable PR interval. The QT interval is approximately 480 ms (QTc 403 ms).

WAVE MORPHOLOGY
There are no visible P waves. The QRS complexes are narrow and are tall in leads V_4–V_6, exceeding 30 mm in V_4 and V_5. There is T-wave inversion in leads I, aVL and V_4–V_6.

 In Summary

This ECG shows a narrow-complex bradycardia with absent P waves and is consistent with a junctional escape rhythm.

A thorough medical history with detailed medication history should be undertaken and blood tests should be measured for electrolytes and thyroid function. However, the most likely cause of this presentation is the sick sinus syndrome, resulting in a junctional escape rhythm.

This patient should be assessed for permanent pacemaker insertion as definitive management of her underlying sick sinus syndrome.

✴ ANSWERS FOR CANDIDATES

1. Which of the following may give rise to sick sinus syndrome?

The correct answers are: **(c) idiopathic fibrosis of the SAN; (d) myocardial infarction; and (e) surgical damage to the SAN.**

The most common aetiology of sick sinus syndrome is idiopathic degeneration of the SAN. However, anything that disrupts SAN structure or function may potentially cause reversible or irreversible sick sinus syndrome.

(a) Atropine – incorrect: atropine blocks muscarinic cholinergic receptors in the heart, reducing parasympathetic tone and promoting increased heart rate. It therefore does not tend to cause SAN dysfunction. However, drugs that depress SAN function, such as beta-blockers or digoxin, may cause sick sinus syndrome.

(b) Hypertension – incorrect: there is some evidence that hypertension is associated with sick sinus

syndrome, perhaps related to increased fibrosis of the atria. However, it is not an established aetiology of SAN dysfunction.

(c) **Idiopathic fibrosis of the SAN – correct: this is a frequent cause of sick sinus syndrome and is associated with increasing age. This is an irreversible cause of SAN dysfunction that warrants permanent pacemaker insertion.**

(d) **Myocardial infarction – correct: myocardial infarction, and particularly inferior myocardial infarction, is associated with sinus bradycardia and SAN dysfunction. This is because the SAN is usually supplied by the right coronary artery. This effect is usually transient but may result in permanent sick sinus syndrome.**

(e) **Surgical damage to the SAN – correct: sick sinus syndrome can occur due to damage to the SAN from cardiac surgery, particularly in procedures that involve the right atrium.**

 Key Points

Sick sinus syndrome may arise due to a number of causes, including:
- Idiopathic fibrosis of the SAN
- Ischaemia and myocardial infarction (especially inferior myocardial infarction)
- Myocarditis
- Infiltrative disease, including sarcoidosis and amyloidosis
- Surgical damage to the SAN
- Electrolyte abnormalities, e.g. hyperkalaemia
- SAN-depressing drugs, e.g. beta-blockers, calcium channel blockers and digoxin

---

2. Which of the following ECG patterns may feature in sick sinus syndrome?

The correct answer is: (e) all of the above.

Sick sinus syndrome is an umbrella term for a group of SAN abnormalities that affect formation of the wave of depolarisation in the heart.

(a) **Alternating bradycardia and tachycardia – correct: this is known as tachycardia–bradycardia syndrome (or tachy–brady syndrome) and is related to periods of atrial arrhythmia, such as atrial flutter or atrial fibrillation, followed by periods of sinus bradycardia. This affects over 50% of patients with sick sinus syndrome.**

(b) **Asystole – correct: sick sinus syndrome can cause periods of sinus arrest of greater than 3 s.**

(c) **Intermittently dropped sinus beats – correct: this manifestation is caused by sinus exit block, where the SAN is able to generate beats but the impulse cannot exit the SAN. This may present as regularly 'absent' P waves on the ECG.**

(d) **Sinus bradycardia – correct: sinus bradycardia is a common feature of sick sinus syndrome.**

(e) **All of the above – correct: each of the above presentations may occur in sick sinus syndrome.**

An additional manifestation includes chronotropic intolerance (inability to increase heart rate in response to stimulus, such as exercise).

Sick sinus syndrome describes a group of disorders of SAN function with heterogeneous ECG features, including:

- Sinus bradycardia
- Sinus arrest (asystole)
- Tachycardia–bradycardia syndrome
- SAN exit block:
  - Mobitz type I
  - Mobitz type II
  - Wenckebach exit block
- Chronotropic intolerance

---

3. How should the junctional rhythm be managed?

The correct answer is: (c) no treatment is necessary as the rhythm is required to maintain cardiac output.

Escape rhythms such as junctional escape rhythms have an important protective function in SAN or atrio-ventricular node (AVN) dysfunction by taking over rhythm generation for the heart. This prevents fatal asystolic cardiac arrest occurring.

(a) Anticoagulation with warfarin to prevent risk of thromboembolism – incorrect: escape rhythms are not generally associated with thromboembolism risk, although concomitant atrial flutter or fibrillation (such as tachycardia–bradycardia syndrome) may require anticoagulation.

(b) Catheter ablation of the junctional rhythm focus – incorrect: this would involve ablating a portion of the cardiac conduction system, which may cause bundle branch block or complete heart block, in addition to terminating the life-sustaining escape rhythm and risking fatal asystole.

(c) No treatment is necessary as the rhythm is required to maintain cardiac output – correct: termination of a junctional rhythm may cause another rhythm in the distal conduction system or ventricles to take over at a slower rate, or cause complete asystole. Neither of these outcomes is desirable, so the junctional rhythm should be preserved and the underlying cause of the bradycardia treated.

(d) Suppression with amiodarone to reduce symptoms – incorrect: amiodarone may further reduce the rate of the escape rhythm, leading to severe bradycardia, or terminate it completely, leading to asystole and death.

(e) Vagal manoeuvres such as Valsalva to terminate the arrhythmia – incorrect: vagal manoeuvres exert their effects by increasing parasympathetic tone, predominantly at the SAN and AVN. Junctional rhythms arise distal to the AVN, so will be unaffected by vagal manoeuvres.

Escape rhythms sustain life by preventing asystole and must not be suppressed. Instead, investigation and treatment of the underlying cause of bradycardia should be initiated, but the definitive treatment would be a permanent pacemaker.

CASE 14 – ANSWERS

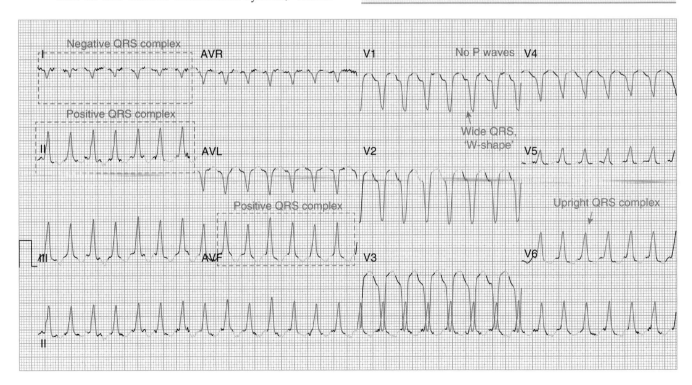

Present Your Findings

BASIC DETAILS
This is an anonymised ECG of unknown date and time.
I would like to ensure that this is calibrated to the usual 25 mm/s paper speed and 1 mV/cm gain.

KEY FEATURES
There is a regular wide-complex tachycardia at a rate of 168 bpm.

HEART RATE AND RHYTHM
The patient is tachycardic with a heart rate of 168 bpm.

CARDIAC AXIS
There is right-axis deviation (cardiac axis is between +90° and +180°).

PR AND QT INTERVAL
There is no visible PR interval. QT interval is normal (approximately 300 ms).

WAVE MORPHOLOGY
There is no visible P wave. The QRS complex is wide (approximately 130 ms). T waves are inverted in leads II and III.

 In Summary

This ECG is suggestive of ventricular tachycardia. The right axis deviation and the R wave progression in the chest leads (which resembles left bundle branch block) is suggestive of a ventricular tachycardia originating in the right ventricle. The positive R waves in the inferior leads (II,aVF,III) suggests the origin is high up in the right ventricle i.e. the right ventricular outflow tract.

As with any ventricular arrhythmia, this is a medical emergency and the patient should be assessed with an ABCDE approach with senior help sought immediately to inform further management. Urgent blood tests for electrolyte disturbances are appropriate to rule out possible causes of VT.

If the patient becomes haemodynamically unstable or progresses to cardiac arrest, immediate DC cardioversion should be carried out. Intravenous amiodarone may be appropriate in a stable patient to attempt to terminate the arrhythmia. Once stable, an urgent cardiology opinion should be obtained to make ongoing management decisions.

★ **ANSWERS FOR CANDIDATES**

1. What are the possible causes of VT in this patient?
The correct answer is: (b) Arrhythmogenic cardiomyopathy; and (c) idiopathic VT.

In young patients without a history of structural damage to the heart, such as a previous myocardial infarction or heart failure, arrhythmogenic cardiomyopathy should be considered. This is a rare genetic form of cardiomyopathy where the heart muscle is replaced by fat and fibrous tissue, predisposing the patient to ventricular arrhythmias; in the early stages this arises from the right ventricle, particularly the outflow tract. Patients with a genetic cause of VT may have relatives who have died suddenly at a young age.

(a) Brugada syndrome – incorrect: although possible, the lack of family history of known Brugada syndrome or sudden death makes this diagnosis unlikely. However, it may be appropriate to test the patient for channelopathies such as Brugada syndrome.

(b) Arrhythmogenic Cardiomyopathy – Correct: Right ventricular VT is associated with this condition and imaging with echocardiography and cardiac MRI should be performed to exclude this condition.

(c) Idiopathic VT – correct: in younger patients without a history of cardiac disease or family history of sudden death, idiopathic VT is a strong possibility for the cause of VT. Most idiopathic VT presents with a right ventricular outflow tract focus.

(d) Ischaemic heart disease – incorrect: in a 40-year-old patient with no known cardiac history, ischaemic heart disease is an unlikely cause of VT.

(e) Long QT syndrome – incorrect: long QT syndrome tends to present with polymorphic torsades de pointes VT as opposed to a regular monomorphic VT, as in this patient. There may be a family history of sudden death.

 Key Points

VT is commonly caused by structural heart disease and genetic or acquired problems with ion channels, or it may be idiopathic. In younger patients without evidence of structural cardiac disease, idiopathic or genetic causes are most likely and should be the focus of history and investigations. However, right ventricular VT can be associated with structural heart disease, such as arrhythmogenic cardiomyopathy and cardiac sarcoid.

2. Why does the blood pressure drop in VT?
The correct answer is: (a) decrease in myocardial contractility due to decreased ventricular filling.

At very high heart rates, diastolic filling time is reduced. This reduces the end-diastolic volume in the ventricles and reduces myocardial stretch. As a result of the Frank–Starling mechanism, reduced stretch of cardiomyocytes leads to reduced stroke volume and reduced cardiac output, and may result in a complete loss of cardiac output.

(a) Decrease in myocardial contractility due to decreased ventricular filling – correct: the Frank–Starling mechanism dictates that increased ventricular filling leads to increased stroke volume and therefore cardiac output. Rapid heart rates reduce filling time and therefore lead to a decline in cardiac output.

(b) Decrease in myocardial contractility due to depletion of calcium from the cardiomyocyte – incorrect: at high heart rates, calcium tends to accumulate in cardiac cells, leading to an increase in contractility as opposed to a decrease. This is known as the Bowditch effect.

(c) Decreased duration of systole causing a decrease in stroke volume – incorrect: the ejection of blood during systole is predominantly affected by the contractility of the heart and is not markedly affected by the duration of systole.

(d) Failure of excitation–contraction coupling – incorrect: this is not normally an acute occurrence and is not a major determinant of blood pressure in VT. However, failing excitation–contraction coupling is a feature of heart failure and may increase the occurrence of arrhythmias.

(e) Reflex vasodilation due to the excessively rapid heart rate – incorrect: the rapid heart rate normally impairs cardiac output and therefore leads to reflex vasoconstriction in order to maintain blood pressure.

¹²₃ Key Points

Blood pressure may drop, often precipitously, during VT, as a result of reduced ventricular filling time and a consequent decrease in cardiac output.

---

3. Which of the following clinical features suggest a good prognosis in VT?

The correct answer is: (e) VT with no known cause (idiopathic VT).

VT carries a poor prognosis when associated with structural heart disease with a high risk of sudden death. This has been greatly reduced with the advent of implantable cardiac defibrillators which may reduce the risk of sudden death by up to 30%.

(a) Family history of sudden death – incorrect: this is suggestive of a genetic cause of VT and is therefore associated with a poor prognosis.

(b) Reduced left ventricular systolic function – incorrect: reduced left ventricular function is one of the most important prognostic indicators of poor outcome.

(c) The presence of known channelopathy – incorrect: patients with channelopathies have a higher rate of sudden death independently of their ventricular function.

(d) The presence of structural heart disease – incorrect: VT in structural heart disease can be difficult to manage and is associated with high rates of cardiac arrest. As such, it is indicative of a poor prognosis, although implantable cardiac defibrillators have improved this considerably.

(e) VT with no known cause (idiopathic VT) – correct: idiopathic VT has a good prognosis if there is no associated structural heart disease and can often be controlled with beta-blockers or calcium channel blockers alone. Some idiopathic VTs, such as right ventricular outflow tachycardia, can be treated by catheter ablation, which is often curative.

¹²₃ Key Points

Underlying structural disease, heart failure or genetic causes of VT are all associated with poor outcomes, while idiopathic VT has a good prognosis. Left ventricular systolic function measures such as ejection fraction are very useful for assessing the prognosis of patients who are at risk of VT.

CASE 15 – ANSWERS

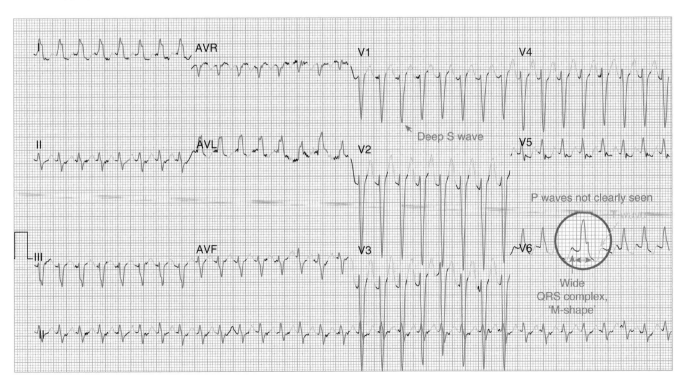

Present Your Findings

BASIC DETAILS

This is an anonymised ECG of unknown date and time.

I would like to ensure that this is calibrated to the usual 25 mm/s paper speed and 1 mV/cm gain.

KEY FEATURES

There is a regular wide-complex tachycardia at a rate of 190 bpm and left-axis deviation.

HEART RATE AND RHYTHM

The patient is tachycardic with a heart rate of 190 bpm.

CARDIAC AXIS

There is left-axis deviation (cardiac axis is between −30° and −90°).

PR AND QT INTERVAL

QT interval is normal (260 ms).

WAVE MORPHOLOGY

There is no visible P wave. QRS complex is wide (approximately 125 ms). T-wave morphology is normal.

In Summary

This ECG is suggestive of either a tachycardia of ventricular origin or a supraventricular tachycardia (SVT) with aberrant conduction. In a patient with a known history of bundle branch block, SVT should be strongly considered. However, senior help should be sought immediately to guide management. If in any doubt or the patient deteriorates, treat as ventricular tachycardia (VT).

Investigations in the acute phase should be similar to those for any tachycardia, including blood tests for electrolytes (including potassium, calcium and magnesium) and thyroid function tests. If the arrhythmia terminates, either spontaneously or with active management, a post-termination ECG will aid with diagnosis and ongoing management.

★ ANSWERS FOR CANDIDATES

1. Which clinical features may point to a diagnosis of SVT with aberrant conduction as opposed to VT?

The correct answer is: (a) a history of left bundle branch block.

It is often very difficult to distinguish between SVT with aberrant conduction and VT and if there is any diagnostic doubt a senior should be contacted and the patient treated as having VT. However, there are some features in both the ECG and in the clinical history that may support the diagnosis.

(a) **A history of left bundle branch block – correct: if there is known pre-existing bundle branch block, this may support a diagnosis of SVT with aberrancy. However, care must be taken as risk factors for bundle branch block and VT (such as myocardial infarction) often coexist.**

(b) Age more than 35 years old – incorrect: in patients over the age of 35, VT is more likely than SVT with aberrancy.

(c) Atrioventricular dissociation – incorrect: while P waves are often absent in wide-complex tachycardias, visible P waves that are independent of the QRS complexes are strongly supportive of VT.

(d) Extreme axis deviation – incorrect: bundle branch block may lead to left- or right-axis deviation but very rarely lead to extreme axis deviation. VT with an apical focus, by contrast, will almost invariably lead to extreme axis deviation.

(e) QRS complex of greater than 160 ms in duration – incorrect: a wider QRS is more suggestive of VT than SVT with aberrancy.

Key Points

The patient's medical history and baseline ECGs, if available, are highly important factors in distinguishing VT from SVT with aberrant conduction. However, ECG features alone may help to distinguish between these two arrhythmias. VT is more likely with the following ECG features:

- Concordance in the chest leads: all positive or all negative chest leads
- Markedly wide QRS complexes: QRS >160 ms
- Brugada sign: the start of the R wave to the deepest point of the S wave >100 ms in duration
- Atrioventricular dissociation: visible P waves that are independent of ventricular contraction
- Presence of fusion or capture beats
- Extreme axis deviation: rarely present in SVT but common in VT

2. The medical registrar attends to the patient rapidly and confirms that this patient has an AVNRT with aberrant conduction. What first-line treatments could be attempted in this patient while in the emergency department?

The correct answers are: (a) adenosine bolus; and (e) vagal manoeuvres.

The treatment of AVNRT with aberrant conduction, if confirmed, does not differ from that of AVNRT with normal conduction.

(a) **Adenosine bolus – correct: a bolus of adenosine may abruptly terminate the arrhythmia by blocking propagation of the arrhythmia through the atrioventricular node (AVN).**

(b) Catheter ablation – incorrect: catheter ablation is an appropriate management of SVTs such as AVNRT in the long term but is not used in the acute setting for SVTs.

(c) Synchronised DC cardioversion – incorrect: this would be an appropriate management in a haemodynamically unstable present or if there was still diagnostic doubt about VT. However, in a stable patient, other interventions should be attempted first.

(d) Transcutaneous pacing – incorrect: transcutaneous pacing is not routinely used as first line for management of SVTs.

(e) Vagal manoeuvres – correct: vagal manoeuvres, such as the Valsalva manoeuvre or carotid sinus massage, act in a similar way to adenosine; they block AVN conduction and prevent propagation of the arrhythmia. Of note, it is not uncommon for patients to report the tachycardia terminating previously with breath holding.

123 Key Points

AVNRT with aberrant conduction can be treated as any other AVNRT, which involves vagal manoeuvres such as Valsalva as a first-line treatment, with adenosine bolus as a first-line pharmacological intervention. Antiarrhythmic therapy or synchronised DC cardioversion may be considered in refractory cases. Following discharge, the patient should be referred to cardiology for consideration for an ablation procedure, which is potentially curative.

---

3. What symptoms may be associated with AVNRT?
The correct answer is: (e) all of the above.
AVNRT may present with standard symptoms associated with tachyarrhythmias, with palpitations being a common feature. However, additional symptoms such as polyuria may also be present.

(a) Chest pain – correct: chest pain may be a feature of myocardial ischaemia, especially in patients with pre-existing coronary artery disease. Patients may also complain of a sensation of fullness or pounding in the chest or neck, which is a relatively specific symptom for AVNRT.

(b) Palpitations – correct: this is a very common symptom of AVNRT, and is a crucial feature of the patient's clinical history and can sometimes be felt in the neck due to the simultaneous atrial and ventricular contraction.

(c) Polyuria – correct: this unexpected symptom of AVNRT is caused by increased atrial pressures leading to increased production of atrial natriuretic peptide from the atria and subsequent diuresis. It is more frequent in AVNRT than in other supraventricular arrhythmias.

(d) Shortness of breath – correct: dyspnoea is also very common in AVNRT and may be associated with poor exercise tolerance and fatigue.

(e) All of the above – correct: all of these symptoms may occur in AVNRT.

123 Key Points

AVNRT may present with a variety of different symptoms, including:
- Shortness of breath
- Fatigue
- Poor exercise tolerance
- Palpitations
- Chest pain
- Pounding sensation in the neck
- Fullness in the chest or neck
- Light-headedness
- Anxiety
- Polyuria

CASE 16 – ANSWERS

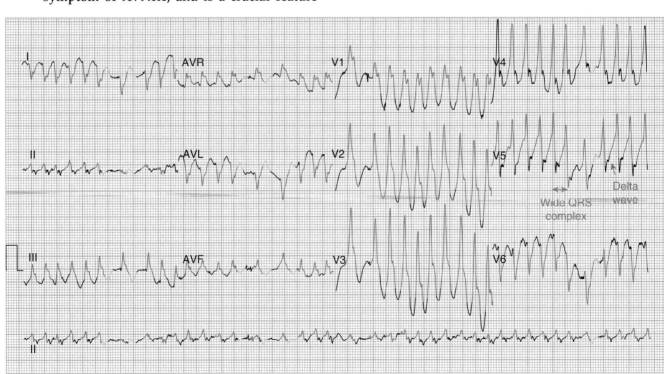

Present Your Findings

BASIC DETAILS

This is an anonymised ECG of unknown date and time.

I would like to ensure that this is calibrated to the usual 25 mm/s paper speed and 1 mV/cm gain.

KEY FEATURES

There is an irregularly irregular wide-complex tachycardia at a rate of 240 bpm. No P waves are clearly visible.

HEART RATE AND RHYTHM

The patient is severely tachycardic with a heart rate of 240 bpm. The rhythm is irregularly irregular.

CARDIAC AXIS

There is right-axis deviation (cardiac axis is between +90° and +180°).

PR AND QT INTERVAL

The PR interval is not appreciable in this ECG. There is no prolongation of the QT interval.

WAVE MORPHOLOGY

No P waves are appreciable in this ECG. The QRS complex is wide with evidence of a slurred upstroke (delta waves) in V_4 and V_5. T waves are intermittently visible but appear inverted in the inferior leads.

In Summary

This ECG is consistent with an irregularly irregular tachycardia with evidence of delta waves, suggesting atrial fibrillation (AF) in a patient with pre-excitation syndrome.

This patient is at very high risk of degenerating into ventricular fibrillation; this should therefore be treated as a medical emergency and a crash team or equivalent sought urgently. Treatment of pre-excited AF is with a synchronised DC cardioversion to terminate the arrhythmia, although anti-arrhythmic medications can be used under guidance of a specialist.

Early emergent investigations should aim to identify possible underlying causes of AF, including blood tests for electrolytes (including potassium, calcium and magnesium levels) and thyroid function tests.

★ ANSWERS FOR CANDIDATES

1. What condition is characterised by the presence of an accessory pathway between the atria and the ventricles?

The correct answer is: (d) Wolff–Parkinson–White syndrome.

(a) Arrhythmogenic right ventricular cardiomyopathy – incorrect: arrhythmogenic right ventricular cardiomyopathy is a genetic inherited condition characterised by replacement of normal myocardium with fibrofatty tissue, which increases the risk of sudden ventricular arrhythmias.

(b) Atrial flutter – incorrect: atrial flutter is characterised by cyclical depolarisation of the atria leading to a supraventricular tachycardia, usually associated with some element of atrioventricular (AV) block. Accessory pathways are not a characteristic feature.

(c) Ebstein anomaly – incorrect: this is a congenital malformation of the tricuspid valve and right ventricle commonly associated with lithium use during pregnancy. Although accessory pathways are common in Ebstein anomaly (in around 10% of cases), these are not a characteristic feature of the condition.

(d) Wolff–Parkinson–White syndrome – correct: Wolff-Parkinson-White syndrome is characterised by the presence of one or more accessory pathways between the atria and the ventricles causing ventricular pre-excitation, together with either symptoms suggestive of an arrhythmia or a documented arrhythmia.

(e) None of the above – incorrect: The presence of one or more accessory pathways between the atria and ventricles is found in patients with Wolff-Parkinson-White syndrome.

2. Which antiarrhythmic drugs could be considered in pre-excited AF?

The correct answer is: (d) flecainide.

The mechanism of action of common antiarrhythmic drugs is particularly important in the treatment of pre-excited AF, as drugs that act preferentially on the AV node may increase conduction via the accessory pathway and predispose to ventricular fibrillation

(a) Adenosine – incorrect: adenosine blocks the AV node, and therefore may increase conduction via the accessory pathway and increase ventricular rate, which increases the risk of ventricular fibrillation.

(b) Amiodarone – incorrect: amiodarone is a class III antiarrhythmic (according to the Vaughan–Williams classification model), although it also has a broad range of other antiarrhythmic properties. In the context of pre-excited AF, amiodarone may enhance accessory pathway conduction and therefore increase the risk of ventricular fibrillation. It may also cause drug-induced hypotension and promote catecholamine release, which may also increase VF risk.

(c) Digoxin – incorrect: digoxin is a cardiac glycoside that acts as a sodium–potassium co-transporter blocker. It promotes vagal activity and therefore acts on the AV node, which may predispose to accessory pathway conduction. It also decreases refractoriness of the accessory pathway, which further increases ventricular rate.

(d) Flecainide – correct: flecainide is a class Ic antiarrhythmic drug, and acts by blocking sodium channels to reduce the upstroke of cardiac action potentials. It acts on cardiac myocytes and decreases conduction across the accessory pathway. Flecainide should be avoided in patients with structural heart disease as it may increase the risk of ventricular fibrillation. Other class I antiarrhythmic drugs may also be used in this setting.

(e) Verapamil – incorrect: verapamil is a class IV antiarrhythmic drug that acts by blocking calcium channels. It has a preferential effect on the AV node and therefore can increase conduction across the accessory pathway. It may also cause hypotension and an increase in catecholamines, which predisposes to AF.

1₂₃ Key Points

Although antiarrhythmic drugs can be used in the treatment of pre-excited AF, treatment is complex and should be guided by specialist input. As all antiarrhythmic treatments carry a risk of triggering ventricular fibrillation, a defibrillator should be available at all times when treating such patients.

---

3. What long-term management options should be considered for pre-excited AF?

The correct answers are: (a) catheter ablation of accessory pathway; and (e) oral flecainide.

(a) Catheter ablation of accessory pathway – correct: this is the mainstay of long-term management of pre-excited AF. It prevents conduction of the rapid atrial rate into the ventricles with a high rate of success (around 95%). Additionally, AF in younger patients is generally a direct result of the accessory pathway, and catheter ablation often prevents AF recurrence.

(b) Insertion of an ICD – incorrect: ICDs are generally inserted for primary or secondary prevention of sudden arrhythmogenic cardiac arrest in cases where the cause of the arrhythmia is not treatable or reversible, such as in heart failure, ischaemic heart disease or inherited channelopathies. Treating the underlying cause of the

ventricular fibrillation risk in pre-excited AF by ablation of the accessory pathway would be preferred in this instance.

(c) Oral adenosine – incorrect: adenosine is used intravenously for rapid termination of an acute supraventricular arrhythmia and does not have a role in long-term management.

(d) Oral anticoagulation – incorrect: although oral anticoagulation is the mainstay of management of permanent AF in older patients, in patients with AF and an accessory pathway there is a very high risk of development of ventricular fibrillation and sudden cardiac death – treatment must therefore focus on preventing the arrhythmia or eliminating the accessory pathway.

(e) Oral flecainide – correct: class Ic antiarrhythmic drugs such as flecainide can be used if patients do not want or cannot have catheter ablation. However, these drugs carry an arrhythmia risk in patients with structural heart disease and should be avoided in such cases.

1₂₃ Key Points

The primary focus on AF in Wolff–Parkinson–White syndrome and other pre-excitation syndromes is to prevent conduction of the rapid atrial rate into the ventricles. The first-line method to achieve this is generally by catheter ablation, which is safe and effective. However, pharmacological blockade of the accessory pathway using class I antiarrhythmic drugs is an option, although this comes with associated risks and is therefore not first line.

CASE 17 – ANSWERS

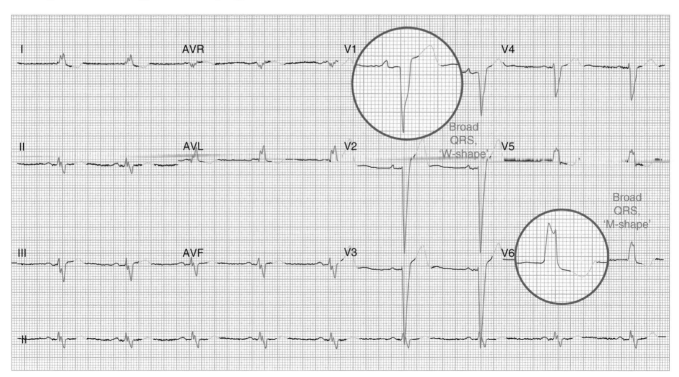

Present Your Findings

BASIC DETAILS
This is an anonymised ECG of unknown date and time.
I would like to ensure that this is calibrated to the usual 25 mm/s paper speed and 1 mV/cm gain.

KEY FEATURES
The most pertinent abnormality is wide QRS complexes; deep S waves in V_1–V_4 and notched R waves in V_5–V_6 can be seen. ST elevation is present in leads V_1–V_3.

HEART RATE AND RHYTHM
The heart rate is 54 bpm with a sinus rhythm.

CARDIAC AXIS
The cardiac axis is normal (between –30° and +90°).

PR AND QRS INTERVAL
The PR interval is normal (200 ms). The QT interval is normal (400 ms).

WAVE MORPHOLOGY
The P waves are normal in morphology. The QRS complexes are wide with deep S waves in V_1–V_4 and notched R waves in V_5–V_6. There is no evidence of ventricular hypertrophy. There is ST elevation in V_1–V_3. T waves cannot be accurately assessed in view of the aberrant ventricular conduction.

 In Summary

This ECG is consistent with a left bundle branch block in a patient with raised venous pressures and bibasal crepitations, so pulmonary oedema should be considered. The patient should be urgently managed on a cardiac ward and a chest X-ray and echocardiogram should be requested to confirm the diagnosis. Blood tests including troponin levels, FBC, U&E, lipid profile and coagulation profile should be requested.

Acute management of pulmonary oedema includes A to E assessment, oxygen (if low oxygen saturation) and intravenous diuretics. Further options include intravenous nitrates, particularly when coexisting hypertension is present.

★ **ANSWERS FOR CANDIDATES**

1. Which of the following conditions are associated with an LBBB?
The correct answers are: **(a) aortic stenosis; (c) cardiomyopathy;** and **(e) ischaemic heart disease.**

LBBBs are usually caused by underlying cardiac conditions that affect the left ventricle.

(a) **Aortic stenosis – correct: the increased left heart pressure produced by aortic stenosis can lead to LBBB.**

(b) Atrial septal defect – incorrect: atrial septal defects produce right bundle branch blocks.

(c) **Cardiomyopathy – correct: LBBB is associated with cardiomyopathy and is a common finding in dilated cardiomyopathy. In these conditions, LBBB may also be a causative factor for the cardiomyopathy.**

(d) Hypokalaemia – incorrect: Hyperkalaemia, not hypokalaemia, can lead to bundle branch blocks.

(e) **Ischaemic heart disease – correct: ischaemic heart disease is one of the commonest causes of LBBB. A new LBBB may indicate a STEMI.**

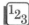 **Key Points**

Causes of LBBBs include:
- Ischaemic heart disease
- Systemic hypertension
- Cardiomyopathy
- Aortic stenosis
- Left ventricular hypertrophy
- Idiopathic conduction system fibrosis

2. Which of the following ECG changes can be produced by an LBBB?
The correct answer is: **(a) left axis deviation;** and **(e) wide QRS complexes.**

The most pertinent change in LBBBs is the development of wide, deep S waves in V_1–V_3 and wide, notched R waves in V_5–V_6 (remembered as 'WiLLiaM' from the mnemonic 'WiLLiaM MaRRoW').

(a) **Left axis deviation - Correct: left axis deviation can rarely occur with LBBB and when present is associated with more significant myocardial disease. Left axis deviation is more commonly associated with left anterior fascicular block, which is a partial block of the left bundle branch.**

(b) Prolonged PR interval – incorrect: bundle branch blocks do not affect the PR interval.

(c) Right-axis deviation – incorrect: right-axis deviations occur in left posterior fascicular block, which is a partial block of the left bundle branch.

(d) RSR' pattern in V_1–V_3 – incorrect: right bundle branch blocks produce an RSR' pattern in V_1–V_3. LBBB produces wide, deep S waves in V_1–V_3.

(e) **Wide QRS complexes – correct: ventricular depolarisation takes longer to spread in LBBB, producing wide QRS complexes. The right bundle branch conducts impulses to the right ventricle, which then propagate through the myocardium to the left ventricle.**

ECG findings of LBBB may include:

- Widened QRS
- Wide, deep S waves in V_1–V_3
- Wide, monophasic or notched ('M'-shaped) R waves in V_5–V_6
- Inverted T waves

---

3. Which of the following are appropriate treatment options for this patient?

The correct answers are: **(a) ACE inhibitors; (d) biventricular pacing; and (e) Diuretics.**

LBBBs should be managed by initially looking for the underlying cause. Appropriate antihypertensives will reduce risk factors of LBBBs and if it does not resolve, surgical treatment of pacemaker or biventricular pacing may be indicated.

(a) **ACE inhibitors – Correct: Anti-hypertensive medications which are not rate limiting, such as ACE-inhibitors, can help to manage symptoms related with hypertension and heart failure.**

(b) Adenosine – Incorrect: Adenosine is usually used in acute management of supraventricular tachycardia.

(c) Calcium channel blockers – Incorrect: Calcium channel blockers are negatively inotropic and can potentially exacerbate heart failure.

(d) Biventricular pacing – Correct: This is especially useful for patients with both bundle branch blocks and poor cardiac function (LV Ejection Fraction <35%) who are symptomatic despite optimal medical therapy. Cardiac resynchronisation treatment or biventricular pacing will help re-coordinate the contraction of both ventricles by pacing them at the same time.

(e) Diuretics – Correct: diuretics are important to diurese the patient and treat his pulmonary oedema.

Management of patients with left bundle branch block should be aimed at treating its underlying cause. Management may include:

- Conservative: stop smoking, reduce alcohol intake, reduce weight, active lifestyle, healthy diet
- Medical: anti-hypertensives, such as ACE-inhibitors, and starting on heart failure medication if there is evidence of a cardiomyopathy
- Surgical: Biventricular pacing if there is evidence of heart failure and poor cardiac function

CASE 18 – ANSWERS

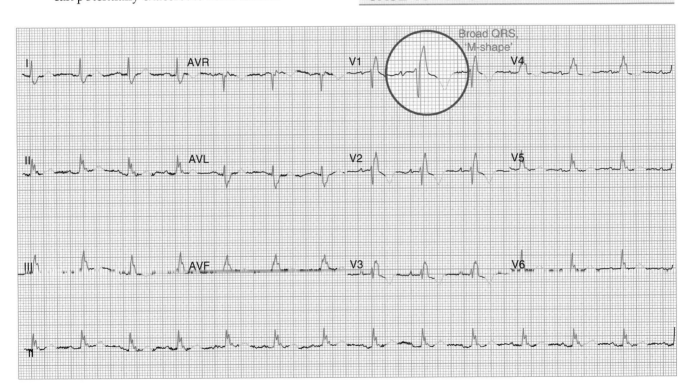

Present Your Findings

BASIC DETAILS
This is an anonymised ECG of unknown date and time.
   I would like to ensure that this is calibrated to the usual 25 mm/s paper speed and 1 mV/cm gain.

KEY FEATURES
The most pertinent abnormality is wide QRS complexes; an RSR' pattern in V_1–V_3 can be seen.

HEART RATE AND RHYTHM
The heart rate is approximately 80 bpm with a sinus rhythm.

CARDIAC AXIS
The cardiac axis is normal (between –30° and +90°).

PR AND QRS INTERVAL
The PR interval is normal (180 ms). The QT interval is normal (360 ms).

WAVE MORPHOLOGY
The QRS complexes are wide and RSR' pattern can be seen in V_1–V_3. There is no evidence of ventricular hypertrophy. T waves cannot be accurately assessed in view of the aberrant ventricular conduction.

 In Summary

This ECG is consistent with a right bundle branch block (RBBB). Given her history and examination findings, it is likely that the patient has a congenital heart defect, which may be an atrial septal defect, given the characteristics of the murmur. Blood tests (including full blood count and urea and electrolytes) and an echocardiogram should be arranged, and the patient should be referred to the cardiology team for further management.

⭐ **ANSWERS FOR CANDIDATES**

1. Which of the following may produce an RBBB?
The correct answers are: (a) atrial septal defect; Change to incorrect answer and (d) pulmonary embolus.

   RBBBs are usually associated with pathologies affecting the right side of the heart, including right ventricular hypertrophy and pulmonary embolism. However, RBBBs may also be seen in healthy individuals.
   (a) **Atrial septal defect – correct: This patient has an atrial septal defect, which is likely to have led to the development of a RBBB.**
   (b) Brugada syndrome – Incorrect: A rare syndrome associated with coved ST elevation in V_1-V_3 which can look like RBBB.

   (c) Systemic hypertension – incorrect: systemic hypertension tends to produce left bundle branch block rather than RBBB. However, pulmonary hypertension is associated with RBBB.
   (d) **Pulmonary embolism – correct: the raised right heart pressure caused by pulmonary embolism can produce RBBB.**
   (e) All of the above – incorrect: systemic hypertension does not usually produce RBBB.

 Key Points

Causes of RBBB include:
* Right ventricular hypertrophy
* Pulmonary embolus
* Congenital heart disease, e.g. atrial septal defect
* Ischaemic heart disease
* Idiopathic – benign finding

2. Which of the following ECG changes can be produced by an RBBB?
The correct answers are: (a) RSR' pattern in V_1–V_3; and (c) widened QRS complex.

   The most pertinent change in left bundle branch blocks is the development of RSR' pattern in V_1–V_3 and wide, slurred S waves in V_5–V_6 (remembered as 'MaRRoW' from the mnemonic 'WiLLiaM MaRRoW').
   (a) **RSR' pattern in V_1–V_3 – correct: an RSR' pattern in V_1–V_3 is one of the classic findings of RBBB. This is represented by the 'M' in the mnemonic 'MaRRoW'.**
   (b) Right-axis deviation – incorrect: isolated RBBBs do not cause axis deviations.
   (c) **Widened QRS complex – correct: as the wave of depolarisation takes longer to spread across the ventricles in RBBB, the QRS complex becomes wide (>120 ms; <3 small squares).**
   (d) Left-axis deviation – incorrect: isolated RBBBs do not cause axis deviations.
   (e) ST elevation in V_1–V_3 – incorrect: RBBBs can produce ST depression in leads V_1–V_3, not ST elevation.

 Key Points

ECG findings of RBBB may include:
* Widened QRS
* RSR' pattern in V_1–V_3 ('M-shaped' QRS complex)
* ST depression and T-wave inversion in V_1–V_3
* Wide, slurred S wave in the V_5–V_6, I, aVL

3. Which of the following statements is/are true with regard to RBBB?

The correct answers are: **(a) bifascicular blocks involve the right bundle; (b) cardiac resynchronisation may be used in patients with heart failure and RBBB; and (e) trifascicular blocks involve the right bundle.**

RBBB can be a normal variant in young healthy people. The left bundle branch is divided into anterior and posterior fascicles. Bifascicular block refers to RBBB and block of one of the left bundle branch fascicles. Trifascicular block is bifascicular block with a first-degree heart block.

(a) **Bifascicular blocks involve the right bundle – correct:** bifascicular block can be defined as RBBB and either left anterior fascicular block or left posterior fascicular block.

(b) **Cardiac resynchronisation may be used in patients with heart failure and RBBB – correct:** Although cardiac resynchronisation therapy has a greater benefit in patients with LBBB and heart failure, there is evidence to show it can help some patients with RBBB, particularly when associated with a wide QRS >150ms.

(c) RBBBs are always benign findings – incorrect: New RBBB is seen in 3-7% of acute myocardial infarctions and can occur in patient with acute heart strain due to a pulmonary embolism.

(d) RBBBs in young individuals are usually indicative of organic heart disease – incorrect: RBBB patterns with a normal duration of QRS complex are quite common in healthy people.

(e) **Trifascicular blocks involve the right bundle – correct:** 'trifascicular' block refers to the presence of first-degree heart block, RBBB and either left anterior or left posterior fascicular blocks.

$^1_{2_3}$ Key Points

Trifascicular block refers to the presence of the following three abnormalities on ECG:

- First-degree heart block
- RBBB
- Left anterior or left posterior fascicular block

CASE 19 – ANSWERS

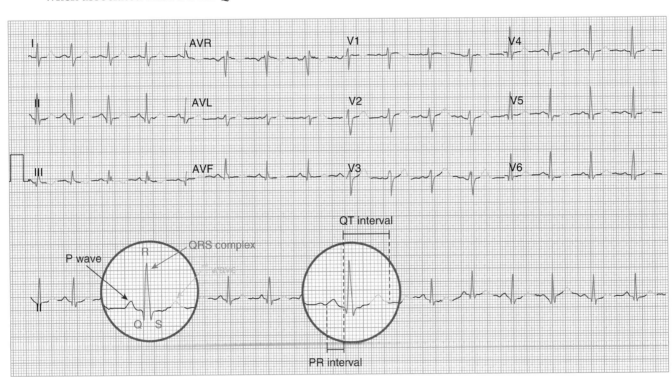

Present Your Findings

BASIC DETAILS

This is an anonymised ECG recorded at an unknown date and time.

I would like to ensure that this is calibrated to the usual 25 mm/s paper speed and 1 mV/cm gain.

KEY FEATURES

There are no obvious abnormalities in this ECG.

HEART RATE AND RHYTHM

The heart rate is 96 bpm with a sinus rhythm.

CARDIAC AXIS

The cardiac axis is normal (between –30° and +90°).

PR AND QT INTERVAL

The PR interval is normal (between 120 and 200 ms) and the QT interval is normal (between 400 and 440 ms).

WAVE MORPHOLOGY

The P waves are normal in morphology. The QRS complexes are narrow and of normal amplitude. The ST segments and I waves are normal.

 In Summary

This is a normal ECG. It is normal sinus rhythm and there are no abnormal waves. This suggests that this man's chest pain is likely to be non-cardiac in origin.

Due to the history and examination findings suggesting a lower respiratory tract infection, blood tests, including full blood count and C-reactive protein, should be arranged and a chest X-ray done.

⋆ ANSWERS FOR CANDIDATES

1. On a standard ECG trace what amount of time is represented by one small square?

The correct answer is (b) 0.04 s

Each small square represents 40 ms of time on the x-axis.

(a) 0.01 s – incorrect: 0.01 s (10 ms) is less time than is represented by a single small square.

(b) 0.04 s – correct: a standard ECG is calibrated to 25 mm/s. A single small square is 1 mm, so this represents 0.04 s, or 40 ms.

(c) 0.1 s – incorrect: this is longer than a single small square.

(d) 0.4 s – incorrect: 0.4 s, or 400 ms would be 10 small squares, or two large squares.

(e) 1 s – incorrect: a standard ECG is calibrated to 25 mm/s, so a single second is 25 small squares, or five large squares.

 Key Points

A standard ECG runs at a rate of 25 mm/s. This means that one small square represents 0.04 s (40 ms), while one large square made up of five small squares represents 0.2 s (200 ms).

2. What is the maximum normal duration for a QRS complex?

The correct answer is (b) 120 ms.

A normal QRS complex should have a width less than 120 ms.

(a) 50 ms – incorrect: a QRS complex of 50 ms would be shorter than average.

(b) 120 ms – correct: a normal QRS complex has a maximum duration of 120 ms. This is represented by three small squares.

(c) 150 ms – incorrect: a QRS complex of 150 ms is wider than normal. This can be seen in conditions such as bundle branch block or if the beats are ventricular in origin.

(d) 200 ms – incorrect: as above, a QRS complex of 200 ms would be abnormally long and could indicate pathology.

(e) 1 s – incorrect: a QRS complex of 25 small squares or five large squares is not possible as this would be extremely wide-complex.

 Key Points

The width of a normal QRS complex is less than 120 ms; this is equivalent to three small squares on a trace calibrated to 25 mm/s. Rhythms with narrow QRS complexes tend to be supraventricular in origin, whereas wide complexes tend to be ventricular in origin. The exception to this is bundle branch block, where a supraventricular rhythm can have a wide complex.

3. Which of the following can be a normal variant on an ECG?

The correct answers are (b) prominent Q waves in aVR; (c) prominent Q waves in lead III; and (e) small Q waves (<2 small squares) in V_4-V_6.

Small Q waves can be normal variants in most leads, particularly in leads aVR and III. Large Q waves are expected in V_5 and V_6.

(a) No Q waves in any leads – incorrect: small Q waves should be seen in V_5 and V_6 and the absence of these is abnormal.

(b) Prominent Q waves in aVR – correct: aVR is one of the leads in which prominent Q waves (>2 mm) can be normal.

(c) Prominent Q waves in lead III – correct: As with aVR, prominent Q waves in lead III can be normal.

(d) Prominent Q waves in V_1–V_3 – incorrect: Q waves >2 mm in leads V_1, V_2 or V_3 are abnormal and indicate pathology, such as previous ischaemia.

(e) Small Q waves (<2 small squares) in V_4–V_6 – correct: small Q waves (<2 mm) are normal and may be seen in any leads, including V_4, V_5 and V_6.

 Key Points

Small Q waves (<2 mm or two small squares) are normal and may be present in any lead. They should always be present in leads V_5 and V_6. Larger Q waves (>2 mm) are normal in leads aVR and III but are abnormal in other leads. The presence of pathological Q waves may indicate:

- Previous ischaemia
- Cardiomyopathy, e.g. hypertrophic obstructive cardiomyopathy
- Extreme rotation of the heart
- Lead misplacement

CASE 20 – ANSWERS

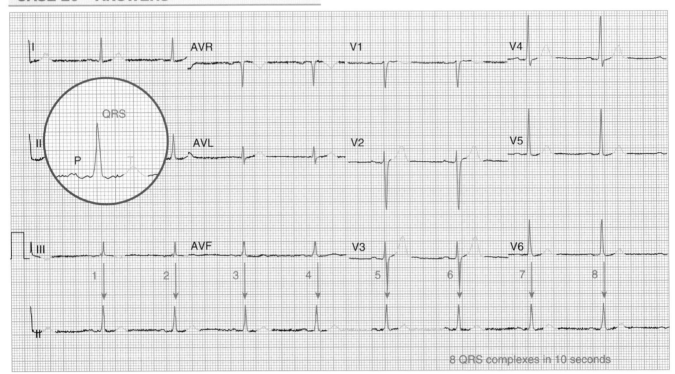

8 QRS complexes in 10 seconds

 Present Your Findings

BASIC DETAILS

This is an anonymised ECG recorded at an unknown date and time.

I would like to ensure that this is calibrated to the usual 25 mm/s paper speed and 1 mV/cm gain.

KEY FEATURES

The most pertinent feature of this ECG is a low heart rate.

HEART RATE AND RHYTHM

The heart rate is 54 bpm with a sinus rhythm.

CARDIAC AXIS

The cardiac axis is normal (between –30° and +90°).

PR AND QT INTERVAL

The PR interval is normal (between 120 and 200 ms) and the QT interval is normal (between 400 and 440 ms).

WAVE MORPHOLOGY

The P waves are normal in morphology. The QRS complexes are narrow and of normal amplitude. The ST segments and T waves are normal.

In Summary

This ECG shows sinus bradycardia. Aside from the low heart rate, there are no abnormalities – all waves are of normal morphology and intervals are normal.

No specific treatment is necessary as this is likely to be the man's normal heart rate, particularly if he is physically fit.

★ ANSWERS FOR CANDIDATES

1. Which of the following are possible causes of sinus bradycardia?

The correct answer are (b) beta-blockers; and (e) increased vagal tone.

Any process that slows down the heart rate can produce sinus bradycardia, including increased vagal tone in athletes or the use of beta-blockers.

(a) ACE inhibitors – incorrect: while ACE inhibitors are antihypertensives, their mechanism of action does not affect heart rate. ACE inhibitors inhibit the conversion of angiotensin I to angiotensin II, which is both a vasoconstrictor and stimulates the release of aldosterone. Neither of these actions directly affects heart rate.

(b) **Beta-blockers – correct: Beta-blockers block the effect of adrenaline on the heart, mainly via beta-1 adrenergic receptors. Adrenaline acts to increase both heart rate and contractility, so blocking its effect can cause sinus bradycardia.**

(c) Hyperthyroidism – incorrect: hyperthyroidism is a possible cause of sinus tachycardia. Hypothyroidism could cause sinus bradycardia.

(d) Hypoglycaemia – incorrect: hypoglycaemia is a cause of sinus tachycardia rather than bradycardia.

(e) **Increased vagal tone – correct: the vagus nerve supplies the heart with parasympathetic fibres which act to decrease heart rate. Increased vagal tone is seen in athletes who can maintain a low resting heart rate.**

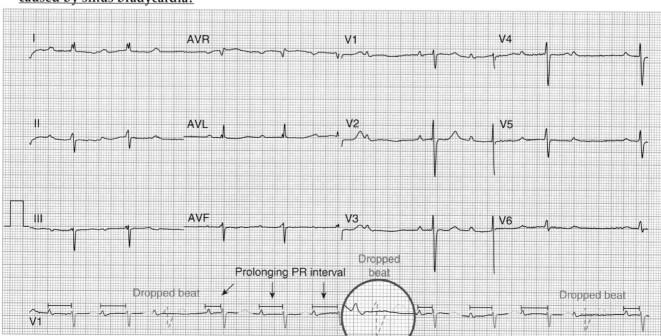
Sinus bradycardia is a relatively common finding on ECGs. There are many causes, including:

- Sleep (the heart rate naturally drops during sleep)
- Increased vagal tone
- Hypothermia
- Hypothyroidism
- Electrolyte disturbances, e.g. hyperkalaemia
- Myocarditis
- Drugs, such as:
  - Beta-blockers
  - Calcium channel blockers
  - Digoxin
  - Amiodarone
  - Opiates

2. What symptoms is this patient likely to be experiencing because of the ECG changes seen?

The correct answer is (b) none.

Most patients with sinus bradycardia are asymptomatic.

(a) Chest pain – incorrect: chest pain is not caused by sinus bradycardia. Pain is likely to produce tachycardia rather than bradycardia.

(b) None – correct: sinus bradycardia is often completely asymptomatic.

(c) Orthopnoea – incorrect: orthopnoea is a possible symptom of heart failure. This ECG shows no evidence of heart failure.

(d) Shortness of breath on exertion – incorrect: as with orthopnoea, shortness of breath on exertion is a possible symptom of heart failure. This patient does report feeling more tired than usual but that is unlikely to be from a cardiac cause.

(e) Syncope – incorrect: syncope can be caused by multiple cardiac issues, such as aortic stenosis and heart block, but is unlikely to be caused by sinus bradycardia.

Key Points

Sinus bradycardia is almost always asymptomatic.

3. Which of the following ECG changes can be caused by sinus bradycardia?

The correct answer is (b) increased QT interval.

As the heart rate slows down, the QT interval prolongs as repolarisation takes a longer time. Therefore, the QT interval should be corrected to account for heart rates.

(a) Increased PR interval – incorrect: an increased PR interval (>200 ms) is defined as first-degree heart block. This can cause bradycardia but is not caused by sinus bradycardia.

(b) Increased QT interval – correct: the QT interval is affected by heart rate and can increase in bradycardia. Therefore, corrected QT (QTc) is a more accurate measure. The QTc is prolonged if >450 ms in males and >470 ms in females

(c) Large Q waves in the inferior leads – incorrect: Q waves are not present in sinus bradycardia. Their presence can indicate an old myocardial infarction.

(d) Presence of a delta wave – incorrect: a delta wave is seen in Wolff–Parkinson–White syndrome, which can cause tachycardia. It is not seen in bradycardia.

(e) Widened QRS complex – incorrect: a widened QRS complex can be seen in bundle branch block as well as some tachycardias (such as ventricular tachycardia). Bradycardia has no effect on the QRS complex.

Key Points

The QT interval is the interval between the beginning of the Q wave and the end of the T wave. This interval is affected by heart rate, so Bazett's formula (shown below) can be used to calculate QTc. The QTc should be <450 ms in men and <470 ms in women. A long QT interval carries a risk of ventricular tachyarrhythmias caused by the 'R on T phenomenon', which occurs when depolarisation (R wave) interrupts repolarisation (T wave) of the previous beat.

QTc is calculated by Fridericia formula:

$$QTc = \frac{QT \ (s)}{\sqrt[3]{RR \ interval \ (s)}}$$

CASE 21

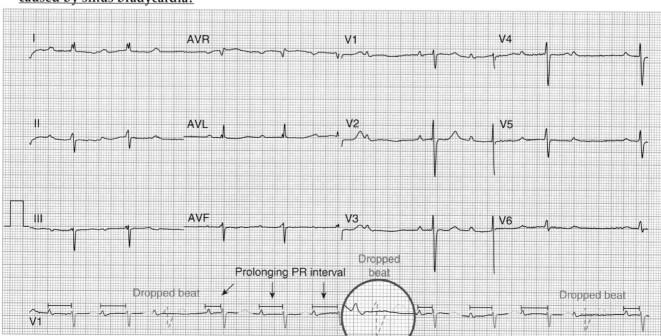

Present Your Findings

BASIC DETAILS

This is an anonymised ECG recorded at an unknown date and time.

I would like to ensure that this is calibrated to the usual 25 mm/s paper speed and 1 mV/cm gain.

KEY FEATURES

The most pertinent abnormality on this ECG is a regularly irregular heart rate with a pause between every 3 beats.

HEART RATE AND RHYTHM

The heart rate is 54 bpm. The rhythm is regularly irregular, with three closely spaced QRS complexes preceded by a P wave and then a P wave followed by no QRS complex.

CARDIAC AXIS

There is left-axis deviation (cardiac axis is between −30° and −90°).

PR AND QT INTERVAL

The PR interval is variable. It is shortest in the first beat of each cycle, then lengthens in the subsequent beats until there is a dropped beat. The QT interval is normal (between 400 and 440 ms).

WAVE MORPHOLOGY

The P waves are normal in morphology. The QRS complexes are narrow and of normal amplitude. ST segment and T waves are normal in morphology.

In Summary

This is an ECG that shows second-degree heart block, specifically Wenckebach block. This can be seen by the progressively lengthening PR interval before a beat is dropped and the cycle repeats.

This patient should be treated according to his presentation, i.e. increasing confusion. The Wenckebach rhythm is unlikely to be the underlying cause of his symptoms. The patient should undergo a full work-up for his confusion, including tests for infection and electrolyte abnormalities.

★ ANSWERS FOR CANDIDATES

1. What is the cause of this arrhythmia?

The correct answer is: (c) AV node conduction disease.

Wenckebach is caused by progressive fatigue of AV node cells until an impulse is not conducted and the AV node cells reset.

(a) Accessory pathways between the atria and the ventricles – incorrect: accessory pathways between the atria and ventricles can cause tachyarrhythmias (atrioventricular re-entrant tachycardia and atrioventricular nodal re-entrant tachycardia) rather than heart block.

(b) Electrolyte disturbances – incorrect: while electrolyte disturbances can cause many arrhythmias, they do not tend to cause this arrhythmia.

(c) **AV node conduction disease – correct: the progressive increase in the time taken for atrioventricular conduction is caused by progressive fatigue of AV node cells. This occurs until they are unable to conduct an impulse, after which they reset and the pattern repeats.**

(d) Malfunction of cells in the Purkinje fibres – incorrect: the fault in Mobitz type I block is at the level of the AV node. In contrast, Mobitz type II block can be caused by failure of cells in the His–Purkinje system.

(e) Ventricular ischaemia – incorrect: ischaemia of the AV node can cause this arrhythmia. However, ischaemia of the ventricle(s) alone would not cause this arrhythmia.

 Key Points

Mobitz I second-degree heart block is also known as Wenckebach. It is caused by progressive fatigue of cells of the AV node, which take longer and longer to conduct an impulse between the atria and the ventricles until they are unable to conduct one and they reset. This results in a progressively lengthening PR interval before a P wave is not conducted and the pattern resets.

2. Which of the following would be appropriate acute investigations and management for this patient?

The correct answer is: (c) no management necessary.

There is no acute intervention necessary for a patient with this arrhythmia who is haemodynamically stable.

(a) Administration of atropine – incorrect: atropine can be used to treat this rhythm if patients are symptomatic with it. In this case, treatment of the acute MI is initially more important than treating the heart block as the patient has a normal heart rate.

(b) Administration of clopidogrel and aspirin – incorrect: while use of dual antiplatelet therapy with aspirin and another antiplatelet, such as clopidogrel or ticagrelor, is recommended in the treatment of acute MI, this patient is not currently suffering an acute MI. The patient presented initially with an NSTEMI, and is being managed medically, so they should already be having dual antiplatelet therapy.

(c) **No management necessary – correct: there is no acute management necessary for this arrhythmia.**

(d) PCI – incorrect: PCI is indicated in the acute management of a STEMI. This patient is currently not experiencing a STEMI so PCI is not indicated.

(e) Thrombolysis using alteplase – incorrect: alteplase is a thrombolytic drug that acts by breaking down blood clots. If PCI is not available, thrombolysis may be used to manage a STEMI. As with PCI, there is no role for thrombolysis in the management of this patient as they are not experiencing a STEMI.

Key Points

Wenckebach is usually a benign arrhythmia that does not cause complications in itself. This patient is experiencing minor symptoms but is haemodynamically stable. Therefore, no management is necessary for this arrhythmia.

3. **Which of the following are potential complications arising from this heart block?**

The correct answers are: (b) hypotension; (d) progression to third-degree heart block; and (e) syncope secondary to bradycardia.

Complications due to Wenckebach are rare but can sometimes occur.

(a) Asystole – incorrect: there is no risk of sudden asystole in Mobitz type I block.

(b) **Hypotension – correct: although rare, Mobitz type I block can cause hypotension. This is unusual though as normally this rhythm is asymptomatic.**

(c) MI – incorrect: Mobitz type I block can occur secondary to an inferior MI that damages the AV node. An MI will not occur due to Mobitz type I block.

(d) **Progression to third-degree heart block – correct: there is a small risk that second-degree heart block can progress to third-degree heart block. This will occur if the AV node becomes damaged further.**

(e) **Syncope secondary to bradycardia – correct: as above, this can rarely occur.**

Key Points

In most cases, Mobitz type I block is asymptomatic and causes no issues. Very rarely, it can cause haemodynamic instability, such as hypotension or bradycardia, and these patients usually respond well to treatment with atropine. Pacemaker insertion is only required if haemodynamic instability persists or the patient has symptoms due to the bradycardia. There is also a small risk of progression to complete heart block if the AV node becomes damaged.

CASE 22 – ANSWERS

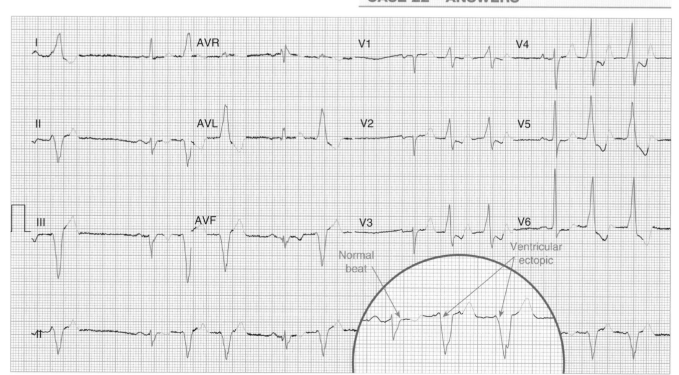

Present Your Findings

BASIC DETAILS
This is an anonymised ECG recorded at an unknown date and time.

I would like to ensure that this is calibrated to the usual 25 mm/s paper speed and 1 mV/cm gain.

KEY FEATURES
The most pertinent abnormality is the presence of multiple abnormal QRS complexes, each followed by an abnormal T wave.

HEART RATE AND RHYTHM
The heart rate is 72 bpm and is irregularly irregular. There are occasional sinus beats with P waves followed by QRS complexes, although most QRS complexes do not have a P wave preceding them.

CARDIAC AXIS
There is left-axis deviation (cardiac axis is between –30° and –90°).

PR AND QT INTERVAL
The PR interval in sinus beats is normal (between 120 and 200 ms) and the QT interval is normal (between 400 and 440 ms).

WAVE MORPHOLOGY
The P waves are normal in morphology.

There are occasional P waves followed by narrow QRS complexes, although most QRS complexes are wide (>120 ms) and followed by abnormal T waves. The ST segments and T waves show appropriate discordance, whereby they are directed in opposite directions to the QRS complex.

In Summary
Although there are sinus beats present, there are also multiple beats of wide QRS complexes with abnormal ST segment and T-wave morphology. As the wide QRS complex beats are not preceded by P waves, these appear to be ventricular ectopics.

A thorough history of her symptoms is required, particularly in view of her symptomatic presentation. This includes asking about chest pain, as myocardial ischaemia may present with frequent ventricular ectopics. Blood tests, including urea and electrolytes, calcium and magnesium, should be performed to rule out electrolyte abnormalities in addition to troponin levels. An echocardiogram should be arranged to assess ventricular function and presence of structural heart disease, and the patient referred to cardiology.

★ ANSWERS FOR CANDIDATES

1. What is the name for the condition where every third beat is a ventricular ectopic?
The correct answer is: (e) ventricular trigeminy.

An ECG in which every third beat is a ventricular ectopic is known as ventricular trigeminy.
- (a) Atrial bigeminy – incorrect: in atrial bigeminy every second beat is an atrial ectopic.
- (b) Atrial trigeminy – incorrect: in atrial trigeminy every third beat is an atrial ectopic.
- (c) Non-sustained ventricular tachycardia – incorrect: non-sustained ventricular tachycardia is the name given to a run of between three and 30 beats of ventricular origin.
- (d) Ventricular bigeminy – incorrect: in ventricular trigeminy every second beat is a ventricular ectopic.
- **(e) Ventricular trigeminy – correct: ventricular trigeminy is the name given when every third beat is a ventricular ectopic, as is the case in this ECG.**

Key Points
If either atrial or ventricular ectopics occur regularly then they are referred to as bigeminy, trigeminy or quadrigeminy (depending on whether the ectopics are every second, third or fourth beats, respectively). Ventricular ectopics may also occur as couplets if two occur together and runs of between three and 30 are known as non-sustained ventricular tachycardia.

2. In which of the following conditions may ventricular ectopic beats induce other arrhythmias?
The correct answers are: (d) ischaemic heart disease; and (e) Wolff–Parkinson–White.

Ventricular ectopics are usually benign, although they can trigger arrhythmias in certain conditions.
- (a) Aortic stenosis – incorrect: aortic stenosis alone would not give a risk of complications from ventricular ectopics.
- (b) Atrial fibrillation – incorrect: a ventricular ectopic would cause no complications in a patient with atrial fibrillation.
- (c) Cor pulmonale – incorrect: cor pulmonale is right-sided heart failure secondary to pulmonary disease. Provided there were no significant structural changes in the heart, ventricular ectopics would be benign in cor pulmonale.
- **(d) Ischaemic heart disease – correct: the dead tissue in a heart with severe ischaemic heart disease could conduct the electrical current from a ventricular ectopic abnormally and, depending on the location of the dead tissue, there could be a risk of re-entrant tachycardia and monomorphic ventricular tachycardia.**
- **(e) Wolff–Parkinson–White – correct: in patients with WPW, the electrical current from a ventricular ectopic may pass through the accessory pathway and trigger a re-entrant tachycardia.**

Key Points

Ventricular ectopics are relatively common and ordinarily there is no risk of complications. There is a slight risk of arrhythmias in people with accessory pathways, such as Wolff–Parkinson–White syndrome, or myocardial infarction. In these patients, a ventricular ectopic may initiate a re-entrant tachycardia. However, the presence of frequent ventricular ectopics, as in this case, should direct investigations with an echocardiogram and cardiac MRI to ensure there is no underlying structural heart disease.

3. Which of the following would a patient with a long QTc be at risk of developing from frequent ventricular ectopics?

The correct answers are: (d) torsades de pointes; and (e) ventricular fibrillation.

If a patient with a long QTc has frequent ventricular ectopics, s/he is at risk of developing ventricular tachyarrhythmias.

(a) Asystole – incorrect: asystole results from a complete lack of electrical activity in the heart. There is no risk of a ventricular ectopic causing this.

(b) Bundle branch block – incorrect: ventricular ectopics do not cause bundle branch blocks.

(c) Pulseless electrical activity – incorrect: in PEA there is normal electrical activity in the heart but there is no pulse. A ventricular ectopic can

disrupt the electrical activity in a patient with a long QTc, so this is incorrect.

(d) **Torsades de pointes – correct: in a patient with a long QTc, there is a risk that the R wave of a ventricular ectopic will fall on the T wave of the preceding normal beat. This is known as 'R on T phenomenon' and can cause ventricular tachyarrhythmias due to disruption of ventricular electrical activity. One example of a tachyarrhythmia caused by this is torsades de pointes.**

(e) **Ventricular fibrillation – correct: as with torsades de pointes, VF is a ventricular tachyarrhythmia that can be caused by the R on T phenomenon, so patients with a long QTc are at increased risk of this.**

 Key Points

As well as patients with an accessory pathway, patients with a long QTc are at risk of arrhythmia if they have frequent ventricular ectopics. If the R wave of a ventricular beat falls on the T wave of the preceding beat, then a ventricular tachyarrhythmia may occur, such as torsades de pointes of ventricular fibrillation. This is more likely to occur if repolarisation is prolonged, as represented by the long QTc interval.

CASE 23 – ANSWERS

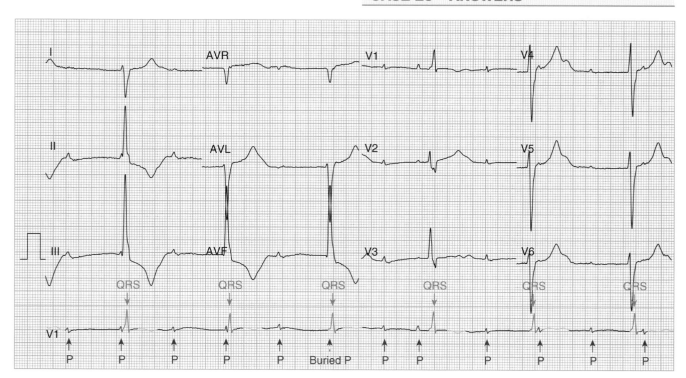

Present Your Findings

BASIC DETAILS

This is an anonymised ECG recorded at an unknown date and time.

I would like to ensure that this is calibrated to the usual 25 mm/s paper speed and 1 mV/cm gain.

KEY FEATURES

The most pertinent abnormalities are the slow heart rate and absence of a relationship between the P waves and the QRS complexes.

HEART RATE AND RHYTHM

The patient is bradycardic with a heart rate of 36 bpm. There is dissociation of atrial and ventricular activity with an atrial rate of approximately 70 bpm.

CARDIAC AXIS

There is right-axis deviation (cardiac axis is between +90° and +180°).

PR AND QT INTERVAL

The PR interval is impossible to assess as there is no relationship between the P waves and the QRS complexes. The QT interval is normal (between 400 and 440 ms).

WAVE MORPHOLOGY

P waves are normal in morphology. QRS complexes are wide (>120 ms) and followed by appropriate ST and T-wave discordance, whereby they are directed in opposite directions to the QRS complex.

In Summary

The atrioventricular dissociation and bradycardia in this ECG are supportive of complete heart block. This occurs as no atrial activity is conducted to the ventricles, so there is no relationship between P waves and QRS complexes.

The wide QRS complex and abnormal T waves suggest an underlying ventricular source of rhythm. The ST and T waves are appropriately discordant to the QRS complex; there is ST depression and T-wave inversion when the R wave is dominant, while ST elevation and upright T waves are present when the S wave is dominant.

The patient's fall may have occurred because of the complete heart block, especially given his bradycardia. Given the history of syncope and the wide ventricular escape rhythm, the patient should be reviewed urgently by Cardiology and be considered for an emergency pacemaker. Concurrent investigations should include an echocardiogram and blood tests for electrolytes (including potassium, calcium and magnesium) and thyroid function.

★ **ANSWERS FOR CANDIDATES**

1. Why are there still QRS complexes in complete heart block?

The correct answers are: (c) the AV node can generate an escape rhythm; and (e) the ventricles can generate an escape rhythm.

Both the AV node and the ventricles are able to generate an escape rhythm to maintain cardiac output if conduction is disrupted.

(a) Conduction through the AV node still occurs but is just delayed – incorrect: the definition of complete heart block is that no conduction occurs through the AV node.

(b) P waves are sporadically conducted through the AV node – incorrect: as above, in complete heart block, there is no conduction between the atria and the ventricles.

(c) **The AV node can generate an escape rhythm – correct: the AV node is capable of generating an escape rhythm known as a 'junctional escape rhythm'. This typically has a rate of 40–60 bpm.**

(d) There are accessory pathways between the atria and the ventricles – incorrect: there is no conduction between the atria and the ventricles via the AV node or any accessory pathways in complete heart block.

(e) **The ventricles can generate an escape rhythm – correct: similarly to the AV node, the ventricles are capable of generating their own 'escape rhythm' of about 20–40 bpm. This allows contraction to continue despite no conduction through the AV node.**

 Key Points

The definition of complete heart block is that there is no conduction between the atria and the ventricles. An ECG with complete heart block will still show P waves but these will not be related to the QRS complexes. The QRS are present because both the AV node and the ventricles can generate 'escape rhythms' to stimulate ventricular contraction despite the absence of atrioventricular conduction. These are typically quite slow, at between 40–60 and 20–40 bpm, respectively.

---

2. Which of the following are causes of complete heart block?

The correct answers are: (a) digoxin toxicity; (c) Lev disease; (d) Inferior myocardial infarction; and (e) septal myocardial infarction.

There are multiple causes of complete heart block.

(a) **Digoxin toxicity – correct: digoxin acts by slowing conduction at the AV node. If digoxin levels become too high, conduction at the AV node can be completely prevented, producing complete heart block.**

(b) Hyperkalaemia – incorrect: hyperkalaemia does not interfere with conduction at the AV node and therefore does not cause complete heart block.

(c) **Lev disease – correct: Lev disease is idiopathic fibrosis of the conducting system of the heart, leading to complete heart block. It is most commonly seen in the elderly.**

(d) **Inferior myocardial infarction – correct: An inferior MI can affect the conducting system of the heart.**

(e) **Septal myocardial infarction – correct:** a septal myocardial infarction would damage the conducting system and could cause complete heart block.

The most common causes of complete heart block are ischaemia, drugs and fibrosis.

---

3. If complete heart block is symptomatic, what treatment may be required?

The correct answers are: (a) atropine; (c) permanent pacemaker insertion; and (e) transcutaneous pacing.

Patients with symptomatic complete heart block require stabilising if they are haemodynamically unstable, and then permanent pacemaker insertion is the definitive treatment.

(a) **Atropine – correct:** in the acute phase, atropine can be used to treat bradycardias resulting from complete heart block. Atropine decreases vagal stimulation on the AV node, so can increase conductivity. This is a temporary measure and only used in the acute phase.

(b) **No treatment required – incorrect:** complete heart block has a high risk of asystole and sudden cardiac death, so urgent treatment is required.

(c) **Permanent pacemaker insertion – correct:** the definitive treatment for complete heart block is a dual-chamber pacemaker. This can deliver an electrical impulse to the ventricles if it senses a long pause in heart rate, thereby reducing the risk of ventricular asystole.

(d) **Regular outpatient follow-up with no acute treatment – incorrect:** there is a high risk of sudden cardiac death with complete heart block, so treatment is required.

(e) **Transcutaneous pacing – correct:** transcutaneous pacing is a temporary measure that can be used to treat acute complete heart block that is causing haemodynamic compromise.

1₂₃ Key Points

Patients symptomatic with complete heart block are likely to suffer haemodynamic compromise. Atropine and transcutaneous pacing can be used acutely to stabilise the patient before admitting him for monitoring. The definitive treatment of complete heart block is permanent pacemaker insertion in view of the high risk of asystole and death.

CASE 24 – ANSWERS

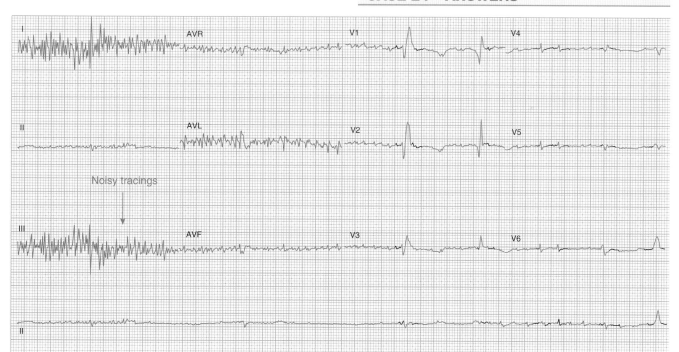

Present Your Findings

BASIC DETAILS
This is an anonymised ECG recorded at an unknown date and time.

I would like to ensure that this is calibrated to the usual 25 mm/s paper speed and 1 mV/cm gain.

KEY FEATURES
The obvious abnormality of this ECG is an irregular baseline in all leads.

HEART RATE AND RHYTHM
The heart rate is hard to assess due to the irregular baseline but appears to be around 60 bpm.

CARDIAC AXIS
The axis is impossible to assess.

PR AND QT INTERVAL
The intervals are impossible to assess due to the irregular baseline obscuring many of the waves.

WAVE MORPHOLOGY
Morphology of the P and T waves is difficult to assess. The QRS complexes are narrow and of normal amplitude.

In Summary
This is an ECG with an irregular baseline. While this makes the ECG difficult to assess, other than this it appears grossly normal. There are multiple possible causes for this; a repeat ECG would be beneficial to interpret the trace more accurately and guide further management, although this should not delay other urgent investigations.

★ ANSWERS FOR CANDIDATES

1. Which of the following are possible causes for an irregular baseline in this patient's ECG?
The correct answers are: **(b) confusion/agitation; (c) electrical interference from nearby equipment; and (d) hypothermia.**

There are multiple possible causes for an irregular baseline on an ECG.

(a) Acute MI – incorrect: an acute MI would not cause an irregular baseline on an ECG. ECG changes associated with acute MI include ST elevation, ST depression, T-wave inversion and Q waves.

(b) **Confusion/agitation – correct: an ECG does not specifically record electrical activity in the heart. Activity in muscles is also recorded on an ECG trace. While it is likely that an agitated patient would make large movements, an agitated patient may be unable to keep completely still and cause an irregular baseline due to muscle activity.**

(c) **Electrical interference from nearby equipment – correct: an ECG measures electrical activity. Nearby electrical machinery/equipment can** interfere with an ECG, especially if there is a problem with the plug preventing it from being grounded properly.

(d) **Hypothermia – correct: as described above, an ECG trace will pick up all muscle activity. Shivering is a response to hypothermia as the body tries to create heat and would show up on an ECG trace due to rapid muscle activity.**

(e) Rhabdomyolysis – incorrect: rhabdomyolysis is the breakdown of muscle fibres and their release into the blood. Following a long lie, this patient may be experiencing rhabdomyolysis; however, it would not cause these ECG changes. ECG changes in rhabdomyolysis may be those of hyperkalaemia, such as tented T waves.

Key Points
An ECG records electrical activity. While ECGs aim to record the electrical activity of the heart, it is not specific for this. Muscle contractions and nearby electrical equipment may also be picked up by an ECG and can make it very difficult to interpret. For this reason, a patient should lie as still as possible while an ECG is recorded.

2. What immediate further investigations will this patient require?
The correct answers are: **(b) bloods, including creatinine kinase and U&Es; and (c) CT head.**

Following a fall and possible long lie, a patient requires investigations, including bloods and, if indicated, a CT head.

(a) 24-h tape – incorrect: the cause of this patient's fall is unclear and it is possible that it was caused by cardiac syncope. A 24-h tape can be useful to pick up arrhythmias over a longer time than measured by a single 12-lead ECG; however, it is not urgent and should not be part of the immediate management.

(b) **Bloods, including creatinine kinase and U&Es – correct: it is likely that this patient has experienced a long lie. Creatinine kinase should be measured to assess whether she is experiencing rhabdomyolysis. Risks of rhabdomyolysis include acute kidney injury and hyperkalaemia, so U&Es should also be measured.**

(c) **CT head – correct: this patient has experienced a fall and is now acutely confused. This and the fact that the patient takes warfarin are indications for an urgent CT head to assess whether the confusion is caused by an intracranial haemorrhage.**

(d) CT pulmonary angiogram – incorrect: a CT pulmonary angiogram is indicated for investigation of a suspected pulmonary embolism. There is no indication that this patient has experienced a pulmonary embolism in this instance.

(e) Echocardiogram – incorrect: as with a 24-h tape, this may be indicated in the future if cardiac syncope is the suspected cause of this patient's fall. As such an echo may be indicated in the future, however, there are other investigations that should be performed more urgently.

 Key Points

Rhabdomyolysis is caused by muscle breakdown and the release of myoglobin, which can damage the kidneys. Creatine kinase is the most helpful investigation to identify this.

3. What should be done before repeating this patient's ECG?

The correct answers are: (a) attempt to make her more comfortable and less agitated; (d) slowly warm her up; and (e) turn off any nearby machinery/equipment.

There are various causes of an irregular baseline on an ECG. These causes should be corrected as much as possible before repeating the ECG to obtain a high-quality ECG.

(a) **Attempt to make her more comfortable and less agitated – correct: it may be difficult to obtain a high-quality ECG in an agitated patient as she is unlikely to lie still long enough to get a good-quality trace. Therefore, the patient's agitation should be minimised before repeating the ECG.**

(b) Change the ECG machine as it is likely to be faulty – incorrect: a faulty ECG machine is not usually the cause of an ECG with an irregular baseline. It should be ensured that the machine is calibrated correctly but it is not necessary to replace the machine.

(c) Give a beta-blocker to slow the heart rate – incorrect: this ECG shows an irregular baseline, not tachycardia. Indeed, if she were tachycardic, it would be important to acquire an accurate ECG trace before treating as the ECG will guide treatment.

(d) **Slowly warm her up – correct: this patient is hypothermic and the irregular baseline may be caused by shivering. A more accurate ECG will be obtained if she is warmed up and shivering is reduced.**

(e) **Turn off any nearby machinery/equipment – correct: another possible cause for this ECG is electrical interference. This can be minimised by turning off any nearby non-essential equipment before repeating the ECG.**

 Key Points

The causes of this ECG's irregular baseline should be addressed before repeating it. Muscle movements should be minimised; if the patient is agitated then she should be made comfortable to reduce agitation, and if she is shivering, she should slowly be warmed. If electrical interference is suspected, nearby equipment could be turned off to prevent this. Once all these steps have been done, the ECG should be repeated to obtain a higher-quality trace.

CASE 25 – ANSWERS

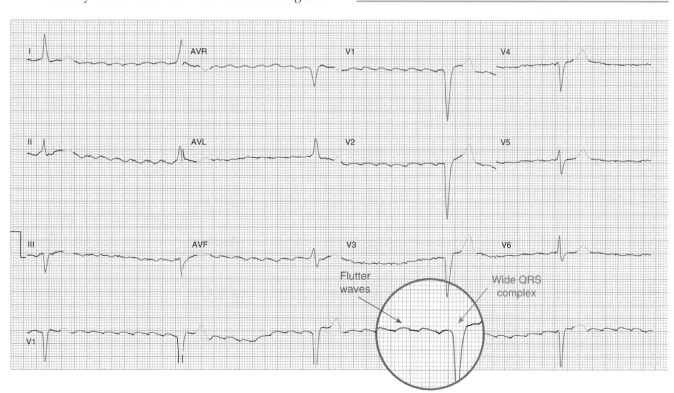

Present Your Findings

BASIC DETAILS
This is an anonymised ECG recorded at an unknown date and time.

I would like to ensure that this is calibrated to the usual 25 mm/s paper speed and 1 mV/cm gain.

KEY FEATURES
The most obvious abnormalities on this ECG are bradycardia, saw-tooth P waves and wide QRS complexes

HEART RATE AND RHYTHM
The rate is 30 bpm. There is a 'sawtooth' pattern of P waves and the QRS complexes are regular and slow.

CARDIAC AXIS
The axis is normal (between −30° and +90°).

PR AND QT INTERVAL
The PR interval cannot be assessed as there is no P wave. The QT interval is marginally prolonged at 480ms, but as there is profound bradycardia, the QTc is normal at 340ms.

WAVE MORPHOLOGY
'P' waves have a 'sawtooth' pattern. The QRS complexes are wide (>120 ms) and of normal amplitude. The ST segments and T waves are normal.

In Summary
This ECG shows a regular ventricular rhythm with wide QRS complexes. The 'sawtooth' pattern of P waves would be consistent with atrial flutter. This would suggest atrial flutter with complete heart block given the slow heart rate and wide QRS (ventricular escape rhythm).

It is important to find out what medication he is on and, as he is unsure, it may be necessary to contact his GP surgery to find out. The acute issue in this patient is the fall, so further assessments should be carried out regarding this. From a cardiac point of view it is important to ensure the bradycardia does not cause any haemodynamic compromise, so the patient requires continuous cardiac rhythm monitoring.

⭐ ANSWERS FOR CANDIDATES

1. Why are the QRS complexes wide?
The correct answer is: (a) he also has complete heart block.

This ECG shows both atrial flutter and complete heart block with a ventricular escape rhythm.

(a) **He also has complete heart block – correct: The wide QRS complexes suggests a ventricular origin of ventricular depolarisation and, therefore, a ventricular escape rhythm. These rhythms are usually slow which is what is seen on this ECG.**

(b) He has been successfully rhythm-controlled – incorrect: once atrial flutter has been rhythm-controlled the ECG will show normal sinus rhythm. This ECG does not show sinus rhythm, so he has not been successfully rhythm-controlled.

(c) He has had electrophysiological ablation – incorrect: similar to rhythm control, successful electrophysiological ablation will give an ECG showing normal sinus rhythm.

(d) The man was wrong about his previous diagnosis – incorrect: this ECG does show atrial flutter with 'sawtooth' pattern of P waves.

(e) The atrial flutter is paroxysmal – incorrect: the man has flutter waves at the time of this ECG, so the atrial flutter being paroxysmal does not explain the regular QRS complexes.

Key Points
This patient has atrial flutter as evidenced by the 'saw-tooth' pattern of P waves in the ECG. The slow and wide QRS complexes suggests a ventricular escape rhythm due to complete heart block.

2. Based on this ECG, which of the following drugs is this patient most likely to be taking?
The correct answer is: (c) digoxin.

Digoxin has many side effects, including complete heart block.

(a) Amiodarone – incorrect: amiodarone is usually used for rhythm control and this patient has not been successfully rhythm-controlled, making other drugs more likely.

(b) Amlodipine – incorrect: this is mainly used as an antihypertensive rather than for rate control and is unlikely to cause complete heart block.

(c) **Digoxin – correct: digoxin can be used to rate control atrial flutter. Digoxin decreases conduction through the atrioventricular (AV) node and digoxin toxicity can cause complete heart block. Therefore, this patient could have atrial flutter combined with digoxin toxicity.**

(d) Pravastatin – incorrect: pravastatin, a statin, can cause muscle toxicity but is not commonly known to cause conduction blocks.

(e) Ramipril – incorrect: ramipril is an angiotensin-converting enzyme inhibitor that can be used for hypertension. However, it is unlikely to cause complete heart block.

Key Points
There are multiple drugs that can be used to rate control a patient with atrial flutter. Digoxin is a commonly used drug and it works by reducing conduction through the AV node by inhibiting sodium-potassium ATPase. In fast atrial flutter, this has the desired effect of reducing heart rate. However, if conduction is inhibited too much (digoxin toxicity), AV node conduction could be completely blocked and result in complete heart block.

3. If he is not already on an equivalent medication, which of the following medications would it be most appropriate to start this patient on?

The correct answer is: (b) apixaban.

It is important that patients with atrial flutter are anticoagulated to reduce the risk of stroke.

(a) Amiodarone – incorrect: amiodarone can be used to rhythm control patients in atrial flutter but this is not the top priority in this patient, who has presented with a stroke.

(b) **Apixaban – correct: apixaban is a direct oral anticoagulant (DOAC) that can be used in this patient once haemorrhagic stroke is excluded. DOACs have been shown in several studies to be at least as effective as warfarin at preventing strokes in patients with atrial flutter and they have a lower risk of bleeding. They also do not require monitoring, whereas warfarin requires occasional international normalised ratio (INR) checks, even when patients are well established on the therapy. The only downside of DOACs compared to warfarin is that most of them do not have antidotes, whereas warfarin does (vitamin K). The other DOACs are rivaroxaban, edoxaban and dabigatran.**

(c) Aspirin – incorrect: aspirin is an antiplatelet agent. It does not provide sufficient anticoagulation to prevent strokes in patients with atrial flutter.

(d) Clopidogrel – incorrect: clopidogrel is also an antiplatelet agent. Even combined with aspirin, antiplatelets are not sufficient to prevent strokes in atrial flutter.

(e) Low-molecular-weight heparin – incorrect: anticoagulation is very important to prevent strokes in atrial fibrillation. Treatment dose low-molecular-weight heparin (as opposed to prophylactic dose) is effective at preventing strokes but it is not ideal for long-term use as it must be injected subcutaneously.

1 2 3 Key Points

Patients with atrial flutter are at increased risk of stroke as the lack of coordinated atrial contractions can lead to blood pooling and thrombus formation in the atria. This thrombus can then become dislodged, travel to the brain and cause a stroke. The CHA_2DS_2-VASc score can be used to calculate a patient's risk of stroke and anybody with a score ≥1 (≥2 in females) should be initiated on anticoagulation. Studies have shown that DOACs are just as effective as warfarin at preventing stroke, have a lower risk of bleeding and do not require regular monitoring.

CASE 26 – ANSWERS

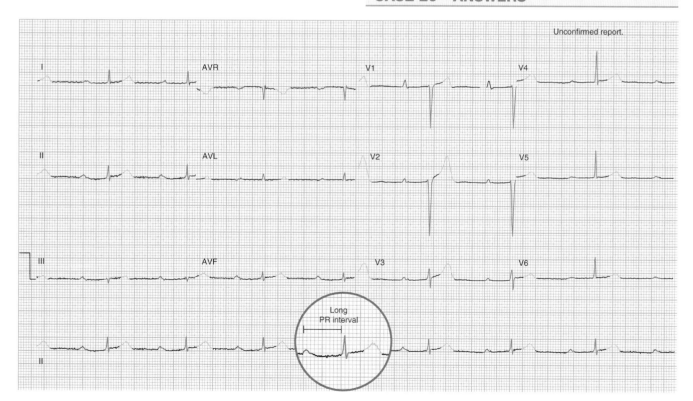

Present Your Findings

BASIC DETAILS

This is an anonymised ECG recorded at an unknown date and time.

I would like to ensure that this is calibrated to the usual 25 mm/s paper speed and 1 mV/cm gain.

KEY FEATURES

The obvious abnormality on this ECG is a prolonged PR interval.

HEART RATE AND RHYTHM

The heart rate is 48 bpm with a sinus rhythm.

CARDIAC AXIS

The axis is normal (between –30° and +90°).

PR AND QT INTERVAL

The PR interval is 400 ms, which is prolonged. The QT interval is normal (360 ms).

WAVE MORPHOLOGY

The P waves are normal in morphology. The QRS complexes are narrow and of normal amplitude. The ST segments and T waves are normal.

In Summary

This is an ECG that shows first-degree heart block (an increased PR interval). While this may be asymptomatic and is likely not relevant to this patient's acute presentation, it may be useful to take a thorough history to assess the cause and whether treatment for it is necessary. Although it is unlikely that this will need urgent intervention, it should be discussed with the anaesthetist before taking the patient to theatre.

★ ANSWERS FOR CANDIDATES

1. What is the normal PR interval?

The correct answer is: (b) 0.12–0.20 s.

The normal PR interval is between 0.12 and 0.20 s.

(a) 0.10–0.15 s – incorrect: a PR interval of 100 ms would be slightly shorter than expected, which could suggest pre-excitation. A PR interval of 150 ms would be normal but a longer PR interval would also be within normal limits.

(b) 0.12–0.20 s – correct: the normal PR interval is between 120 and 200 ms. This is equivalent to between 3 and 5 small squares on a trace calibrated to 25 mm/s.

(c) 0.15–0.25 s – incorrect: while a PR interval of 150 ms is within normal limits, a PR interval of 250 ms would be abnormally long.

(d) 0.20–0.30 s – incorrect: the upper limit of a normal PR interval is 200 ms. Any longer than this is considered to be first-degree heart block. A PR interval of 300 ms would be abnormally long.

(e) 0.30–0.38 s – incorrect: the upper limit of a normal PR interval is 200 ms. A PR interval of between 300 and 380 ms would be extremely prolonged and would be classified as first-degree heart block.

Key Points

The PR interval is the time between the start of the P wave and the start of the subsequent QRS complex. This should be between 0.12 and 0.20 s, or 3–5 small squares. Any less than this can indicate pre-excitation, while longer than this is first-degree heart block.

2. Which of the following can cause first-degree heart block?

The correct answers are: (a) athletic training; (b) digoxin; and (c) electrolyte disturbances.

There are multiple causes of first-degree heart block, including physiological changes.

(a) **Athletic training – correct: it is not unusual to see first-degree heart block in athletic people. This is completely normal in isolation.**

(b) **Digoxin – correct: digoxin works by blocking the atrioventricular (AV) node. It delays conduction through the AV node, which can cause first-degree heart block.**

(c) **Electrolyte disturbances – correct: electrolyte disturbances, such as hyperkalaemia, can interfere with normal conduction through the AV node and cause first-degree heart block.**

(d) Pericarditis – incorrect: inflammation of the pericardium would not affect conduction through the AV node and would not cause heart block.

(e) Posterior myocardial infarction – incorrect: a posterior MI would not be expected to cause heart block. An inferior MI could cause AV heart block.

Key Points

There are multiple causes of first-degree heart block and some of them are physiological. First-degree heart block can be seen as a normal variant in young healthy people. Causes include:

- Increased vagal tone (e.g. athletic training)
- Inferior MI
- Myocarditis
- Electrolyte disturbances (hyperkalaemia)
- Drugs that block the AV node:
  - Digoxin
  - Calcium channel blockers
  - Beta-blockers
  - Amiodarone

3. Assuming this patient has no underlying heart disease, what treatment is indicated?

The correct answer is: (d) no treatment.

First-degree heart block is usually benign and does not require treatment.

(a) Atropine – incorrect: atropine is an antimuscarinic agent that decreases the effects of the parasympathetic nervous system on the heart. Atropine is indicated in the treatment of bradycardias.

(b) Dual-chamber pacemaker – incorrect: a dual-chamber pacemaker is indicated in conditions where there is no conduction between the atria and the ventricles (such as complete heart block). In first-degree heart block, there is still conduction between the atria and the ventricles.

(c) Catheter ablation – incorrect: catheter ablation can be used to ablate accessory pathways, such

as those causing atrial fibrillation or atrioventricular re-entrant tachycardia. It does not play a role in improving AV node function.

(d) **No treatment – correct: if there is no underlying heart disease, first-degree heart block alone does not require treatment and is asymptomatic.**

(e) Ventricular pacemaker – incorrect: a ventricular pacemaker is indicated in certain conditions where the ventricles do not receive electrical current from the atria. It is not indicated in this condition.

Key Points

In the absence of underlying heart disease, treatment of first-degree heart block is not usually required.

CASE 27 – ANSWERS

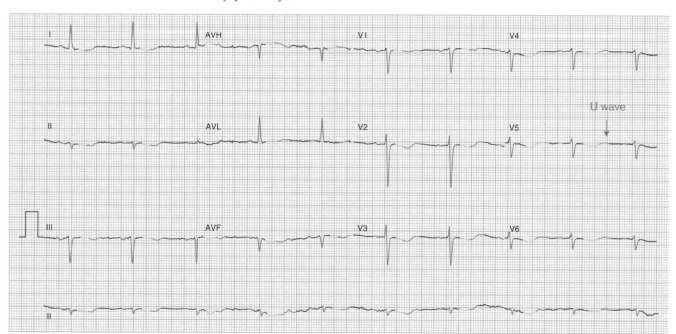

Present Your Findings

BASIC DETAILS

This is an anonymised ECG recorded at an unknown date and time.

I would like to ensure that this is calibrated to the usual 25 mm/s paper speed and 1 mV/cm gain.

KEY FEATURES

The most obvious abnormalities in this ECG are the presence of U waves in multiple leads and widespread T-wave flattening.

HEART RATE AND RHYTHM

The heart rate is 60 bpm with a sinus rhythm.

CARDIAC AXIS

The axis is normal (the combination of positive lead I, negative aVF and equivocal lead II puts the axis between 0° and +30°).

PR AND QT INTERVAL

The PR interval is normal (160 ms) and the QT interval is difficult to assess due to T-wave flattening but appears around 440 ms.

WAVE MORPHOLOGY

The P waves are normal in morphology. The QRS complexes are narrow and of normal amplitude. There is T-wave flattening in all leads. Additionally, there are U waves present, most apparent in leads V_1, V_2 and V_3.

In Summary

This is an ECG showing flattened T waves and the presence of U waves. These are signs of hypokalaemia, which is consistent with the patient's history of vomiting and diarrhoea. Due to its risk of complications, hypokalaemia requires urgent treatment. Further investigations, including full blood count, urea and electrolytes (U&E) and C-reactive protein, should be arranged and treatment for hyperkalaemia initiated.

★ ANSWERS FOR CANDIDATES

1. Which of the following would be appropriate in the initial management of this patient?

The correct answers are: **(a) bloods, including U&Es and magnesium; (d) IV fluids, including potassium chloride; and (e) IV magnesium replacement.**

Management of hypokalaemia includes both the measurement and replacement of potassium and magnesium.

(a) Bloods, including U&Es and magnesium – correct: this patient's ECG shows signs of hypokalaemia, so it is important to measure the potassium. Venous or arterial blood gas can give a rapid reading, although this is less accurate than a biochemistry sample sent to the laboratory. Hypokalaemia may be associated with hypomagnesaemia, so an accurate measure of both the potassium and magnesium is necessary.

(b) Give calcium gluconate 10% – incorrect: calcium gluconate is used to protect from arrhythmias in hyperkalaemia. It is not used to treat hypokalaemia.

(c) Give IV insulin and dextrose 20% – incorrect: as above, this is used to treat hyperkalaemia. Insulin shifts potassium from the extracellular fluid into cells, thus decreasing serum potassium.

(d) IV fluids, including potassium chloride – correct: in moderate or severe hypokalaemia, or in a patient who is not drinking, IV potassium should be given.

(e) IV magnesium replacement – correct: if there is hypomagnesaemia, it is very difficult to rectify the hypokalaemia without also rectifying the hypomagnesaemia. Low magnesium levels should be treated with IV magnesium replacement.

Key Points

Do not forget to check magnesium in a patient with very low potassium, or whose low potassium is not responding to treatment. Low magnesium increases renal excretion of potassium, meaning it is very hard to correct hypokalaemia without also correcting hypomagnesaemia.

2. Which of the following are complications of hypokalaemia?

The correct answers are: **(b) supraventricular tachycardia; (c) torsades de pointes; (d) ventricular fibrillation; and (e) ventricular tachycardia.**

Complications of hypokalaemia include both supraventricular and ventricular tachyarrhythmias.

(a) Left bundle branch block – incorrect: new left bundle branch block can be a sign of myocardial infarction. It is not a sign of hypokalaemia.

(b) Supraventricular tachycardia – correct: hypokalaemia can cause supraventricular tachycardia, such as atrial fibrillation/flutter.

(c) Torsades de pointes – correct: hypokalaemia can cause ventricular tachyarrhythmias, such as torsades de pointes.

(d) Ventricular fibrillation – correct: ventricular fibrillation is another ventricular tachyarrhythmia that can be caused by severe hypokalaemia.

(e) Ventricular tachycardia – correct: ventricular tachycardia is a ventricular tachyarrhythmia that can be caused by severe hypokalaemia.

Key Points

The possibility of developing severe arrhythmias is the reason why hypokalaemia is dangerous and requires urgent management. The most concerning of these is ventricular tachyarrhythmias, which can cause severe haemodynamic compromise and cardiac arrest.

3. Which of the following are risk factors for hypokalaemia?

The correct answers are: (a) burns; (b) diarrhoea; (c) hypomagnesaemia; and (d) increased sweating.

There are multiple risk factors for hypokalaemia. Most causes include increased loss of potassium from the body.

(a) **Burns – correct: the skin is an important barrier in regulating electrolyte balance in the body. Burns victims can rapidly lose large amounts of fluid and electrolytes over the area where this barrier is damaged. This can lead to many electrolyte imbalances, including hypokalaemia.**

(b) **Diarrhoea – correct: as is the case with the above patient, people with diarrhoea are at risk of hypokalaemia. They lose large volumes of fluid and electrolytes (including potassium) through their stools and this excess excretion of potassium can cause levels in the body to fall.**

(c) **Hypomagnesaemia – correct: low magnesium levels lead to increased excretion of potassium by the kidneys.**

(d) **Increased sweating – correct: similarly to patients with burns, excess sweating can cause increased fluid and electrolyte loss via the skin. One of the electrolytes that can be lost is potassium, leading to hypokalaemia.**

(e) Vitamin D deficiency – incorrect: vitamin D deficiency can cause hypocalcaemia rather than hypokalaemia. Vitamin D does not have an effect on potassium.

[1,2,3] Key Points

As with many electrolytes, low potassium levels can be caused by decreased intake, increased loss or transcellular shift. Causes of hypokalaemia include:

- Decreased intake:
  - Poor dietary intake
  - Starvation
- Increased loss:
  - Diarrhoea
  - Vomiting
  - Increased sweating
  - Burns
  - Mineralocorticoid excess
  - Diuretics
- Transcellular shift:
  - Insulin
  - Beta-agonists
  - Respiratory/metabolic alkalosis

Additionally, it is important to remember that low magnesium levels cause increased renal excretion of potassium. This means that it is very hard to correct hypokalaemia without also correcting hypomagnesaemia.

CASE 28 – ANSWERS

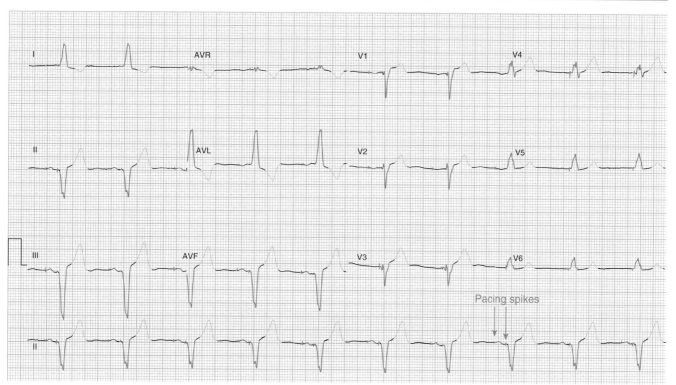

Present Your Findings

BASIC DETAILS

This is an anonymised ECG recorded at an unknown date and time.

I would like to ensure that this is calibrated to the usual 25 mm/s paper speed and 1 mV/cm gain.

KEY FEATURES

The obvious abnormality on this ECG is that there are multiple pacing spikes in all leads preceding both the P waves and QRS complexes.

HEART RATE AND RHYTHM

The heart rate is 60 bpm. The rhythm is regular with P waves before every QRS complex. However, there are pacing spikes before every P wave and every QRS complex.

CARDIAC AXIS

There is left-axis deviation (cardiac axis is between –30° and –90°).

PR AND QT INTERVAL

The PR interval is normal (200 ms). The QT interval is normal (440 ms).

WAVE MORPHOLOGY

The P waves are normal in morphology. Before every P wave and QRS complex, there is a single spike, consistent with a pacing spike. The QRS complexes are widened and there is evidence of left bundle branch block. The ST segments are normal. The T waves are normal.

In Summary

This is an ECG that shows a pacemaker in situ pacing both the P waves and QRS complexes. The ECG shows that the pacemaker is working well and, as the man is asymptomatic, there are no acute concerns regarding this patient.

★ **ANSWERS FOR CANDIDATES**

1. **Which chamber(s) are being paced?**

The correct answer is: **(d) right ventricle and one atrium.**

This ECG is consistent with pacing of the right ventricle and one atrium (it is impossible to tell which atrium). Right ventricular pacing produces a left bundle branch block pattern as the right ventricle is activated before the left ventricle.

(a) Both ventricles only – incorrect: biventricular pacing can produce a number of QRS morphologies. However, this ECG has pacing spikes before the P waves, indicating that the atrium is also paced.

(b) Left ventricle and one atrium – incorrect: if an atrium and the left ventricle were paced, there would be pacing spikes before the P waves and QRS complexes as well as a right bundle branch block. This ECG has a left bundle branch block.

(c) Left ventricle only – incorrect: if the left ventricle alone were paced, there would be pacing

spikes before the QRS complexes and right bundle branch block would be seen.

(d) **Right ventricle and one atrium – correct: this ECG shows pacing spikes before both P waves and QRS complexes, as well as left bundle branch block. This is consistent with a dual-chamber pacemaker in the right ventricle and one atrium.**

(e) Right ventricle only – incorrect: the right ventricle is paced and this can be seen by the pacing spikes preceding the QRS complexes that show left bundle branch block. However, there are also pacing spikes preceding the P waves, showing that an atrium is also paced.

 Key Points

There are two things to look for when assessing which chamber(s) are paced:

• Are there P waves following the pacing spikes? If yes, then an atrium is being paced. If not, then only a ventricle is being paced. In this case, there are both P waves and QRS complexes following the pacing spikes, so this pacemaker is pacing both an atrium and a ventricle.

• Check for the presence of a left or right bundle branch block. Ventricular pacemakers give the opposite bundle branch block to the ventricle they are in; a left ventricular pacemaker will give right bundle branch block, while a right ventricular pacemaker will give left bundle branch block.

2. **Which of the following is/are an indication for this type of pacemaker?**

The correct answers are: **(b) complete heart block; and (d) sick sinus syndrome.**

Both complete heart block and sick sinus syndrome are indications for a dual-chamber pacemaker.

(a) Atrial flutter – incorrect: a ventricular pacemaker may be used in this condition but it is not an indication for a dual-chamber pacemaker.

(b) **Complete heart block – correct: dual-chamber pacemaker insertion is indicated in patients with complete heart block.**

(c) Ischaemic heart disease – incorrect: ischaemic heart disease on its own is not an indication for pacemaker insertion.

(d) **Sick sinus syndrome – correct: dual-chamber pacing is indicated in sick sinus syndrome with impaired atrioventricular conduction. If there is no evidence of atrioventricular conduction delay, single-chamber atrial pacing could be considered, particularly if they are young.**

(e) Wolff–Parkinson–White – incorrect: Wolff–Parkinson–White is a type of re-entrant tachycardia characterised by the presence of an accessory pathway and episodes of tachyarrhythmia. Treatment options depend on whether the patient is haemodynamically stable but this does not include pacemaker insertion. If the patient is unstable, DC cardioversion is required acutely.

Key Points

Dual-chamber pacing is preferred in conditions where there is atrioventricular block and the atria are able to contract (unlike in atrial fibrillation/flutter). This gives a more physiological contraction of the heart, with the atria contracting first to maximise ventricular filling. Therefore, conditions such as complete heart block and sick sinus syndrome with atrioventricular block benefit from dual-chamber pacing by removing the risk of asystole and improving cardiac output.

3. Which of the following investigations should be routinely performed following pacemaker insertion?

The correct answers are: (c) chest X-ray; and (e) device check.

There are a number of investigations that should be performed following pacemaker insertion. Routine investigations are chest X-ray, to assess lead position and possible complications, as well as a device check to ensure correct pacing function.

(a) 24-h tape – incorrect: a 24-h ECG tape is performed to detect paroxysmal arrhythmias that may not be picked up on a single ECG. This may be used before pacemaker insertion to detect an arrhythmia that requires pacing, but it is not indicated after pacemaker insertion.

(b) Bloods, including CRP – incorrect: one possible complication of pacemaker insertion is infection. Bloods, including inflammatory markers such as CRP, are not routinely done post-procedure but can be used to assess for possible infection if clinically indicated.

(c) **Chest X-ray – correct: another potential complication of pacemaker insertion is pneumothorax. A chest X-ray should always be done following pacemaker insertion to rule out pneumothorax.**

(d) CT chest – incorrect: while a chest X-ray is necessary, a CT chest is not necessary. A chest X-ray is sufficient to detect pneumothorax and is a significantly lower dose of radiation.

(e) **Device check – correct: a device check is necessary after pacemaker insertion to assess that the pacemaker is functioning and able to generate electrical impulses that stimulate the heart to beat.**

Key Points

There are a number of complications related to pacemaker insertion, including lead dislodgement, pneumothorax and infection. Investigations should be carried out following insertion to assess whether these complications have occurred and to ensure that the pacemaker is able to function.

CASE 29 – ANSWERS

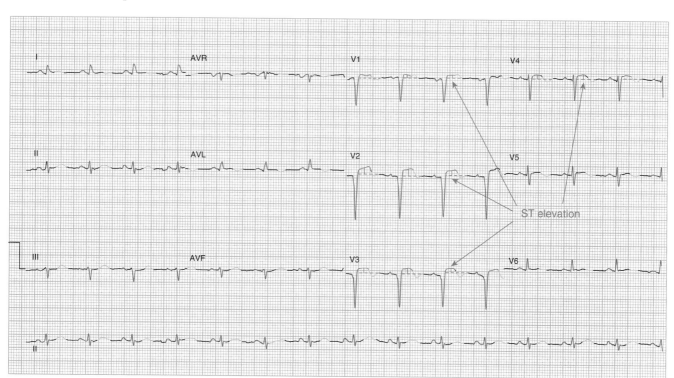

Present Your Findings

BASIC DETAILS
This is an anonymised ECG recorded at an unknown date and time.

I would like to ensure that this is calibrated to the usual 25 mm/s paper speed and 1 mV/cm gain.

KEY FEATURES
The obvious abnormality on this abnormality is prominent Q waves and ST elevation in leads V_1, V_2 and V_3.

HEART RATE AND RHYTHM
The heart rate is 90 bpm with a sinus rhythm.

CARDIAC AXIS
The axis is normal (between $-30°$ and $+90°$).

PR AND QT INTERVAL
The PR interval is normal (160 ms) and the QT interval is slightly shortened due to the tachycardia (280 ms).

WAVE MORPHOLOGY
The P waves are normal in morphology. The QRS complexes are narrow and of normal amplitude. There are large Q waves in leads V_1, V_2 and V_3. The ST segments are elevated ≥ 2 mm in V_1, V_2 and V_3 and T waves are normal.

 In Summary

This is an ECG showing ST elevation and deep Q waves in the anterior leads, V_1, V_2, and V_3. Given the patient's history of several days of chest pain, this is consistent with anterior infarction. Treatment for ACS should be started urgently, including dual antiplatelets and fondaparinux. If the patient had presented sooner, then urgent PCI would have also been considered; however, the presence of Q waves indicates that the infarcted myocardium is already dead, so revascularisation is unlikely to be of benefit. An angiogram +/- stenting should be considered in view of continuing symptoms. A cardiac MRI can also be useful to determine myocardial viability to assess the likelihood that revascularisation will be beneficial.

★ ANSWERS FOR CANDIDATES

1. What size of Q waves are the minimum to be considered significant?
The correct answer is: (b) 2 mm.

Q waves are only considered significant if they are greater in size than 2 mm.
   (a) 1 mm – incorrect: Q waves of 1 mm are too small to be considered significant.
   (b) 2 mm – correct: Q waves of greater than 2 mm are considered significant.
   (c) 3 mm – incorrect: Q waves of 3 mm are above the threshold to be considered significant. While

they are significant, slightly smaller Q waves would also be considered significant.
   (d) 4 mm – incorrect: as above, Q waves of 4 mm are significant, but smaller Q waves are also significant.
   (e) 5 mm – incorrect: as above, Q waves of 5 mm would be very large, so much smaller Q waves would also be considered significant.

 Key Points

Q waves of at least 2 mm are considered significant. Q waves smaller than this can be normal if seen in most leads, but Q waves larger than this should not be seen in any leads except III and aVR.

2. Which of the following can cause significant Q waves?
The correct answers are: (b) cardiomyopathy; (c) lead misplacement; (d) previous ischaemia; and (e) rotation of the heart.

There are many causes of Q waves, including previous myocardial infarction.
   (a) Acute ischaemia – incorrect: ischaemic Q waves occur due to scarring from dead cardiac tissue. In acute ischaemia, the tissue has not yet died, so Q waves will not be seen.
   (b) Cardiomyopathy – correct: cardiomyopathies such as hypertrophic obstructive cardiomyopathy (HOCM) can give Q waves. These are typically seen in the lateral leads.
   (c) Lead misplacement – correct: if the upper limb leads are accidentally placed on the lower limbs, the QRS complexes will be inverted. Therefore, what would normally be R waves would appear as Q waves.
   (d) Previous infarction – correct: the dead tissue that is responsible for ischaemic Q waves typically takes a few hours to days to form. Therefore, previous infarction would produce Q waves.
   (e) Rotation of the heart – correct: if the heart is extremely rotated, the direction that current moves relative to the leads will be abnormal, so Q waves may be seen.

Key Points

There are multiple causes of Q waves, including HOCM, lead misplacement and rotation of the heart. It is important to remember that only old rather than acute myocardial infarcts will give Q waves. Ischaemia that has been ongoing for less than a few hours will not produce Q waves.

3. Which of the following are risk factors for this patient's presentation?

The correct answers are: (a) diabetes mellitus; (b) hypertension; (c) hypercholesterolaemia; (d) family history of ischaemic heart disease.

This patient has presented following a myocardial infarction, which has multiple risk factors.

(a) **Diabetes mellitus – correct: this patient has suffered a myocardial infarction. Diabetes is a risk factor for atheroma formation and ischaemic heart disease, particularly if blood sugars are not well controlled.**

(b) **Hypertension – correct: poorly controlled hypertension is another risk factor for ischaemic heart disease.**

(c) **Hypercholesterolaemia – correct: high cholesterol is a risk factor for atheroma formation and, consequently, increases the risk of ischaemic heart disease.**

(d) **Family history of ischaemic heart disease – correct: family history of ischaemic heart disease is a known risk factor for ischaemic heart disease.**

(e) Pulmonary artery hypertension – incorrect: pulmonary artery hypertension can cause cardiac conditions, such as cor pulmonale, but it does not directly increase the risk of ischaemic heart disease.

Key Points

Risk factors for ischaemic heart disease include:
- Diabetes mellitus
- Hypertension
- Hypercholesterolaemia
- Family history
- Smoking
- Obesity

Most of these risk factors can be modified to reduce an individual's risk of developing ischaemic heart disease or its risk of recurrence.

CASE 30 – ANSWERS

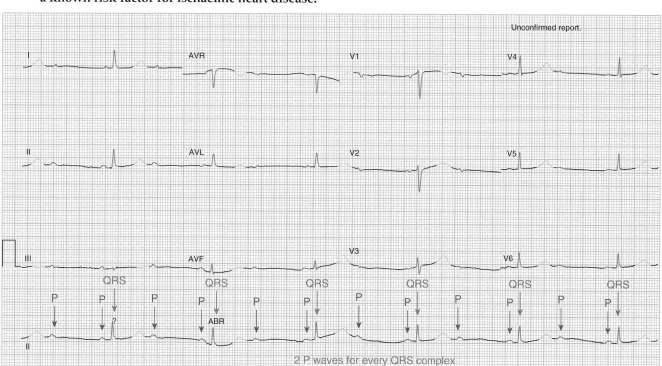

Present Your Findings

BASIC DETAILS
This is an anonymised ECG recorded at an unknown date and time.

I would like to ensure that this is calibrated to the usual 25 mm/s paper speed and 1 mV/cm gain.

KEY FEATURES
The obvious abnormality on this ECG is that every second P wave is not followed by a QRS complex.

HEART RATE AND RHYTHM
The heart rate is 36 bpm. Every QRS complex is preceded by a P wave, but every second P wave is not followed by a QRS complex.

CARDIAC AXIS
The axis is normal (between –30° and +90°).

PR AND QT INTERVAL
The PR interval is normal (160 ms) when a P wave is followed by a QRS complex. The QT interval is normal.

WAVE MORPHOLOGY
The P waves are normal in morphology. The QRS complexes are narrow and of normal amplitude. The ST segments and T waves are normal.

In Summary
This ECG shows every 2nd P wave not being followed by a QRS complex. This is 2:1 heart block, where there are 2 P waves for every 1 QRS complex. Associated with this, the ventricular rate is very low, which could account for this patient's presenting symptoms. As his heart rate was extremely low with the ambulance crew, this patient should be put on a cardiac monitor and be considered for cardiac pacing.

★ ANSWERS FOR CANDIDATES

1. Which of the following may be the site of the lesion in 2:1 heart block?
The correct answers are: (a) AV node; (b) bundle of His; and (c) Purkinje fibres.

2:1 heart block can be due to a lesion in either the AV node or the His–Purkinje conducting system.

(a) **AV node – correct: a lesion in the AV node can cause only alternate beats to conduct to the ventricles, producing 2:1 heart block.**
(b) **Bundle of His – correct: a lesion below the AV node in the bundle of His can cause only alternate beats to be conducted and lead to 2:1 heart block.**
(c) **Purkinje fibres – correct: a lesion in the Purkinje fibres can produce 2:1 heart block as only alternate beats may be conducted.**
(d) Sinoatrial node – incorrect: there is normal P-wave activity, showing that the sinoatrial node and the atria are functioning properly. The lesion is below the level of the sinoatrial node.

(e) Ventricular myocardium – incorrect: a lesion in the ventricular myocardium would not prevent conduction of P waves to QRS complexes, although it may change the morphology of the QRS complex or ST segment.

Key Points
Lesions in either the AV node or His–Purkinje system can cause 2:1 heart block. Since it is difficult to determine if the PR interval is prolonging or constant in 2:1 blocks, they are given a separate term to Mobitz I and Mobitz II blocks. Typically, AV node disease will produce a narrow QRS complex while a lesion in the His–Purkinje system will produce a wide QRS complex, although this is not always the case.

2. Which of the following treatment options may be appropriate in an asymptomatic patient with 2:1 heart block?
The correct answer is: (d) no treatment may be necessary.

2:1 block may require treatment with pacemaker insertion in symptomatic cases or if there is a high likelihood it may progress.

(a) Daily beta-blockers – incorrect: beta-blockers act to slow the heart rate, so would have no place in the management of this arrhythmia.
(b) DC cardioversion – incorrect: DC cardioversion can be used to treat tachyarrhythmias. 2:1 block is a pathology of either the AV node or the conducting system, neither of which would be treated by DC cardioversion.
(c) Cardiac catheter ablation – incorrect: ablation can be used to ablate aberrant conduction pathways in conditions such as atrial fibrillation of atrioventricular re-entrant tachycardia. As 2:1 block is not caused by the presence of an aberrant pathway, ablation is not indicated.
(d) **No treatment may be necessary – correct: If the 2:1 block is asymptomatic, no treatment may be needed, particularly if it is paroxysmal and nocturnal. However, the likelihood is that this will progress and therefore the patient needs to be aware of the symptoms to look out for, with a low threshold for a permanent pacemaker.**
(e) Permanent pacemaker insertion – incorrect: pacemaker insertion is indicated if a patient is symptomatic with AV conduction block. The patient in this case reports no symptoms.

Key Points
2:1 atrioventricular block can be a benign arrhythmia, particularly if the level of block is at the AV node, is paroxysmal, nocturnal and patients are asymptomatic. However, a pacemaker is indicated in symptomatic cases.

3. Which of the following would be the appropriate treatment for this patient?

The correct answers are: (b) isoprenaline infusion; (d) permanent pacemaker insertion; and (e) transcutaneous pacing before urgent permanent pacemaker insertion.

Symptomatic 2:1 heart block has a high risk of progression to complete heart block or ventricular standstill so requires permanent pacemaker insertion.

(a) Amiodarone infusion – incorrect: amiodarone infusion is useful in the treatment of tachyarrhythmias such as fast atrial fibrillation. It is not indicated in the treatment of 2:1 heart block.

(b) Isoprenaline infusion – correct: Isoprenaline is a non-selective beta-adrenoreceptor agonist used in the treatment of bradyarrhythmias and is indicated if the patient is haemodynamically unstable as a temporary measure whilst pacing is being considered.

(c) No treatment is necessary – incorrect: Symptomatic 2:1 heart block has a high risk of progression to complete heart block or even ventricular standstill, so treatment is necessary.

(d) Permanent pacemaker insertion – correct: due to the risk of developing complete heart block, symptomatic 2:1 heart block requires pacemaker insertion.

(e) Transcutaneous pacing before urgent permanent pacemaker insertion – correct: while this patient will require permanent pacemaker insertion, as he is haemodynamically unstable, he may require transcutaneous pacing to maintain adequate cardiac output until a permanent device can be inserted.

Key Points

There is a risk of 2:1 heart block progressing to complete heart block and ventricular standstill. In symptomatic cases, treatment is needed. Haemodynamically unstable patients should be treated as an emergency with inotropes, such as isoprenaline. Transcutaneous/transvenous pacing may also be indicated.

CASE 31 – ANSWERS

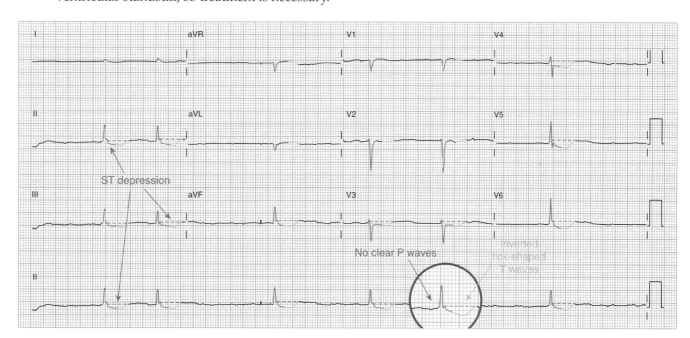

Present Your Findings

BASIC DETAILS
This is an anonymised ECG recorded at an unknown date and time.

    I would like to ensure that this is calibrated to the usual 25 mm/s paper speed and 1 mV/cm gain.

KEY FEATURES
The obvious abnormality in this ECG is widespread ST depression, and an irregularly irregular rhythm.

HEART RATE AND RHYTHM
The heart rate is 36 bpm and is irregularly irregular with no obvious P waves, suggesting atrial fibrillation.

CARDIAC AXIS
The axis is normal (between −30° and +90°).

PR AND QT INTERVAL
There are no P waves present. The QT interval is difficult to assess but appears normal (around 400 ms).

WAVE MORPHOLOGY
The P waves are normal in morphology. The QRS complexes are narrow and of normal amplitude. The ST segments are depressed in multiple leads and T waves are normal.

 In Summary

This is an ECG showing ST depression in multiple leads, and slow atrial fibrillation. The morphology of the ST depression is in keeping with the 'reverse tick' sign, which can be caused by digoxin use. This ECG, together with the patient's clinical features, could indicate digoxin toxicity.

    This patient has chronic kidney disease and is on a relatively high daily dose of digoxin. As digoxin is renally cleared, it is likely that levels in this patient have built up as her kidneys could not adequately excrete the drug. Urgent bloods, including a digoxin level (taken at least 6 h after last dose), should be sent to confirm this.

★ **ANSWERS FOR CANDIDATES**

1. What is the mechanism of action of digoxin?
The correct answer is: **(d) inhibition of Na$^+$/K$^+$-ATPase.**

    Digoxin acts by inhibiting Na$^+$/K$^+$-ATPase as well as stimulating the parasympathetic system.

(a) Activation of Na$^+$/K$^+$-ATPase – incorrect: digoxin acts on Na+/K+-ATPase but it inhibits rather than activates it.

(b) Activation of voltage-gated potassium channels – incorrect: digoxin does not act on these channels. Voltage-gated potassium channels are important in excitable cells in terminating the action potential as they return the depolarised cell to its resting voltage.

(c) Activation of voltage-gated sodium channels – incorrect: digoxin does not act on these channels. Voltage-gated sodium channels play an important role in excitable cells as they initiate the action potential by allowing sodium influx into the cell.

(d) **Inhibition of Na$^+$/K$^+$-ATPase – correct: Na$^+$/K$^+$-ATPase establishes the resting potential of cells. By inhibiting this, digoxin has two effects. Firstly, it increases the time it takes for the AV node to reset, delaying AV conduction. Secondly, it increases intracellular sodium, which inhibits sodium-dependent calcium transport out of cells. This increases intracellular calcium, which increases contractility of cardiac myocytes.**

(e) Inhibition of voltage-gated calcium channels – incorrect: digoxin does not affect these channels. Voltage-gated calcium channels play an important role in all types of muscle (smooth, striated and cardiac) in causing contraction.

 Key Points

Digoxin is a cardiac glycoside which acts by binding to Na$^+$/K$^+$-ATPase and inhibiting it. Inhibition of this enzyme increases the refractory period of cardiac myocytes, which decreases AV node conduction. This also increases intracellular sodium, which in turn inhibits sodium-dependent transport of calcium out of the cell. This increases intracellular calcium, which increases the contractility of cardiac myocytes. By these two mechanisms, digoxin both slows the heart rate in arrhythmias and increases cardiac contractility.

2. Which of these can be caused by digoxin toxicity?
The correct answers are: **(a) complete heart block; (b) hyperkalaemia; (d) ventricular fibrillation; and (e) xanthopsia.**

    Digoxin toxicity has multiple side effects, including arrhythmias and xanthopsia.

(a) **Complete heart block – correct: digoxin acts to decrease AV node conduction. In toxicity, this can be excessively decreased to produce bradycardias, including complete heart block.**

(b) **Hyperkalaemia – correct: Na$^+$/K$^+$-ATPase acts to transport sodium out of cells and potassium into cells. Disruption of this can increase extracellular potassium levels.**

(c) Hypokalaemia – incorrect: digoxin toxicity causes hyperkalaemia rather than hypokalaemia. However, hypokalaemia does exacerbate the effects of digoxin toxicity.

(d) **Ventricular fibrillation – correct: digoxin can cause several fatal arrhythmias, including ventricular fibrillation.**

(e) **Xanthopsia – correct: digoxin can cause xanthopsia, which is yellowing of vision. The** mechanism behind this is complex and not fully understood but involves disruption of cone cell function in the retina.

Digoxin toxicity can cause a wide range of symptoms. There are non-specific symptoms such as nausea, vomiting, diarrhoea and abdominal pain. Despite being an antiarrhythmic drug, its side effects include a wide range of both bradyarrhythmias and tachyarrhythmias, some of which can be fatal. Famously, it can also cause yellowing of the vision and there is speculation that the reason why many of the artist Vincent van Gogh later works are yellow is that he was taking digitalis and suffered from xanthopsia.

---

3. Which of the following are appropriate in the management of digoxin toxicity?

The correct answers are: (a) administration of digoxin-specific antibody; (b) discontinue digoxin; (d) intravenous calcium if hyperkalaemia is present; and (e) intravenous fluid resuscitation if hypotension is present.

There are multiple steps that should be undertaken in the management of digoxin toxicity depending on the severity of toxicity.

(a) **Administration of digoxin-specific antibody – correct:** in severe digoxin toxicity with evidence of end-organ damage, digoxin-specific antibody (e.g. Digibind) can be administered to bind digoxin rapidly and reduce its effects.

(b) **Discontinue digoxin – correct:** digoxin should immediately be discontinued if toxicity is suspected.

(c) Immediate transcutaneous pacing – incorrect: while this may be indicated in certain bradyarrhythmias caused by digoxin, digoxin toxicity alone is not an indication for transcutaneous pacing.

(d) **Intravenous calcium if hyperkalaemia is present – correct:** the use of intravenous (IV) calcium in digoxin toxicity is slightly controversial. Digoxin can cause hyperkalaemia; in hyperkalaemia, it is important to give IV calcium to protect against arrhythmias. It was previously thought that IV calcium was contraindicated in digoxin toxicity as digoxin increases intracellular calcium, so additional calcium could induce 'stone heart' – a non-contractile state in which the heart cannot relax. It is now felt that there is minimal evidence for this and the benefits of IV calcium far outweigh the risks if there is significant hyperkalaemia.

(e) **Intravenous fluid resuscitation if hypotension is present – correct:** if hypotension is present, IV fluids should be given to maintain blood pressure and end-organ perfusion.

Treatment of digoxin toxicity includes stopping digoxin and assessing the potassium level to check whether IV calcium is needed. In cases of severe toxicity with life-threatening arrhythmias, digoxin-specific antibody can be used.

CASE 32 – ANSWERS

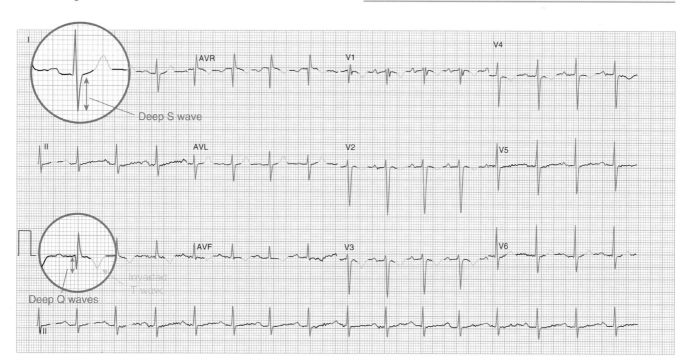

Deep S wave

Deep Q waves

Present Your Findings

BASIC DETAILS
This is an anonymised ECG of unknown date and time.

I would like to ensure that this is calibrated to the usual 25 mm/s paper speed and 1 mV/cm gain.

KEY FEATURES
The most pertinent abnormality is the $S_1Q_3T_3$ pattern, which is defined as an S wave in lead I, and Q wave and T wave in lead III, sinus tachycardia and T wave inversion in leads V_1-V_4.

HEART RATE AND RHYTHM
The heart rate is approximately 100 bpm with a regular sinus rhythm.

CARDIAC AXIS
The cardiac axis is normal (between –30° and +90°).

PR AND QRS INTERVAL
The PR interval is normal (200 ms), and the QT interval is normal (320 ms).

WAVE MORPHOLOGY
The P waves are of normal morphology. The QRS complexes are narrow and of normal amplitude. The ST segments are normal. There are T-wave inversions in the right precordial leads (V_1–V_4) as well as leads III and aVF.

In Summary

The history and ECG finding of $S_1Q_3T_3$, sinus tachycardia and T wave changes over the right ventricular chest leads (V_1-V_3) is consistent with right heart strain due to a pulmonary embolism (PE). The above history suggested multiple risk factors for provoked pulmonary embolism, including reduced mobility (post-orthopaedic surgery) and hypercoagulable state (recovering from surgery, contraceptive pill). Investigations should include routine blood tests, including full blood count, urea and electrolytes, C-reactive protein, clotting screen and (if Wells score is low) D-dimer. The above patient has a high Wells score and, thus, a D-dimer test is not needed prior to computed tomography pulmonary angiogram (CTPA). Imaging studies that are important to diagnose pulmonary embolism include chest X-ray and then CTPA or V/Q scan. Management includes anticoagulants (low-molecular-weight heparin then warfarin or novel oral anticoagulants) and reduction of risk factors for pulmonary embolism. Thrombolysis is indicated if the patient is haemodynamically unstable and has low bleeding risks.

★ ANSWERS FOR CANDIDATES

1. Which of the following is/are a risk factor(s) for developing pulmonary embolism?
The correct answers are: (b) malignancy; (c) oral contraceptive pills; and (d) polycythaemia.

Risk factors of pulmonary embolism are those defined by Virchow triad: increased blood hypercoagulability, increased stasis or intrinsic/extrinsic damage to the vessel wall.

(a) Diabetes mellitus – incorrect: diabetes does not cause a direct increase in the risk of pulmonary embolism. However, diabetes may cause vascular disease which may then increase the chance of blood clot formation.

(b) Malignancy – correct: underlying malignancy or active treatment of the malignancy can cause increased blood coagulability, and in addition to the reduced mobility, these can increase the risk of pulmonary embolism.

(c) Oral contraceptive pills – correct: oral contraceptive pills can cause increased blood coagulability and, consequently, increase the risk of pulmonary embolism. It is one of the side effects that needs to be taken into consideration before starting oral contraceptive pills.

(d) Polycythaemia – correct: polycythaemia causes blood to clot more easily and therefore increases the risk of developing pulmonary embolism.

(e) Previous myocardial infarction – incorrect: previous myocardial infarction does not directly increase the risk of pulmonary embolism.

Key Points

The main risk factors for pulmonary embolism can be categorised into three main causes according to Virchow triad: blood hypercoagulability, stasis and damage to the vessel wall.

Risk factors include:
- Surgery
- Pregnancy
- Reduced mobility
- Malignancy
- Previous venous thromboembolism
- Hypertension
- Congestive cardiac failure
- Combined oral contraceptive pills
- Haematological disorders
- Long-distance travel
- Obesity
- Inflammatory diseases, e.g. Behçet disease

2. Which of the following ECG changes can be produced by a pulmonary embolism?
The correct answers are: (a) deep S wave in lead I; (d) sinus tachycardia; (e) T-wave inversion in V_1–V_4.

The most common ECG change in pulmonary embolism is sinus tachycardia. It is important also to note the classical ECG pattern of $S_1Q_3T_3$.

(a) Deep S wave in lead I – correct: this is part of the classical $S_1Q_3T_3$ pattern, which is pathognomonic of pulmonary embolism. This refers to deep S waves in lead I along with Q waves and T-wave inversion in lead III.

(b) P mitrale – incorrect: pulmonary embolism produces P pulmonale due to increased pressure in the right atrium. P mitrale usually indicates left atrial hypertrophy.

(c) Peaked T wave – incorrect: pulmonary embolism usually causes T-wave inversion rather than T-wave peaking. Peaked T wave classically indicates hyperkalaemia.

(d) **Sinus tachycardia – correct: this is the commonest ECG abnormality among patients with pulmonary embolism.**

(e) **T-wave inversion in V_1–V_4 – correct: this represents increased right heart pressure and a right ventricular 'strain' pattern on ECG, which includes T-wave inversion and ST depression in V_1–V_4 and inferior leads.**

1_23 Key Points

ECG findings of pulmonary embolism reflect increased right heart pressures and may include:
- Sinus tachycardia: the commonest abnormality
- Right bundle branch block
- Right ventricular 'strain' pattern: T-wave inversion and ST depression in leads V_1–V_4, II, III, aVF
- Right-axis deviation
- P pulmonale
- $S_1Q_3T_3$ pattern: an uncommon finding that refers to deep S waves in lead I along with Q waves and T-wave inversion in lead III

---

3. Which of the following is/are true with regard to the management of pulmonary embolism?

The correct answers are: (a) CTPA is the gold-standard diagnostic tool for pulmonary embolism; (c) echocardiography may be used if pulmonary embolism is suspected; and (e) Wells score can be used as a probability scoring tool for diagnosing pulmonary embolism.

Pulmonary embolism is diagnosed using CTPA as gold standard. The D-dimer test is only indicated when there is a low Wells score. Patients with confirmed pulmonary embolism should be treated with anticoagulants, although thrombolytic treatment can be used in haemodynamically unstable patients.

(a) **CTPA is the gold-standard diagnostic tool for pulmonary embolism – correct: CTPA is** widely used to confirm the diagnosis of clinically suspected pulmonary embolism.

(b) D-dimer should be used to diagnose pulmonary embolism – incorrect: D-dimer is a sensitive but non-specific test. It can be raised in inflammatory condition and sepsis. Thus, it is not diagnostic of pulmonary embolism.

(c) **Echocardiography may be used if pulmonary embolism is suspected – correct: Besides CTPA, which is the gold standard to diagnose PE, echocardiography can sometimes be useful to demonstrate right heart strain due to a massive PE.**

(d) Thrombolytic therapy is only indicated in patients with acute pulmonary embolism with low bleeding risk who are haemodynamically stable – incorrect: thrombolytic therapy is only reserved for patients with acute pulmonary embolism who are haemodynamically unstable with a low bleeding risk.

(e) **Wells score can be used as a probability scoring tool to aid diagnosing pulmonary embolism – correct: Wells score can be used to help clinicians predict the probability of pulmonary embolism, thus aiding decision making when investigating pulmonary embolism.**

1_23 Key Points

The management of pulmonary embolism includes:
- Conservative: stop smoking, reduce alcohol
- Acute management: oxygen, intravenous fluids, unfractionated/low-molecular-weight heparin
- Haemodynamically unstable cases: thrombolytic therapy
- Percutaneous pulmonary embolectomy

CASE 33 – ANSWERS

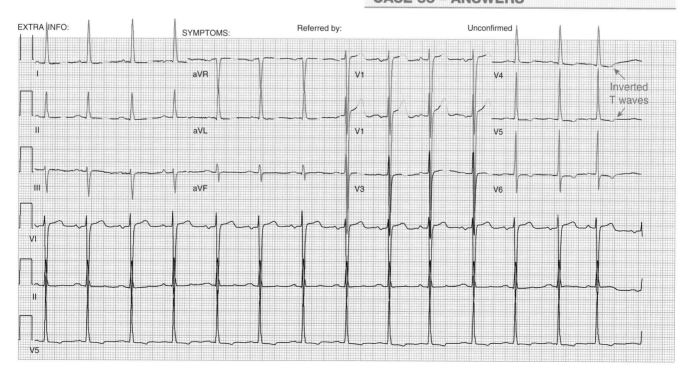

EXTRA INFO: SYMPTOMS: Referred by: Unconfirmed

I aVR V1 V4 Inverted T waves

II aVL V1 V5

III aVF V3 V6

VI

II

V5

Present Your Findings

BASIC DETAILS
This is an anonymised ECG of unknown date and time.
I would like to ensure that this is calibrated to the usual 25 mm/s paper speed and 1 mV/cm gain.

KEY FEATURES
The most pertinent abnormality is the large amplitude of QRS voltage complexes in leads V_1–V_6.

HEART RATE AND RHYTHM
The heart rate is 84 bpm with a regular sinus rhythm.

CARDIAC AXIS
The cardiac axis is normal (between −30° and +90°).

PR AND QRS INTERVAL
The PR interval is normal (120 ms), and the QT interval is normal (320 ms).

WAVE MORPHOLOGY
The P waves are normal in morphology. The QRS complexes are narrow and are of high amplitude. There is also T-wave inversion in V_4–V_6.

In Summary

This ECG is consistent with left ventricular hypertrophy. Her examination findings are consistent with mitral regurgitation, which may have led to symptoms of congestive heart failure. The patient also has risk factors for congestive cardiac failure in her past medical history, including hypertension, diabetes mellitus and ischaemic heart disease. In view of likely mitral regurgitation, a transthoracic echocardiogram should be arranged in addition to routine blood tests (including brain natriuretic peptide levels). Symptom management and treating the cause are key management points. In this case, congestive cardiac failure is likely to be secondary to mitral regurgitation. Hence, surgical management with mitral valve replacement may be offered if the patient's symptoms do not improve with diuretics.

★ **ANSWERS FOR CANDIDATES**

1. Which two of the following are the LEAST likely to be an aetiology of left ventricular hypertrophy?

The correct answer is: (d) mitral regurgitation; and (e) Mitral stenosis.

Left ventricular hypertrophy is usually caused by underlying heart conditions that cause pressure overload in the left ventricles.

(a) Aortic regurgitation – incorrect: the aortic valve is located between the left ventricle and aorta. Hence, when there is aortic regurgitation, there is more blood that returns back into the left ventricle during ventricular systole. This produces volume and pressure overload, which then leads to left ventricular hypertrophy.

(b) Aortic stenosis – incorrect: when the aortic valve is stenosed, the left ventricle will need to pump harder to maintain cardiac output, eventually causing ventricular hypertrophy.

(c) Hypertension – incorrect: when the systemic vascular resistance increases in cases of hypertension, the left ventricle will need to pump harder, leading to hypertrophy.

(d) **Mitral regurgitation – Correct: The mitral valve is located between the left atrium and left ventricle. When there is regurgitation of blood into the left atrium during ventricular systole, this causes increased volume in the left ventricle, usually leading to left ventricular dilatation rather than hypertrophy.**

(e) **Mitral stenosis – correct: when the mitral valve is stenosed, the left atrium will need to pump harder, eventually producing left atrial hypertrophy.**

Key Points

Causes of left ventricular hypertrophy include:
- Hypertension (commonest cause)
- Valvular defects: aortic stenosis, aortic regurgitation
- Coarctation of the aorta
- Hypertrophic cardiomyopathy

2. Which of the following ECG changes can be produced by left ventricular hypertrophy?

The correct answers are: (b) increased R-wave amplitude in V_6; and (c) left-axis deviation.

The most pertinent ECG change in left ventricular hypertrophy is an increase in the amplitude of S and R waves in V_1 and V_6, respectively. However, severe hypertrophy can lead to other ECG changes.

(a) Dominant R wave in V_1 – incorrect: this is observed in right ventricular hypertrophy.

(b) **Increased R-wave amplitude in V_6 – correct: V_6 represents the lateral lead and electrical changes of left ventricle. Thus, R-wave amplitude will be increased during ventricular systole when the left ventricle is hypertrophied.**

(c) **Left-axis deviation – correct: left ventricular hypertrophy can cause left-axis deviation, which can be seen as a more positive deflection of ECG waves in lead I compared to lead II.**

(d) Prolonged PR interval – incorrect: left ventricular hypertrophy has no impact on atrioventricular conduction.

(e) ST elevation in lateral leads – incorrect: ST depression occurs in leads V_5–V_6 in left ventricular strain.

Key Points

ECG changes in left ventricular hypertrophy include:
- Increased S-wave depth in leads V_1–V_3
- Increased R-wave amplitude in leads V_4–V_6
- Left-axis deviation
- T-wave inversion and ST depression in V_5–V_6

3. Which of the following statements is/are true regarding left ventricular hypertrophy?

The correct answers are: (a) a total sum of 22 mm from R-wave amplitude in aVL plus S-wave amplitude in V_3 indicates left ventricular hypertrophy; and (d) left ventricular hypertrophy may be a sign of left ventricular failure.

Left ventricular hypertrophy is usually the result of pressure overload in the left ventricle, resulting in increased R wave in left-sided ECG leads, and increased S-wave depth in right-sided leads.

(a) **A total sum of 22 mm from R-wave amplitude in aVL plus S wave amplitude in V_3 indicates left ventricular hypertrophy – correct: total amplitude greater than 20 mm in women indicates left ventricular hypertrophy.**

(b) Large ventricular amplitude is a normal finding in patients older than 45 years – incorrect: always investigate patients with large ventricular amplitudes, especially in the older demographic.

(c) Left ventricular hypertrophy is diagnosed if the sum of R-wave height in V_1 plus S-wave depth in V_5–V_6 is greater than 35 mm – incorrect: a sum greater than 35 mm of S-wave depth in V_1 plus tallest R-wave height in V_5–V_6 indicates left ventricular hypertrophy.

(d) **Left ventricular hypertrophy may be a sign of left ventricular failure – correct: left ventricular hypertrophy may be a result of aortic stenosis or regurgitation or mitral regurgitation, which may lead to left ventricular failure if left untreated.**

(e) Left-sided heart failure can cause portal hypertension and peripheral oedema – incorrect: left ventricular failure does not produce peripheral oedema, which is a feature of right-sided heart failure.

1 2 3 Key Points

Voltage criteria for left ventricular hypertrophy include:
- S-wave amplitude in V_1 plus R-wave amplitude in V_5/V_6 greater than 35 mm
- R-wave amplitude in aVL plus S-wave amplitude in V_3 greater than 20 mm in women, or greater than 28 mm in men

CASE 34 – ANSWERS

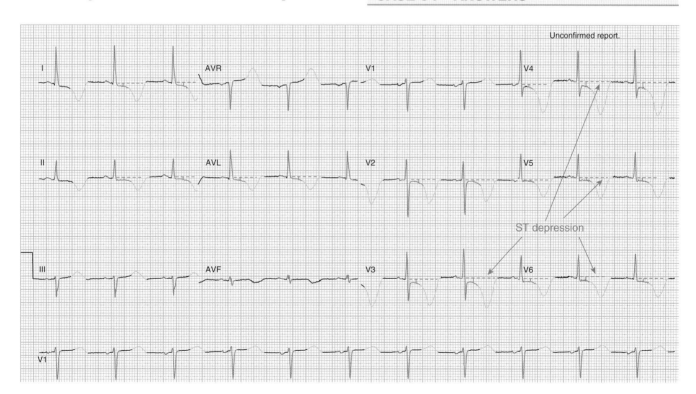
Unconfirmed report.
ST depression

Present Your Findings

BASIC DETAILS
This is an anonymised ECG of unknown date and time.
  I would like to ensure that this is calibrated to the usual 25 mm/s paper speed and 1 mV/cm gain.

KEY FEATURES
The most pertinent abnormality is the T-wave inversion and ST depression in leads I, II, aVL and V_2–V_6. There is also ST depression in V_3–V_6.

HEART RATE AND RHYTHM
The heart rate is 66 bpm with a regular sinus rhythm.

CARDIAC AXIS
The cardiac axis is normal (between –30° and +90°).

PR AND QRS INTERVAL
The PR interval is normal (120 ms), and the QT interval is prolonged (520 ms).

WAVE MORPHOLOGY
The P waves are normal in morphology. The QRS complexes are narrow. There is T-wave inversion in leads I, II, aVL and V_2–V_6, as well as associated ST depression (1 mm in limb leads, 1–2 mm in precordial leads).

In Summary

This ECG is consistent with a non-ST elevation myocardial infarction (NSTEMI). The history of sudden-onset central exertional chest pain radiating to the neck should prompt investigation for myocardial infarction. Blood tests that are essential in this case include full blood count, urea and electrolytes, bone profile, magnesium and troponin. ECG findings in this case additionally confirm the diagnosis of NSTEMI. Acute management of NSTEMI includes A–E assessment, analgesia, oxygen (if low oxygen saturation), nitrate, aspirin and clopidogrel. All NSTEMI patients should also receive a beta-blocker as soon as clinically stable unless contraindicated. Other risk factors such as smoking, hypertension, diabetes mellitus, family history of premature coronary artery disease and hypercholesterolaemia would need to be managed following discharge.

★ **ANSWERS FOR CANDIDATES**

1. <u>Which of the following ECG changes can be produced by an NSTEMI?</u>

The correct answers are: (a) hyperacute T waves; (d) ST depression; and (e) T-wave inversion.

ST depression is the most common ECG change in NSTEMI, usually most prominent in leads V_4–V_6, I, II

and aVL. Other changes include T-wave inversion and hyperacute T waves.

  (a) **Hyperacute T waves – correct: this may be a sign of NSTEMI. Other causes of hyperacute T waves include hyperkalaemia.**
  (b) P-wave flattening – incorrect: this is a sign of left atrial hypertrophy.
  (c) Prolonged PR interval – incorrect: this would indicate atrioventricular conduction block.
  (d) **ST depression – correct: ST depression is the most common ECG change in NSTEMI.**
  (e) **T-wave inversion – correct: causes of T-wave inversion are usually non-specific and a diagnosis of NSTEMI would need to be excluded in cases of new T-wave inversion associated with history of chest pain.**

Key Points

ST depression and T-wave inversion are the commonest ECG findings in NSTEMI.

2. <u>Which of the following treatments should be routinely offered in the acute management of NSTEMIs?</u>

The correct answers are: (a) antiplatelet therapy; and (b) aspirin.

The acute management of an NSTEMI is similar to STEMI, which includes analgesia, beta-blockers, antiplatelets and anticoagulation therapy.

  (a) **Antiplatelet therapy – correct: patients with NSTEMI should be put on antiplatelets such as aspirin. Other antiplatelets that may be considered, in addition to aspirin, include clopidogrel or ticagrelor. Depending on whether there is concurrent non-valvular atrial fibrillation, after assessing the bleeding risks, antithrombotic treatment may be offered.**
  (b) **Aspirin – correct: loading dose of aspirin 300 mg should be offered in the acute management of patients with NSTEMI.**
  (c) Coronary angiography – incorrect: this should be offered to patients with a moderate or higher risk of adverse cardiovascular outcomes.
  (d) Spironolactone – incorrect: spironolactone has no role in the management of myocardial infarctions unless heart failure is present.
  (e) Statin – incorrect: statins have no role in acute management, although they should be offered for secondary prevention of cardiovascular disease following discharge.

Key Points

The management of NSTEMI includes:
- Morphine and antiemetic
- Nitrates
- Beta-blockers
- Antiplatelet therapy
- Anticoagulation
- Coronary revascularisation for patients in high-risk category

---

3. Which of the following would most likely describe the underlying pathology?

The correct answer is: (b) subendocardial infarct due to atherosclerosis.

Ninety per cent of myocardial infarctions are due to coronary artery atherosclerosis and associated vessel occlusion with overlying thrombosis. NSTEMIs results from part-thickness infarction.

(a) Reversible cardiac ischaemia – incorrect: this would represent angina as infarction has not occurred.

(b) **Subendocardial infarct due to atherosclerosis – correct: atherosclerosis leading to subendocardial infarction accounts for most NSTEMIs.**

(c) Subendocardial infarct due to vasospasm – incorrect: this is an uncommon cause for an NSTEMI.

(d) Transmural infarct due to atherosclerosis – incorrect: this is the commonest cause of a STEMI.

(e) Transmural infarct due to vasospasm – incorrect: this is an uncommon cause of a STEMI.

Key Points

An NSTEMI usually results from atherosclerosis, producing subendocardial infarction. This includes the inner third or half of the ventricular wall, which is normally the least perfused region.

CASE 35 – ANSWERS

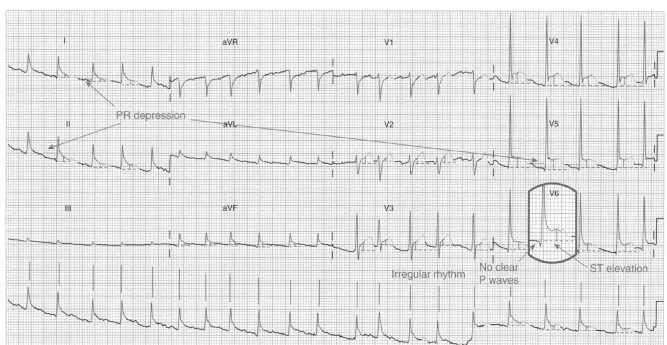

Present Your Findings

BASIC DETAILS

This is an anonymised ECG of unknown date and time.

I would like to ensure that this is calibrated to the usual 25 mm/s paper speed and 1 mV/cm gain.

KEY FEATURES

The most pertinent abnormality is the concave ST elevation in most limb leads of I, II and aVF as well as most chest leads of V_3–V_6 and PR depression.

HEART RATE AND RHYTHM

The heart rate is 126 bpm with an irregularly irregular rhythm.

CARDIAC AXIS

The cardiac axis is normal (between –30° and +90°).

PR AND QRS INTERVAL

There is PR depression. The QT interval is shortened (240 ms).

WAVE MORPHOLOGY

There are no obvious P waves. The QRS complexes are narrow. There are widespread ST changes (elevation 3–4 mm in most leads) but no significant T-wave abnormalities.

⬆ In Summary

This ECG is consistent with pericarditis (ST elevation and PR depression) and atrial fibrillation.

In the context of history, chest pain on leaning forward, recent cold, cough and fever point us towards the diagnosis of pericarditis (likely of viral origin). Widespread ST elevation shown on most leads on ECG strengthens pericarditis as the most likely cause. He mentions he has a history of a 'funny heart rhythm' which likely refers to the atrial fibrillation seen on this ECG; anticoagulation was not used as his CHA_2DS_2-VASc is 0.

Blood tests should include full blood count, urea and electrolytes, C-reactive protein and troponin. Further blood tests may be needed if we are suspecting other causes of pericarditis. Echocardiography may also be useful to identify the presence of pericardial fluid. Initial management of pericarditis includes non-steroidal anti-inflammatory drugs (NSAIDs) and colchicine. In severe cases with pericardial effusions, pericardiocentesis may be considered. Rate control with medication, such as beta-blockers or calcium channel blockers, should be considered for his atrial fibrillation.

★ ANSWERS FOR CANDIDATES

1. Which of the following may produce pericarditis?

The correct answers is: (e) all of the above.

In pericarditis, the pericardium becomes inflamed and blood or fluid can leak into it. Most cases are secondary to viral infection. However, any infection or inflammation of structures neighbouring the pericardium can cause pericarditis.

(a) **Cardiac surgery – incorrect:** cardiac surgery increases the risk of infection, therefore may cause pericarditis.

(b) **Myocardial infarction – incorrect:** pericarditis which occurs around 4–6 weeks after myocardial infarction is also known as Dressler syndrome.

(c) **Rheumatic heart disease – incorrect:** rheumatic fever can affect the heart muscles, eventually causing pericarditis.

(d) **Viral respiratory tract infection – incorrect:** viral infection is one of the main causes of pericarditis.

(e) **All of the above – correct:** there are various causes of pericarditis. All of the above options are known causes of pericarditis.

¹²₃ Key Points

Causes of pericarditis include:
- Viral infection
- Dressler syndrome
- Systemic inflammatory disorders, e.g. rheumatoid arthritis
- Trauma
- Tuberculosis
- Uraemia

2. Which of the following ECG changes can be produced by acute pericarditis?

The correct answers are: (a) PR depression; (b) sinus tachycardia; and (d) ST depression.

The most pertinent ECG finding in pericarditis is widespread ST elevation, which may be accompanied by PR depression and sinus tachycardia.

(a) **PR depression – correct:** PR depression and ST elevation can be caused by pericarditis.

(b) **Sinus tachycardia – correct:** sinus tachycardia is a common finding among patients with pericarditis as part of the normal inflammatory response.

(c) Slurred upstroke in the QRS complex – incorrect: a slurred upstroke in the QRS complex (delta wave) suggest pre-excitation.

(d) ST depression – correct: pericarditis can produce ST depression in lead aVR.

(e) T-wave inversion – incorrect: T-wave inversion is usually caused by coronary artery disease or other pulmonary causes such as pulmonary embolism. It is not usually seen with myocardial inflammatory disorders.

123 Key Points

ECG features suggesting pericarditis include:
- Widespread ST elevation
- Widespread PR depression
- ST depression in aVR
- Sinus tachycardia

---

3. Which of the following are effective in the management of pericarditis?

The correct answer is: (c) NSAIDs.

The mainstay of pericarditis management is rest and NSAID therapy, especially as most cases are of viral origin.

(a) Anticoagulants – incorrect: anticoagulants are usually contraindicated in pericarditis as they may exacerbate cases of haemopericardium.

(b) Beta-blockers – incorrect: there is no role for beta-blockers in the management of pericarditis.

(c) NSAIDs – correct: NSAIDs are useful as first-line treatment of pericarditis.

(d) Pericardiocentesis – Incorrect: Although pericardial effusions can occur with pericarditis, they rarely require drainage. However, pericardiocentesis is performed in some cases for diagnostic purposes or if the effusion is large, especially if it is causing tamponade.

(e) Thiazide diuretics – incorrect: there is no role for thiazide diuretics in the management of pericarditis.

123 Key Points

Management of pericarditis includes:
- Conservative: rest, avoid triggers
- Medical: NSAIDs, colchicine

CASE 36 – ANSWERS

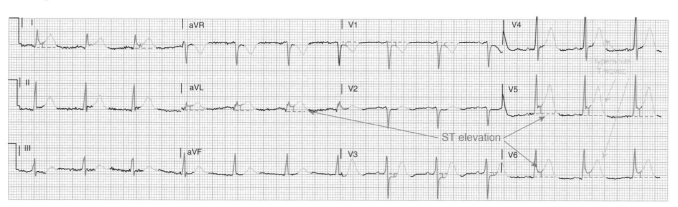

Present Your Findings

BASIC DETAILS

This is an anonymised ECG of unknown date and time. There is artefact with baseline noise present in the first half of the recording that limits interpretation, so a repeat recording would be useful.

I would like to ensure that this is calibrated to the usual 25 mm/s paper speed and 1 mV/cm gain.

KEY FEATURES

The most pertinent abnormality is ST elevation in leads I, aVL, and V_5–V_6. There are also hyperacute T waves in the anterolateral chest leads of V_3–V_6, as well as leads I and II.

HEART RATE AND RHYTHM

The heart rate is 78 bpm with a regular sinus rhythm.

CARDIAC AXIS

The cardiac axis is normal (between −30° and +90°).

PR AND QRS INTERVAL

The PR interval is normal (160 ms), and the QT interval is normal (400 ms).

WAVE MORPHOLOGY

The P waves are normal in morphology, although difficult to see in the first half of the recording due to baseline noise. The QRS complexes are narrow with no evidence of ventricular hypertrophy.

There is 1–2 mm ST elevation in leads I, aVL and V_5–V_6. There is also reciprocal ST depression in V_1 and V_3. There are hyperacute T waves in the anterolateral chest leads of V_3–V_6, as well as subtle T-wave changes in leads I and II.

In Summary

This ECG is consistent with lateral ST elevation myocardial infarction (STEMI). This patient reports a typical history of central crushing chest pain and shortness of breath. Lateral STEMI usually causes ST elevation in lateral chest leads. Blood tests that are essential in this case include full blood count, urea and electrolytes and troponin. ECG findings in this case additionally confirm the diagnosis of STEMI.

Acute management of STEMI includes A–E assessment, analgesia, oxygen (if low oxygen saturation), antiemetic, nitrate and antiplatelet therapy (aspirin and ticagrelor/clopidogrel). All patients who present within 12 h of symptom onset of STEMI should be considered for a reperfusion strategy unless they have severe comorbidities. The ideal treatment for all STEMIs is primary percutaneous coronary intervention (PCI) or, in some cases, emergency coronary artery bypass grafts. Primary PCI is preferred for reperfusion therapy in patients with STEMI if it can be performed within 90 min of first medical contact. If this time frame is not possible, then fibrinolytic therapy is preferred for those without contraindications.

★ ANSWERS FOR CANDIDATES

1. Which of the following is/are a risk factor(s) for developing myocardial infarction?

The correct answers are: (a) diabetes mellitus; (b) male sex; (c) smoking; and (e) use of combined oral contraceptive pill.

Some risk factors for developing myocardial infarction are reversible; others are not. Lifestyle modification is a key part of reducing risk, particularly targeting smoking, alcohol, exercise and dietary habits.

(a) **Diabetes mellitus – correct: diabetes is recognised as a strong risk factor for ischaemic heart disease. Coronary artery disease is the cause of death in half of all patients with diabetes.**

(b) **Male sex – correct: male sex is a recognised risk factor for ischaemic heart disease. This is likely because of the presence of higher risk factor levels at younger ages in men, such as smoking and hyperlipidaemia.**

(c) **Smoking – correct: smoking is recognised as a strong risk factor for ischaemic heart disease. Therefore, all smoking cessation advice should be offered to all patients as associated morbidity and mortality fall immediately after stopping smoking.**

(d) Use of ACE inhibitors – incorrect: ACE inhibitors are used in heart failure, hypertension and after myocardial infarction. They act by inhibiting the conversion of angiotensin I to angiotensin II, reducing vasoconstriction and the secretion of aldosterone. Indeed, they reduce morbidity and mortality following myocardial infarction and also have a role in primary prevention through their antihypertensive effect.

(e) **Use of combined oral contraceptive pill – correct: the combined oral contraceptive pill produces a small increase in risk for developing ischaemic heart disease. This is likely due to the prothrombotic effects of the hormone oestrogen.**

$\begin{smallmatrix}1\\2\\3\end{smallmatrix}$ Key Points

Risk factors for developing myocardial infarction include the following:

- Increasing age
- Smoking
- Male sex
- Diabetes mellitus
- Hypertension
- Hypercholesterolaemia
- Family history of ischaemic heart disease
- Obesity
- Combined oral contraceptive pill
- Alcohol
- Stress

2. What of the following best describes the classic characteristics of chest pain due to myocardial ischaemia?

The correct answer is: (b) central crushing chest pain radiating to the left shoulder.

Patients can present with a variety of symptoms, although the most common is tight, 'band-like' chest pain or discomfort. However, bear in mind that patients may present with atypical clinical pictures or can even be asymptomatic; this is especially common in elderly patients.

(a) Burning, diffuse bilateral chest pain – incorrect: this would suggest a diagnosis of gastro-oesophageal reflux disease. It is typically worse an hour after a meal and exacerbated by lying flat or on bending.

(b) **Central crushing chest pain radiating to the left shoulder – correct: this pain is characteristic of ischaemic heart disease. Anatomically, this is referred chest pain as the visceral sensory nerves of the heart synapse at levels T_1–T_4. The dermatomes of these spinal levels correspond to the chest and arm.**

(c) Sharp, well-localised chest pain with overlying tenderness – incorrect: this would suggest a musculoskeletal cause for the pain. Musculoskeletal causes account for 35% of all cases of chest pain.

(d) Sharp, well-localised right chest pain worse on inspiration – incorrect: these features suggest a pleuritic cause of pain. This includes pneumonia, pulmonary embolus and lung cancer. However, bear in mind the possibility of pericarditis, which also produces sharp, well-localised chest pain and is relieved by leaning forwards.

(e) Tearing chest pain radiating to the back – incorrect: these features suggest an aortic dissection. An aortic dissection is an especially important diagnosis to consider due to its high mortality and ability to produce ischaemic features on an ECG following vessel damage.

Key Points

Myocardial ischaemia classically produces central, crushing chest pain that radiates to the jaw, neck, shoulders or arms. Other symptoms may include a sense of impending doom, nausea and vomiting, dyspnoea and syncope.

3. What is the most likely coronary artery to have been affected in this patient?

The correct answer is: (b) Left circumflex artery.

ST elevation in the lateral leads suggests occlusion of the left circumflex artery. However, it is important to bear in mind that anatomical variants in coronary supply mean that not all patients will present with the classical ECG findings for their particular artery.

(a) Left anterior descending artery – incorrect: Occlusion produces an anterior infarct with ST elevation in leads V_1–V_4.

(b) **Left circumflex artery – correct: Occlusion produces a lateral infarct with ST elevation in leads V_5–V_6 and I, aVL.**

(c) Posterior descending artery – incorrect: occlusion of this artery can produce an inferior infarct with ST elevation in leads II, III and aVF as the posterior descending artery is a branch of the right coronary artery.

(d) Right coronary artery – incorrect: occlusion produces an inferior infarct with ST elevation in leads II, III and aVF.

(e) Right marginal artery – incorrect: occlusion of this artery does not produce specific ECG changes.

Key Points

Classic findings in a STEMI include:
- Anterior infarct: V_1–V_4 ST elevation → left anterior descending artery occlusion
- Lateral infarct: V_5–V_6, I, aVL ST elevation → left circumflex artery occlusion
- Inferior infarct: II, III, aVF elevation → right coronary artery occlusion
- Posterior infarct: ST depression with tall R wave in leads V_1–V_3 → right coronary or left circumflex occlusion
- New left bundle branch block

CASE 37 – ANSWERS

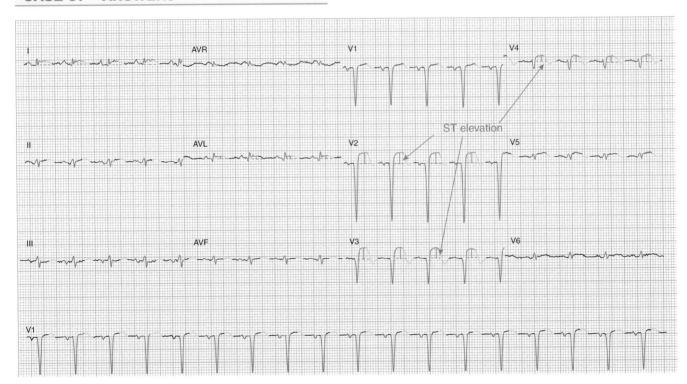

ST elevation

Present Your Findings

BASIC DETAILS
This is an anonymised ECG of unknown date and time.

I would like to ensure that this is calibrated to the usual 25 mm/s paper speed and 1 mV/cm gain.

KEY FEATURES
The most pertinent abnormalities are ST elevation in precordial leads V_2–V_4. There is also subtle ST elevation in I and aVL.

HEART RATE AND RHYTHM
The heart rate is 108 bpm with a regular sinus rhythm.

CARDIAC AXIS
The cardiac axis is normal (between –30° and +90°).

PR AND QRS INTERVAL
The PR interval is normal (120 ms), and the QT interval is normal (320 ms). There are Q waves in V_1–V_3.

WAVE MORPHOLOGY
The P waves are normal in morphology. The QRS complexes are narrow with evidence of high-voltage amplitude in V_1 and V_2.

There is 2–4 mm ST elevation in precordial leads V_2–V_4. There is also subtle ST elevation in I and aVL.

In Summary

This ECG is consistent with anterior ST elevation myocardial infarction (STEMI). Central chest pain radiating to the jaw is classic of chest pain of cardiac nature. ST elevation in V_2–V_4 represents an anterior myocardial infarction, likely due to occlusion of the left anterior descending artery. Subtle ST elevation at I and aVL represents 'collateral damage' at the lateral territory (as diagonal branches of LAD supply this area). Blood tests that are essential in this case include full blood count, urea and electrolytes and troponin.

Acute management of STEMI includes A–E assessment, analgesia, oxygen (if low oxygen saturation), antiemetic, nitrate and antiplatelet therapy (aspirin and a second antiplatelet agent, such as prasugrel, ticagrelor or clopidogrel). All patients who present within 12 h of symptom onset of STEMI should be considered for a reperfusion strategy unless they have severe comorbidities. The ideal treatment for all STEMIs is primary percutaneous coronary intervention (PCI) or, in some cases, emergency coronary artery bypass grafts. Primary PCI is preferred for reperfusion therapy in patients with STEMI if it can be performed within 90 min of first medical contact. If this time frame is not possible, then fibrinolytic therapy is preferred for those without contraindications.

Myocardial infarction in a younger patient, as portrayed in this case, should prompt further investigations and risk factors should be controlled and monitored. Family history is recommended to be elicited in this case.

★ ANSWERS FOR CANDIDATES

1. Which of the following would most likely describe the underlying pathology?

The correct answer is: (d) transmural infarct due to atherosclerosis and plaque rupture.

Ninety per cent of myocardial infarctions are due to coronary artery atherosclerosis and associated vessel occlusion with overlying thrombosis. Ten per cent of cases are non-atherosclerotic, such as vasospasm and intracardial emboli, sometimes referred to as MINOCA (Myocardial Infarction with non-onbstructive coronary arteries).

(a) Reversible cardiac ischaemia – incorrect: this would cause angina.

(b) Subendocardial infarct due to atherosclerosis – incorrect: atherosclerosis leading to subendocardial infarction accounts for most non-ST elevation myocardial infarction (NSTEMIs).

(c) Subendocardial infarct due to vasospasm – incorrect: this is an uncommon cause of an NSTEMI.

(d) **Transmural infarct due to atherosclerosis and plaque rupture – correct: 90% of myocardial infarctions are due to coronary artery atherosclerosis.**

(e) Transmural infarct due to vasospasm – incorrect: a STEMI results from transmural infarction, although most are due to atherosclerosis.

> **1₂₃ Key Points**
>
> A STEMI results from transmural myocardial infarction. Ischaemic necrosis extends throughout the full thickness of the ventricular wall in the distribution of a single coronary vessel.

2. Which of the following can lead to myocardial ischaemia?

The correct answer is: (e) all of the above.

Myocardial ischaemia results from either a reduction in blood supply or an increase in muscular demand.

(a) **Atherosclerosis – incorrect: atherosclerosis leads to vessel narrowing and, if the plaque becomes unstable, overlying thrombus formation. This leads to vessel occlusion and is implicated in 90% of myocardial infarctions.**

(b) **Anaemia – incorrect: anaemia reduces the transport of oxygen via red blood cells. This restricts the oxygen supply to the myocardium and leads to ischaemia, especially if there is underlying atherosclerosis.**

(c) **Cocaine use – incorrect: cocaine use is associated with vasospasm of the vessels. By blocking noradrenaline and dopamine reuptake at synapses, it enhances sympathetic outflow. Consequently, there is myocardial ischaemia due to increased oxygen demands (increased heart rate and stroke volume) as well as reduced supply (vasoconstriction).**

(d) **Infective endocarditis – incorrect: infective endocarditis can produce septic emboli. These can lodge in and occlude coronary vessels, reducing oxygen supply. This may produce myocardial ischaemia in conjunction with the increased workload following valvular pathology.**

(e) **All of the above – correct: as the previous answers suggest, myocardial ischaemia can result from a variety of factors.**

> **1₂₃ Key Points**
>
> Multiple factors can lead to the development of myocardial ischaemia. These can involve either a reduction in coronary blood supply or an increase in myocardial demands. This includes:
> - Atherosclerosis
> - Coronary spasm, e.g. cocaine use
> - Arrhythmias
> - Infective endocarditis
> - Vasculitis
> - Aortic dissection
> - Hypotension

3. Which of the following is/are a diagnostic ECG finding(s) for a STEMI?

The correct answers are: (a) >1 mm ST elevation in two or more limb leads; and (c) new left bundle branch block.

ECG findings are important in differentiating a STEMI from an NSTEMI in the presence of elevated cardiac biomarkers. These changes occur due to changes in the electrophysiology following damage to the myocardium.

(a) **>1 mm ST elevation in two or more limb leads – correct: this suggests a diagnosis of STEMI.**

(b) >1 mm ST elevation in two or more precordial leads (V_1–V_6) – incorrect: ST elevation of >2 mm is required to be diagnostic in the precordial leads.

(c) **New left bundle branch block – correct: extensive myocardial damage involving a large portion of the distal conduction system can cause left bundle branch block.**

(d) New right bundle branch block – incorrect: a right bundle branch block is commonly found in healthy people. In some cases, it may indicate right heart strain or hypertrophy. There is no clear link between myocardial infarction and a right bundle branch block.

(e) T-wave inversion – incorrect: T-wave inversion may result from ischaemia and infarction but is not considered a useful diagnostic marker of a STEMI.

> **1₂₃ Key Points**
>
> UK guidelines suggest considering a diagnosis of STEMI if at least one of following is present:
> - >1 mm ST elevation in two or more limb leads
> - >2 mm ST elevation in two or more precordial leads (V_1–V_6)
> - New left bundle branch block

CASE 38 – ANSWERS

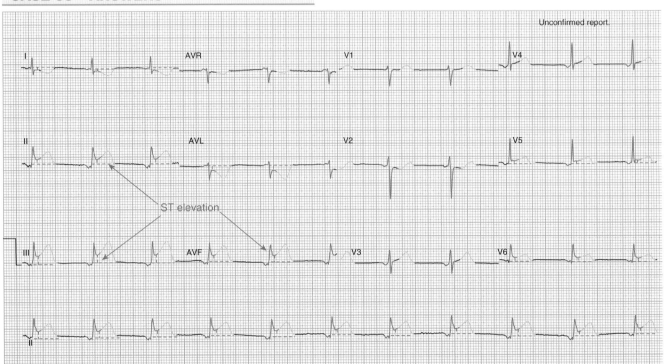

Unconfirmed report.

ST elevation

Present Your Findings

BASIC DETAILS
This is an anonymised ECG of unknown date and time.
I would like to ensure that this is calibrated to the usual 25 mm/s paper speed and 1 mV/cm gain.

KEY FEATURES
The most pertinent abnormalities are ST elevation in leads II, III and aVF, as well as subtle ST elevation in leads V_5–V_6. There is reciprocal ST depression in leads I and aVL with T-wave inversion.

HEART RATE AND RHYTHM
The heart rate is 66 bpm with a regular sinus rhythm.

CARDIAC AXIS
The cardiac axis is normal (between –30° and +90°).

PR AND QRS INTERVAL
The PR interval is shortened (80 ms) and the QT interval is normal (360 ms).

WAVE MORPHOLOGY
The P waves are inverted in most leads. The QRS complexes are narrow with no evidence of ventricular hypertrophy. There is T-wave inversion in leads I and aVL.
There is 3–4 mm ST elevation in leads II, III and aVF as well as subtle ST elevation in leads V_5–V_6. There is reciprocal ST depression in leads I and aVL with T-wave inversion.

In Summary

This ECG is consistent with inferior ST elevation myocardial infarction (STEMI). Classical distribution of ECG changes for inferior STEMI is most obvious on leads II, III and aVF. Epigastric pain is an atypical 'cardiac chest pain' symptom and may be easily confused with other causes such as indigestion. In this case, ECG changes would help to confirm the diagnosis of a cardiac infarct. In addition, a patient with oxygen requirement would also help to lead the clinician towards a chest diagnosis for the presenting complaint. Blood tests that are essential in this case include full blood count, urea and electrolytes and troponin.

★ **ANSWERS FOR CANDIDATES**

1. What is the most appropriate cardiac biomarker for investigating myocardial infarction?
The correct answer is: **(e) troponin I and T.**
Cardiac biomarkers are helpful in confirming whether infarction has occurred. These intracellular proteins are released into the blood stream once cell necrosis occurs. Therefore, a normal biomarker in the context of ischaemic symptoms suggests a diagnosis of angina.
(a) Aspartate aminotransferase – incorrect: not specific for the heart and also used as a biomarker

for liver function. Begins rising after 12 h and normalises within 3 days.

(b) Creatine kinase – incorrect: creatine kinase begins rising after 6 h and normalises within 2 days after infarction but is not cardiac-specific.

(c) Lactate dehydrogenase – incorrect: this begins rising after 12 h of ischaemia and normalises within 14 days. It is a widespread intracellular protein, so is not as specific as troponin.

(d) Myoglobin – incorrect: although the myoglobin level may rise after a myocardial infarction, it is not as specific as troponin I and T in investigating myocardial infarction.

(e) **Troponin I and T – correct: the most sensitive and specific cardiac biomarker. It begins to elevate within a few hours of infarction and normalises after a few weeks.**

> **Key Points**
>
> The following table shows the features that would help differentiate the different acute coronary syndromes.

	UNSTABLE ANGINA	↔	NSTEMI	↔	STEMI
ST elevation	✗		✗		✓
Raised troponin	✗		✓		✓

2. What is the most appropriate immediate treatment for this patient?

The correct answer is: (a) aspirin 300 mg and primary PCI.

Following a diagnosis of a STEMI, patients should be offered aspirin and referred for urgent interventional management.

(a) **Aspirin 300 mg and primary PCI – correct: this is the recommended treatment for STEMI. If PCI cannot be performed within 2 h, provide fibrinolysis instead after consultation with a cardiologist.**

(b) Aspirin, clopidogrel, fondaparinux, beta-blocker and pain relief – incorrect: this is the treatment of choice for patients with unstable angina or non-ST elevation myocardial infarction (NSTEMI). In addition, patients with an intermediate risk of cardiovascular events should be offered coronary angiography (and PCI, if indicated) within 96 h.

(c) CABG – incorrect: a CABG is used to treat severe coronary artery stenosis that produces angina or an NSTEMI. Rarely, CABG is considered in an emergency setting to treat a STEMI if PCI is not possible or has been ineffective.

(d) Heart transplant – incorrect: heart transplants are used for the treatment of refractory end-stage heart failure.

(e) High-flow oxygen and IV atropine – incorrect: this is a recommended treatment for bradyarrhythmias.

> **Key Points**
>
> Patients with a STEMI should be offered aspirin followed by primary PCI as soon as possible. If PCI is not available within 2 h, fibrinolysis should be offered instead.

3. A few days following admission, the patient complained of acute shortness of breath. A new pansystolic murmur and bibasal lung crackles can be heard on auscultation. Which of the following is the most likely complication that the patient has developed?

The correct answer is: (c) papillary muscle rupture.

Myocardial infarction can lead to a range of complications. These can be considered as acute, subacute or chronic. Given the subacute timing in the case above and with severe mitral regurgitation post-myocardial infarction, papillary muscle rupture is the most likely diagnosis.

(a) Complete heart block – incorrect: an area of infarcted cardiac muscle can affect the conduction pathway of the heart, leading to heart block. However, this would not produce a new murmur.

(b) Heart failure – incorrect: heart failure occurs following myocardial infarction due to myocardial scarring, recurrent ischaemia and mechanical complications, such as ventricular aneurysms. It usually leads to pulmonary oedema if it is left-sided heart failure and/or peripheral oedema and hepatomegaly if it is right-sided heart failure.

(c) **Papillary muscle rupture – correct: the occurrence of mitral regurgitation, as suggested by a pansystolic murmur, and pulmonary oedema due to left ventricular dysfunction subacutely post-myocardial infarction should raise suspicion of a diagnosis of papillary muscle rupture.**

(d) Pericarditis – incorrect: pericarditis usually presents with low-grade fever and classically, sharp, well-localised chest pain relieved by leaning forwards. ECG may show widespread ST elevation.

(e) Ventricular aneurysm – incorrect: ventricular aneurysm can occur after a myocardial infarction, usually arising from an area of weakened (or infarcted) tissue in a ventricular wall, causing it to swell and fill with blood. Although also subacute in presentation, it does not usually cause heart failure and it will be picked up using transthoracic echocardiogram.

> **Key Points**
>
> Mechanical complications of myocardial infarction tend to presently subacutely a few days post-myocardial infarction. These include tear or rupture of:
> - Ventricular septum ê ventricular septal defect
> - Papillary muscles ê mitral regurgitation
> - Ventricular free wall ê tamponade

CASE 39 – ANSWERS

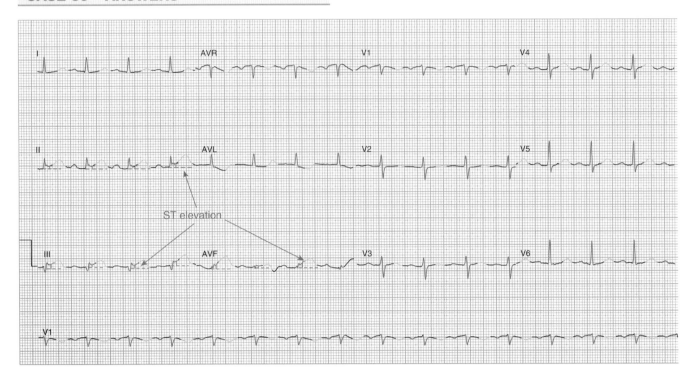

Present Your Findings

BASIC DETAILS

This is an anonymised ECG of unknown date and time.

I would like to ensure that this is calibrated to the usual 25 mm/s paper speed and 1 mV/cm gain.

KEY FEATURES

The most pertinent abnormalities are ST elevation in leads II, III and aVF with associated Q waves.

HEART RATE AND RHYTHM

The heart rate is 95 bpm with a regular sinus rhythm.

CARDIAC AXIS

The cardiac axis is normal (between –30° and +90°).

PR AND QRS INTERVAL

The PR interval is normal (200 ms), and the QT interval is normal (360 ms).

WAVE MORPHOLOGY

The P waves are normal in morphology. The QRS complexes are narrow with no evidence of ventricular hypertrophy. T waves are normal.

There is 1–2 mm ST elevation in leads II, III and aVF with associated Q waves.

In Summary

This ECG is consistent with inferior ST elevation myocardial infarction (STEMI). This represents a case with a classical ECG pattern for an inferior myocardial infarction: ST elevation in leads II, III and aVF with associated Q waves. Blood tests that are essential in this case include full blood count, urea and electrolytes and troponin.

Acute management of STEMI includes A–E assessment, analgesia, oxygen (if low oxygen saturation), antiemetic, nitrate and antiplatelet therapy (aspirin and ticagrelor/clopidogrel). All patients who present within 12 h of symptom onset of STEMI should be considered for a reperfusion strategy unless they have severe comorbidities. The ideal treatment for all STEMIs is acute percutaneous coronary intervention (PCI) or, in some cases, emergency coronary artery bypass grafts. Primary PCI is preferred for reperfusion therapy in patients with STEMI if it can be performed within 90 min of first medical contact. If this time frame is not possible, then fibrinolytic therapy is preferred for those without contraindications.

★ ANSWERS FOR CANDIDATES

1. What drugs should be offered for the following 12 months, assuming no contraindications?

The correct answer is: (b) aspirin, clopidogrel, statin, beta-blocker, ACE inhibitor.

The following drugs are recommended for 12 months after myocardial infarction:

- Two antiplatelet drugs, e.g. aspirin and clopidogrel
- Statin
- Beta-blocker
- ACE inhibitor

(a) Aspirin, clopidogrel, spironolactone, statin, beta-blocker, ACE inhibitor – incorrect: spironolactone is not a recommended routine drug following acute coronary syndrome.

(b) Aspirin, clopidogrel, statin, beta-blocker, ACE inhibitor – correct: these drugs should be offered to patients with STEMI, assuming no contraindications.

(c) Aspirin, statin, ACE inhibitor – incorrect: this option did not have a second antiplatelet agent (such as clopidogrel), which is recommended to be used for up to 12 months after myocardial infarction. A beta-blocker is also recommended to be used lifelong.

(d) Aspirin, statin, beta-blocker – incorrect: this option did not have a second antiplatelet agent (such as clopidogrel), which is recommended to be used for up to 12 months after myocardial infarction. ACE inhibitors are also recommended to be used lifelong.

(e) Aspirin, statin, beta-blocker, ACE inhibitor – incorrect: this option did not have a second antiplatelet agent (such as clopidogrel), which is recommended to be used for up to 12 months after myocardial infarction.

1₂₃ Key Points

After myocardial infarction, aspirin, a statin, a beta-blocker and an ACE inhibitor should be taken for life, and a second antiplatelet agent (such as clopidogrel) for 12 months. All of the recommended drugs have evidence of improved mortality following myocardial infarction.

2. The following medications are matched to drug classes. Which of the following is/are correct?

The correct answer is: (b) bivalirudin – direct thrombin inhibitor.

There are various groups of medications that can be used in the management of myocardial infarction, including ADP platelet receptor inhibitor, glycoprotein IIb/IIIa inhibitors, direct thrombin inhibitors and fibrinolytics.

(a) Abciximab – cyclooxygenase inhibitor – incorrect: abciximab is an example of a glycoprotein IIb/IIIa inhibitor.

(b) Bivalirudin – direct thrombin inhibitor – correct: bivalirudin is an example of a direct thrombin inhibitor.

(c) Clopidogrel – phosphodiesterase inhibitor – incorrect: clopidogrel is an example of an ADP receptor inhibitor.

(d) Prasugrel – non-thienopyridine ADP platelet receptor inhibitor – incorrect: prasugrel belongs to the same group as clopidogrel – thienopyridine ADP receptor inhibitors.

(e) Ticagrelor – thienopyridine ADP platelet receptor inhibitor – incorrect: ticagrelor belongs to non-thienopyridine ADP receptor inhibitors.

1₂₃ Key Points

CLASSES OF MEDICATION USED IN THE TREATMENT OF MYOCARDIAL INFARCTION

	EXAMPLES
Cyclooxygenase inhibitors	Aspirin
Thienopyridine ADP receptor inhibitors	Clopidogrel, prasugrel
Non-thienopyridine ADP receptor inhibitors	Ticagrelor
Glycoprotein IIb/IIIa inhibitors	Abciximab, tirofiban, eptifibatide
Phosphodiesterase inhibitors	Dipyridamole
Direct thrombin inhibitor	Bivalirudin

3. Which of the following statement(s) regarding reperfusion strategy after myocardial infarction is/are false?

The correct answer is: (c) primary PCI is preferred for reperfusion therapy over fibrinolytic therapy in patients with STEMI if it can be performed within 4 h of first medical contact.

Patients with STEMI should be considered for a reperfusion strategy, which is usually primary PCI.

(a) Coronary artery bypass can be considered as a reperfusion strategy when PCI fails – incorrect: this statement is true.

(b) Patients presenting within 12 h of symptom onset of STEMI should be considered for a reperfusion strategy, unless they have severe comorbidities – incorrect: this statement is true.

(c) Primary PCI is preferred for reperfusion therapy over fibrinolytic therapy in patients with STEMI if it can be performed within 4 h of first medical contact – correct: primary PCI is preferred for reperfusion therapy in patients with STEMI if it can be performed within 90 min of first medical contact. There is some evidence that early fibrinolysis can be an effective reperfusion therapy if administered early following the onset of symptoms; this is particularly relevant in areas where access to primary PCI is limited.

(d) The ideal reperfusion therapy for STEMIs is acute PCI – incorrect: this statement is true.

(e) Thrombolysis using alteplase may be considered as a reperfusion strategy after myocardial infarction – incorrect: this statement is true. If there are absolute contraindications to thrombolysis, PCI remains the only option. It is recommended that patients who are treated with fibrinolytic therapy should also be transferred immediately to a PCI centre. If PCI is indicated, it is recommended to be performed within 24 h.

1₂₃ Key Points

Reperfusion strategies for myocardial infarction include:
- PCI (unfractionated or low-molecular-weight heparin may also be given)
- Coronary artery bypass graft
- Thrombolysis

CASE 40 – ANSWERS

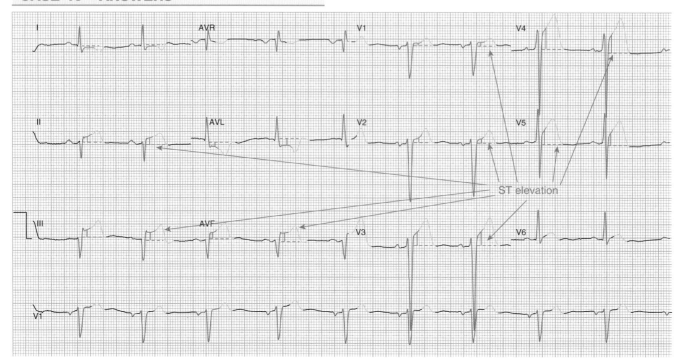

ST elevation

Present Your Findings

BASIC DETAILS

This is an anonymised ECG of unknown date and time.

I would like to ensure that this is calibrated to the usual 25 mm/s paper speed and 1 mV/cm gain.

KEY FEATURES

The most pertinent abnormalities are ST elevation in leads V_2-V_5 as well as in leads II, III and aVF. Q waves are present in the inferior leads. There is ST depression and T wave inversion in leads I and aVL.

HEART RATE AND RHYTHM

The heart rate is 58 bpm with a regular sinus rhythm.

CARDIAC AXIS

There is left-axis deviation (cardiac axis is between –30° and –90°).

PR AND QRS INTERVAL

The PR interval is normal (160 ms), and the QT interval is normal (400 ms). There are Q waves in the inferior leads.

WAVE MORPHOLOGY

The P waves are normal in morphology. The QRS complexes are narrow with high-voltage amplitudes. There is 2–5 mm ST elevation in leads V_2–V_5 as well as in leads II, III and aVF. There is subtle ST elevation in precordial leads V_1. There are hyperacute T waves in V_3–V_5. Q waves are forming in most precordial leads. There is ST depression and T-wave inversion in leads I and aVL.

In Summary

This ECG is consistent with a STEMI. In this ECG, there appears to be ST elevation in 2 territories (inferior and anterior), although it is very unlikely the patient has occluded 2 coronary arteries at the same time. The presence of Q waves in the inferior leads suggests an old inferior MI, with now an acute anterior STEMI.

This elderly lady has multiple comorbidities and risk factors for cardiac disease. The patient also had typical cardiac symptoms of chest pain, shortness of breath and syncope. The patient appears unwell and has a high oxygen requirement. Chest findings on auscultation may also indicate worsening of her pneumonia.

Acute management of STEMI includes A–E assessment, analgesia, oxygen (if low oxygen saturation), antiemetic, nitrate and antiplatelet therapy (aspirin and ticagrelor/clopidogrel). All patients who present within 12 h of symptom onset of STEMI should be considered for a reperfusion strategy unless they have severe comorbidities. The patient should be referred to a percutaneous coronary intervention (PCI) centre for consideration of primary PCI, although her comorbidities may be a limiting factor for intervention. The ideal treatment for all STEMIs is acute PCI or, in some cases, emergency coronary artery bypass grafts. Primary PCI is preferred for reperfusion therapy in patients with STEMI if it can be performed within 90 min of first medical contact. If this time frame is not possible, then fibrinolytic therapy is preferred for those without contraindications.

★ **ANSWERS FOR CANDIDATES**

1. A few days after presenting to the emergency department, the patient developed a drop in blood pressure, raised jugular venous pressure and muffled heart sounds. Which of the following best describes the complication that she has developed?

The correct answer is: **(e) tamponade due to ventricular rupture.**

Myocardial infarction can lead to a range of complications. These can be classified as acute, subacute or chronic. Given the timing of this case, this would represent a subacute complication. Subacute complications include:

- Mechanical complications
- Arrhythmias
- Heart failure
- Cardiogenic shock
- Sudden cardiac death
  (a) Arrhythmia – incorrect: arrhythmias are a common complication of myocardial infarction. An area of infarction and fibrosis can disrupt the electrical conduction of the heart and provide a substrate or setting with which arrhythmias can be maintained. The most common symptom is palpitations, although dyspnoea, angina and syncope may result from the inefficient circulation of blood.
  (b) Left-to-right shunting due to ventricular septal defect – incorrect: rupture of the ventricular septum leads to a ventricular septal defect and left-to-right shunting. This would usually produce cardiogenic shock with hypotension and tachycardia. Auscultation reveals a pansystolic murmur heard loudest on the left sternal edge.
  (c) Pericarditis – incorrect: pericarditis can occur subacutely 2–3 days after myocardial infarction. Symptoms include a low-grade fever and sharp, well-localised chest pain relieved by leaning forwards; the pain may radiate to the shoulder or the arm. Auscultation may reveal a pericardial rub. Note that, unlike Dressler syndrome, non-steroidal anti-inflammatory drugs (NSAIDs) should be avoided in this setting as they promote myocardial remodelling and increase the risk of developing ventricular aneurysms.
  (d) Pulmonary oedema due to mitral regurgitation – incorrect: mitral regurgitation can subacutely occur following papillary muscle rupture. This would lead to pulmonary oedema and shock due to left ventricular dysfunction.
  (e) **Tamponade due to ventricular rupture – correct: ventricular rupture can occur subacutely post-myocardial infarction, allowing blood to collect between the ventricle and pericardium (tamponade). Beck's triad summarises the classic symptoms of a tamponade: hypotension, raised jugular venous pressure and muffled**

heart sounds. **This should be urgently treated with pericardiocentesis.**

 Key Points

Mechanical complications of myocardial infarction tend to presently subacutely a few days post-myocardial infarction. These include tear or rupture of:
- Ventricular septum → ventricular septal defect
- Papillary muscles → mitral regurgitation
- Ventricular free wall → tamponade

2. Following successful treatment, the patient returns 8 weeks later complaining of a fever and a sharp, well-localised chest pain that is relieved by leaning forwards. What complication has this patient developed?

The correct answer is: **(b) Dressler syndrome.**

The patient's symptoms are consistent with pericarditis. Dressler syndrome is pericarditis that develops a few weeks following myocardial infarction.

(a) Arrhythmias – incorrect: arrhythmias are a common complication of myocardial infarction. An area of infarction and fibrosis can disrupt the electrical conduction of the heart and provide a substrate or setting with which arrhythmias can be maintained. The most common symptom is palpitations, although dyspnoea, angina and syncope may result from the inefficient circulation of blood.

(b) **Dressler syndrome – correct: Dressler syndrome is pericarditis that develops 2–10 weeks after myocardial infarction or heart surgery. Symptoms include a low-grade fever and sharp, well-localised chest pain relieved by leaning forwards; the pain can also radiate to the shoulder or the arm. Auscultation may reveal a pericardial rub. An ECG would show ST elevation in all leads. Dressler syndrome is best treated with colchicine.**

(c) Heart failure – incorrect: heart failure can result following myocardial infarction due to myocardial scarring, recurrent ischaemia and mechanical complications, such as ventricular aneurysms. Left-sided heart failure leads to pulmonary oedema with symptoms of dyspnoea, orthopnoea and paroxysmal nocturnal dyspnoea. Right-sided heart failure produces peripheral oedema, raised jugular venous pressure and hepatomegaly. This is best managed with a combination of a beta-blocker, angiotensin-converting enzyme inhibitor, loop diuretic and spironolactone.

(d) New myocardial infarction – incorrect: survivors of myocardial infarction have an increased risk of developing recurrent infarctions. However, the clinical picture does not support this diagnosis. A myocardial infarction would typically present with central crushing chest pain that radiates to the shoulder, neck or jaw.

(e) Reflux oesophagitis – incorrect: reflux oesophagitis can produce burning retrosternal pain. Myocardial infarction is not a risk factor for developing oesophagitis.

> **1₂₃ Key Points**
>
> Medium- to long-term complications after myocardial infarction include:
> - Mural thrombosis
> - Ventricular aneurysm
> - Dressler syndrome

---

3. Twelve months later, the patient returns for a routine check-up at her general practice. What is the most likely finding on the ECG?

The correct answer is: (c) Q waves.

Following myocardial infarction, ECG changes can include ST elevation or depression, T-wave inversion or peaking and Q-wave appearance. However, most of these normalise within a few months and Q waves can be present, particularly in those with delayed reperfusion resulting in a transmural infarct.

(a) Delta waves – incorrect: delta waves are a sign of pre-excitation due to the presence of an accessory electrical pathway. On an ECG, they appear as a slurred upstroke of QRS as there is a combination of two depolarisation sources: a slow accessory pathway followed by fast normal atrioventricular node conduction. Wolff–Parkinson–White syndrome is diagnosed if these signs are present together with symptoms of tachycardia.

(b) PR prolongation – incorrect: a prolonged PR interval indicates first-degree heart block. There is delay in the conduction of impulses from the sinoatrial node to the ventricles, which is reflected in the increased time interval between atrial and ventricular depolarisation. This is found in many normal patients but can be a pathological sign, such as an inferior myocardial infarction. Nevertheless, it is not considered a useful diagnostic marker of a myocardial infarction.

(c) **Q waves – correct: pathological Q waves appear within days. These are typically lifelong and reflect the appearance of scar tissue. A Q wave a deep or wide negative deflection that appears before the R wave. Q waves are the result of absent electrical activity following infarction and scarring.**

(d) ST elevation – incorrect: ST segment and T-wave changes appear within hours. These would usually normalise within weeks or months, although they can be present if there is subsequent development of a left ventricular aneurysm; this is usually present together with pathological Q waves.

(e) ST depression – incorrect: although ST depression may occur following myocardial infarction, these changes usually appear within hours.

> **1₂₃ Key Points**
>
> Myocardial infarction leads to ST segment changes, T-wave inversion and appearance of Q waves. In the long term, most of these normalise, except for the Q waves, which are often the last remaining sign of a previous myocardial infarction.

12

Quick Reference Guide

ECG BASICS (FIGS 12.1–12.3)

- Normal ECG recording speed: 25 mm/s
- An ECG page represents electrical activity over 10 s
- One small square = 40 ms
- One large square = 200 ms

NORMAL VALUES

- Rate: 60–100 bpm

Calculate rate from either:
(a) 6 × number of peaks across rhythm strip in lead II or
(b) 300 ÷ number of big squares between two QRS peaks

- PR interval: 120–200 ms (3–5 small squares)
- QRS width: <120 ms (<3 small squares)
- Normal QRS transition zone: V_3/V_4
- QTc: 350–440 ms

$$QTc = \frac{QT\ (s)}{\sqrt[3]{RR\ interval\ (s)}}$$

Practical note: At normal heart rates, a QT interval that measures less than half the R–R interval can be considered normal.

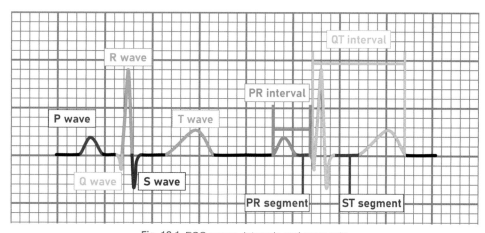

Fig. 12.1 ECG waves, intervals and segments.

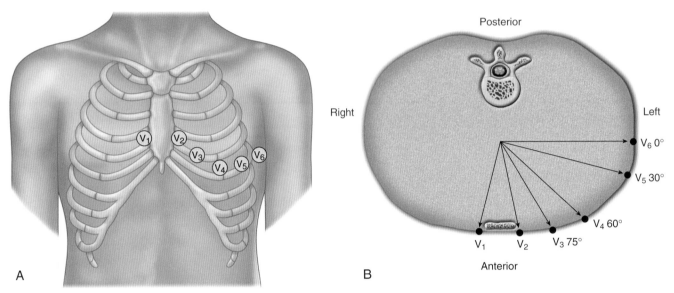

A   B

Fig 12.2 (A, B) Precordial leads measure electrical activity in the transverse plane. (Source: Griffin Perry, A., Potter, P. A., Ostendorf, W., Laplante, N. (2021). Cardiac care. In: *Clinical Nursing Skills & Techniques*, 10th ed. Elsevier. Transverse: Zipes, D. P., Libby, P. (2018). Electrocardiography. In: *Braunwald's Heart Disease: A Textbook of Cardiovascular Medicine*, 11th ed. Elsevier.)

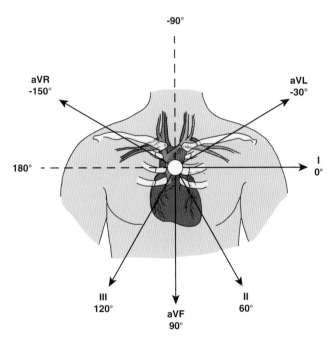

Fig 12.3 Limb leads measure electrical activity in the coronal plane. (Source: Griffin Perry, A., Potter, P. A., Ostendorf, W., Laplante, N. (2021). Health assessment. In: *Clinical Nursing Skills & Techniques*, 10th ed. Elsevier.)

INTERPRETATION STRUCTURE

CARDIAC AXIS (FIG. 12.4)

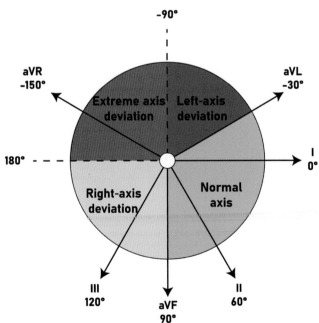

Fig. 12.4 Cardiac axis interpretation.

ARRHYTHMIAS

Tachyarrhythmias

ARRHYTHMIA	TYPICAL ECG FINDINGS
Atrial tachycardia	• Regular P waves with abnormal morphology • Ventricular rate 100–200 bpm
Atrial flutter	• Sawtooth P waves • Usually 2:1 heart block; atrial rate 300 bpm and ventricular rate 150 bpm
Atrioventricular nodal re-entrant tachycardia (AVNRT)	• Regular narrow QRS tachycardia • No P waves before each QRS complex. Retrograde P waves just after the QRS complex
Atrioventricular re-entrant tachycardia Orthodromic AVRT	• Regular narrow QRS tachycardia • No P waves before each QRS complex. Retrograde P waves in ST segment
Atrial fibrillation	• No P waves • Irregularly irregular
Ventricular tachycardia	• Wide QRS • No P waves
Ventricular fibrillation	• No discernible waves

Bradyarrhythmias

ARRHYTHMIA	ECG FINDINGS
Sinus bradycardia	• Normal P wave morphology • Heart rate <60 bpm
Sick sinus syndrome	Includes: • Sinus bradycardia • Sinus arrest (pauses of ≥3 s) • Sinus node exit block • Tachycardia–bradycardia syndrome
Atrioventricular block with escape rhythm	More P wave than QRS complexes with: • Junctional escape: narrow QRS • Ventricular escape: wide QRS, abnormal T wave

INTERVALS AND WAVE MORPHOLOGY

PR Interval

INTERVAL CHANGE	CAUSES
Prolonged PR	Atrioventricular node or His-Purkinje system conduction delay
Short PR	• Pre-excitation, e.g. Wolff–Parkinson–White syndrome • Junctional rhythm

QT Interval

INTERVAL CHANGE	CAUSES
Long QT	• Hypocalcaemia • Hypokalaemia • Hypomagnesaemia • Long QT syndrome
Short QT	• Hypercalcaemia • Wolf–Parkinson–White syndrome • Short QT syndrome

P Wave

MORPHOLOGY CHANGE	CAUSES
Broad, bifid P wave	Left atrial enlargement
Peaked P wave	Right atrial enlargement
Tall, broad P wave	Left and right atrial enlargement

QRS Complex

MORPHOLOGY CHANGE	CAUSES
Wide QRS (>120 ms)	• Bundle branch blocks • Ventricular escape rhythms • Hyperkalaemia • Ventricular rhythms • Pre-excitation
Pathological Q waves	Myocardial infarction
High-voltage QRS	Ventricular hypertrophy
Low-voltage QRS	Pericardial effusion

ST Segment

MORPHOLOGY CHANGE	CAUSES
ST elevation	• ST elevation myocardial infarction (STEMI) • Pericarditis • Brugada syndrome
ST depression	• Myocardial ischaemia • Non-STEMI (NSTEMI) • Posterior myocardial infarction • Digoxin use • Aberrant repolarisation, e.g. left bundle branch block (LBBB), right bundle branch block (RBBB), hypokalaemia

T Wave

MORPHOLOGY CHANGE	CAUSES
Peaked T wave	Hyperkalaemia
T-wave inversion	• Myocardial ischaemia and infarction • Bundle branch blocks • Ventricular hypertrophy • Pulmonary embolism • Cardiomyopathy

Extra Waves

EXTRA WAVES IN ECG	CAUSE
U wave	Hypokalaemia
Delta wave	Pre-excitation, including Wolff–Parkinson–White syndrome
Osborn wave	Hypothermia
Pacing spikes	Pacemakers

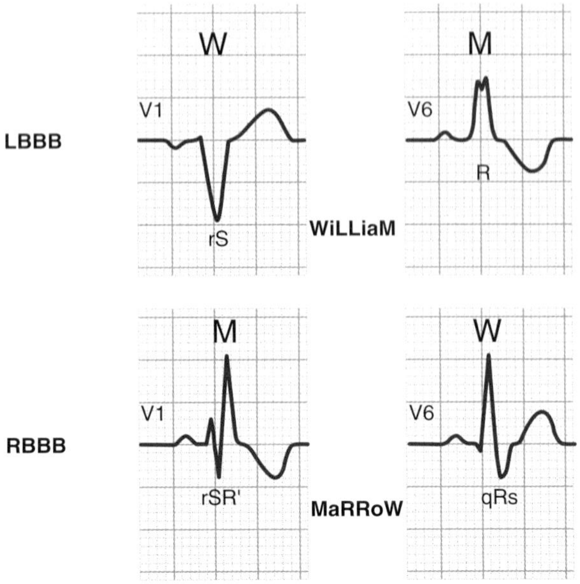

Fig. 12.5 RBBB: wide QRS, RSR' in V$_1$ ('MaRRoW').

IMPORTANT CONDITIONS (TABLES 12.1 AND 12.2)

Table 12.1 Acute Coronary Syndrome

Condition	ECG Changes
STEMI	Consider if at least one of following present: • ≥2 mm ST elevation in at least two contiguous leads in leads V2–V3 • ≥1 mm ST elevation in at least two contiguous leads in all other precordial leads and limb leads • Posterior myocardial infarction (ST depression and dominant R waves in V1–V3)
Myocardial ischaemia and nstemi	ECG changes: • ST depression • T-wave inversion

Table 12.2 Bundle Branch Blocks (Fig. 12.5)

Block	ECG Changes
LBBB	Wide QRS, notched R wave in V6 ('WiLLiaM')
Left anterior fascicular block	Left-axis deviation
Left posterior fascicular block	Right-axis deviation
Bifascicular block	RBBB + left/right-axis deviation
Trifascicular block	RBBB + left/right-axis deviation + first-degree heart block

Atrioventricular Block

ATRIOVENTRICULAR BLOCK TYPE		ECG FEATURES
First-degree heart block		PR interval >200 ms
Second-degree heart block (intermittent blockage of impulses)	Mobitz I (Wenckebach)	Progressive PR prolongation until a P wave is not conducted
	Mobitz II	Intermittent failure to conduct a P wave; conducted P waves have the same PR interval
	2:1 atrioventricular block	Two P waves for every QRS complex
Third-degree heart block		No relation between P waves and QRS complexes

Hypertrophy

CHAMBER HYPERTROPHIED	ECG CHANGES
Left ventricular hypertrophy	S wave in V$_1$ + R wave in V$_5$/V$_6$ is ≥35 mm
Left atrial hypertrophy	Broad, bifid P waves
Right ventricular hypertrophy	Dominant R wave in V$_1$
Right atrial hypertrophy	Peaked P waves

Electrolyte Abnormalities

ELECTROLYTE ABNORMALITY	ECG CHANGES
Hyperkalaemia	• Peaked T waves • Flat P waves • Prolonged PR interval • Wide QRS complex • ST segment depression • Atrial standstill • Sinusoidal waves
Hypokalaemia	• T-wave flattening • U-wave appearance • ST depression • T-wave inversion • PR prolongation • P-wave peaking
Hypercalcaemia	Short QT interval
Hypocalcaemia	Long QT interval

Case List

Case 1   Atrial fibrillation with left bundle branch block

Case 2   Atrial flutter with variable atrioventricular
          conduction

Case 3   Atrial tachycardia

Case 4   STEMI and complete heart block

Case 5   Biventricular pacing

Case 6   Long QT interval

Case 7   Pre-excitation

Case 8   Narrow-complex tachycardia (AVNRT/AVRT)

Case 9   Ventricular tachycardia

Case 10   Complete heart block

Case 11   Bifascicular block

Case 12   Narrow-complex tachycardia (AVNRT/AVRT)

Case 13   Junctional escape rhythm

Case 14   Ventricular tachycardia

Case 15   Tachycardia (SVT with aberrancy versus VT)

Case 16   Atrial fibrillation with pre-excitation

Case 17   Left bundle branch block

Case 18   Right bundle branch block

Case 19   Normal ECG

Case 20   Sinus bradycardia

Case 21   Wenckebach block

Case 22   Ventricular ectopic beats

Case 23   Complete heart block

Case 24   Noisy ECG tracing

Case 25   Atrial flutter and complete heart block

Case 26   First-degree heart block

Case 27   U waves

Case 28   Dual chamber pacemaker

Case 29   Anterior infarction with Q waves

Case 30   2:1 heart block

Case 31   Digoxin toxicity

Case 32   Pulmonary embolism

Case 33   Left ventricular hypertrophy

Case 34   NSTEMI

Case 35   Pericarditis

Case 36   Lateral STEMI

Case 37   Anterior STEMI

Case 38   Inferior STEMI

Case 39   Inferior STEMI

Case 40   Acute anterior STEMI with old inferior infarct

Index

A

ABCD$_2$ score, atrial fibrillation, 143
Abnormal extra waves
  delta waves, 91–93
  normal ECG variants, 96–99
  Osborn wave, 94, 95f
  pacemakers, 94–96
  U waves, 90
Abnormal rhythms, 14
Absent P wave, 41, 43f
Acute coronary syndrome (ACS)
  classification, 75
  definition, 75
  non-ST elevation myocardial
    infarction (NSTEMI), 79–82
  ST elevation myocardial infarction
    (STEMI), 75–77
Acute heart failure, 155
Acute mitral regurgitation, 149
Adenosine bolus, symptoms, 157
Altered automaticity, arrhythmia, 14
Ambulatory monitoring, 5
Amiodarone-related heart block, 161
Anterior infarct, 9f
Anticoagulation therapy, non-ST
  elevation myocardial infarction
  (NSTEMI), 208
Antidromic circuit, atrioventricular
  nodal re-entrant tachycardia
  (AVNRT), 21, 25f
Aortic regurgitation, 147, 149
Aortic stenosis
  atrial fibrillation, 142
  left bundle branch block (LBBB), 175
Apixaban, 191
Apnoea, 158–159
Arrhythmia
  assessment, 14–15
  causes, 182
  investigations and management,
    182
  mechanisms, 14
  termination, 156–157
  Wolff-Parkinson-White (WPW)
    syndrome, 155
Arrhythmogenic right ventricular
  cardiomyopathy, 165
Aspirin, non-ST elevation myocardial
  infarction (NSTEMI), 208
Asystole, sick sinus syndrome, 167

Athletes
  ECG changes, 96–99, 96b, 98f
  first-degree heart block, 192
Atrial ectopic beat, 19, 31f
Atrial escape rhythm, 30, 30f
Atrial fibrillation (AF), 225b
  absent P wave, 41, 43f
  cardiac catheter ablation, 147
  clinical significance, 21
  consequences, 142
  definition, 21, 25f
  ECG findings, 21, 26f
  12-lead ECG, 101f–102f
  management, 22, 26f, 143
  mechanism, 142
  risk factors, 142b
  scoring systems, 143
  Wolff-Parkinson-White (WPW)
    syndrome, 155
Atrial flutter, 225b
  adenosine, 102–103, 144
  definition, 19
  ECG findings, 19
    atrial rate, 19
    4:1 conduction, 21f
    sawtooth appearance, 20f
  management, 19
  risk factors, 145
Atrial pacing, 96f
Atrial septal defect, right bundle
  branch block (RBBB), 177
Atrial tachycardia (AT), 225b
  definition, 17–18
  ECG findings, 18–19, 19f
  inverted P wave, 41, 43f
  lesion, 104, 147
  management, 19
  mechanism, 146
Atrioventricular (AV) block, 226b
  classification, 47
  definition, 46
  with escape rhythm, 225b
  first-degree heart block, 47
  P:QRS ratios, 50b
  second-degree heart block, 47–50
  third-degree heart block, 50–52
Atrioventricular nodal re-entrant
  tachycardia (AVNRT), 225b
  clinical significance, 20
  definition, 19

Atrioventricular nodal re-entrant
  tachycardia (AVNRT) *(Continued)*
  depolarisation, 21
  ECG findings, 20, 23f
  first-line treatment, 116
  management, 20
  mechanism, 22f
  RP intervals, 23f
  symptoms, 172
Atrioventricular reentrant tachycardia
  (AVRT), 155, 225b
  vs. atrioventricular nodal re-entrant
    tachycardia (AVNRT), 24f
  cardiac condition and mechanism,
    112–113, 165–166
  ECG findings, 24f
  long-term management, 166
  myocardial infarction, 155
  orthodromic and antidromic circuits,
    25f
  RP intervals, 23f
Atropine
  complete heart block, 187

B

Beta-blockers, sinus bradycardia,
  180–181
Bifascicular block, 68, 68f, 111–112,
  163–164, 178
Bigeminy, 32f
Bivalirudin, 219
Biventricular pacemaker, 151
Bowel ischaemia, atrial fibrillation, 143
Bradyarrhythmias, 225b
Bradycardias
  escape rhythm, 30–31
  pathological, 26
  sick sinus syndrome, 29–30
  sinus, 27–28
Brugada syndrome, 151, 165
  clinical features, 84
  definition, 84
  ECG findings, 84, 85f
  management, 85
  right bundle branch block (RBBB), 177
Bundle branch blocks (BBB)
  aetiologies, 111–112, 163
  classification, 62
  left bundle branch block (LBBB),
    64–65

Note: Page numbers followed by 'f' indicate figures those followed by 't' indicate tables and 'b' indicate boxes.

Bundle branch blocks (BBB) (Continued)
   right bundle branch block (RBBB),
      62–64
Bundle of His, 2:1 heart block, 200
Burns, hypokalaemia, 195

C

Cardiac anatomy, 1, 1f–2f
Cardiac arrest, 109–110
   absent carotid pulse, 158–159
   apnoea, 158–159
   electrical defibrillation, 159
Cardiac axis, 35f, 224f
   definition, 34
   electrophysiology, 34, 34f
   extreme axis deviation, 39–40, 39f
   interpretation, 34–35, 35f
   left-axis deviation, 38, 38f
   left ventricular hypertrophy (LVH), 59f
   normal, 34
   QRS complexes, 34–35, 36t–37t
   right-axis deviation, 38–39, 39f
Cardiac biomarker, myocardial
      infarction, 138–139, 216
Cardiac resynchronisation, right
      bundle branch block (RBBB), 178
Cardiac syncope, 106–107
   long QT syndrome, 153
   loss of consciousness, 152–153
Cardiac tamponade, 147
Cardiomyopathy
   left bundle branch block, 175
   significant Q waves, 198
Carotid sinus massage, 156–157
Catheter ablation, pre-excited AF, 174
Central crushing chest pain, 213
CHA$_2$DS$_2$-VASc score, atrial
      fibrillation, 143
Chest pain, atrioventricular nodal
      re-entrant tachycardia (AVNRT), 172
Chest tightness, 157
Chest X-ray, pacemaker insertion, 197
Clinical cases
   adenosine bolus, symptoms, 157
   arrhythmia termination, 108–109,
      156–157
   atrial fibrillation, 101–102
   atrial flutter, adenosine, 102–103, 144
   atrial tachycardia, 103–104, 146–147
   bifascicular block, 111–112, 163
   bundle branch block, 111–112, 163
   cardiac arrest, 109–110
   cardiac syncope, 106–107, 152–153
   complete heart block, 123–124,
      186–187
   2:1 conduction block, 102–103, 145
   coronary artery occlusion, 104–105,
      148–149
   digoxin toxicity, 131–132, 202–203
   heart block, 110–111, 160–162
   2:1 heart block, 130–131, 200
   hypokalaemia, 127–128, 193–195
   LBBB, 117–118, 174–176

Clinical cases (Continued)
   left ventricular hypertrophy,
      133–134, 206–207
   myocardial infarction, 136–137
   negative deflection, QRS complex,
      109, 157
   NSTEMIs, 207–209
   pacemaker insertion, 128–129, 195–197
   pacemaker insertion complications,
      105–106
   pericarditis, 135–136, 209–211
   pre-excited AF, 116–117, 173
   pulmonary embolism, 132–133,
      204–205
   right bundle branch block (RBBB),
      118–119, 176–178
   second-degree heart block, 121–122,
      181–183
   sick sinus syndrome, 113–114, 167–168
   sinus bradycardia, 120–121, 180–181
   SVT diagnosis, 171
   ventricular ectopics, 122–123,
      183–185
   ventricular tachycardia, 114–115,
      168–170
   Wolff-Parkinson-White (WPW)
      syndrome, 107–108, 154–155
Complete heart block, 151, 155, 164
   causes, 186
   digoxin toxicity, 202–203
   pacemaker insertion, 196
   QRS complexes, 186
   treatment, 187
2:1 Conduction block, 102–103, 145
Confusion/agitation, irregular
      baseline ECG, 188
Congenital cardiac abnormalities, 155
Coronary artery occlusion, 104–105,
      148–149
Coronary sinus dissection, 151
Corrected QT interval (QTc), 71

D

Deep-vein thrombosis, 143
Delta waves and pre-excitation, 92f
   cause of, 92f
   clinical findings, 93
   definition, 91
   ECG findings, 91, 92b, 94f
      resting, 91
      tachycardias, 91–93
   management, 93
Depolarisation, 13
Device-related endocarditis, 151
Diabetes mellitus, 145, 155, 199, 212
Diarrhoea, hypokalaemia, 195
Digoxin
   first-degree heart block, 192
   heart block, 161
   toxicity
      causes, 202
      clinical features, 85
      complete heart block, 186

Digoxin (Continued)
   definition, 85
   ECG findings, 85, 85f–86f
   management, 85, 203
   mechanism of action, 202
   severe, 86f
Dressler syndrome, 149, 221
Dual-chamber pacemaker, 96f, 196, 197b

E

Echocardiography, pulmonary
      embolism, 205
Ectopic beats
   clinical significance, 32
   definition, 31–32
   ECG findings, 31–32
   management, 32
Electrical conduction, 1–2, 2f
Electrical interference, irregular
      baseline ECG, 188
Electrocardiogram (ECG)
   changes, pathologies, 1b
   conventional tracing, 10f
   electrode placement, 3, 6f
      chest, 5f
      limbs, 5f
   exercise, 8–11
   heart conduction, 1–2
   Holter/ambulatory monitoring, 5
   leads, 3–4
   normal heart beat, 4f
   normal pacemakers, 1–2
   paperaxes, 3f
   presentation, 11–12, 11f
   recording types, 4–11
   smartphone apps, 11, 11f
   three-lead, 5, 10f
   utility, 1
Electrolyte abnormalities, 192, 227b
Erythromycin, QT interval, 153
Escape rhythm, 168
   clinical significance, 31
   definition, 30–31
   ECG findings, 30–31
   management, 31
Excessive alcohol consumption, atrial
      fibrillation, 142
Exercise electrocardiogram, 8–11
Extra waves, 226b. See also Abnormal
      extra waves.
Extreme axis deviation
   clinical significance, 39–40
   definition, 39
   ECG findings, 39, 40f
   management, 40

F

Femoral vein pseudoaneurysm, 147
First-degree heart block, 47, 192–193
   clinical features, 47
   management, 47
   PR interval, 47f–48f
Flecainide, 173

G

GRACE score, atrial fibrillation, 143

H

HAS-BLED score, atrial fibrillation, 143
Head-up tilt test, 156
Heart
   anatomy, 1, 1f–2f
   electrical conduction, 2f
Heart block
   2:1, 130–131, 200, 201b
      lesion site, 200
      treatment, 200–201
   first-degree, 47
   high-grade, 162
   medication-related, 160–161
   risk factors, 50b
   second-degree, 47–50, 162
   third-degree, 50–52, 162
Heart conduction, 1–2
Heart failure, 143, 151
Heart rate
   calculation, 14–15, 14f, 14b
   definition, 13–15
High-amplitude QRS complex, 55, 56f, 57b
Holter monitoring, 5, 10f
Hypercalcaemia, 73f
Hypercholesterolaemia, 199
Hyperkalaemia
   clinical features, 89
   definition, 88
   digoxin toxicity, 202–203
   ECG findings, 88, 88f
      sine wave appearance, 89f
      tented T waves, 88
   management, 89
   severe, 89f
Hypertension, 145, 157, 163, 199
Hypertrophy, 226b
Hypocalcaemia
   clinical features, 74
   definition, 72
   ECG findings, 72, 73f
   management, 74
   QT interval, 153
Hypokalaemia, 90–91, 91f
   causes, 195b
   complications, 194
   management, 194
   QT interval, 153
   risk factors, 195
Hypomagnesaemia, 195
Hypothermia, irregular baseline ECG, 188
Hypothyroidism, atrial fibrillation, 142

I

Idiopathic fibrosis, bundle branch block, 163
Implantable loop recorders (ILRs), 5, 10f
Increased vagal tone, sinus bradycardia, 180–181

Inferior infarct, 9f
Intermittently dropped sinus beats, sick sinus syndrome, 167
Intervals and wave morphology, 225
Intracranial haemorrhage, 143
Inverted P wave, 41, 43f
Irregular baseline ECG, 188
Irregular broad-complex tachycardia, ventricular fibrillation (VF), 25–26
Irregular narrow-complex tachycardia, 21–22
Ischaemic heart disease
   left bundle branch block (LBBB), 175
   ventricular ectopics, 184
Isoprenaline infusion, 2:1 heart block, 201

J

Junctional ectopic beat, 19, 31f
Junctional escape rhythm, 30, 30f, 168

L

Lateral infarct, 9f
Leads
   and anatomical correlation, 4
   and arteries, 9f
   electrical activity measure
      direction, 8f
      limbleads, 7f
      pracordial leads, 8f
   12-lead ECG, 3–4
   misplacement, significant Q waves, 198
Left-axis deviation, bifascicular block, 38, 38f
Left bundle branch block (LBBB), 65f
   causes, 65b
   clinical features, 64
   conditions, 175
   ECG changes, 175
   ECG findings, 64
   management, 65
   treatment options, 176
Left fascicular block
   anterior, 65, 66f
   posterior, 67f
Left ventricular aneurysm, 149
Left ventricular hypertrophy (LVH), 38
   aetiology, 206
   cardiac axis, 59f
   clinical features, 59–60
   definition, 57
   ECG findings, 58–59, 59f, 206
   management, 60
   pressure overload, 207
   voltage criteria, 59b
Lev disease, 186
Limb leads, 224f
Long PR Interval, 46
Long QT syndrome, 153, 153b
Loss of consciousness, 152–153
Low-amplitude QRS morphology, 56, 57f

M

Malignancy, pulmonary embolism, 204
Medication-related heart block, 160–161
Metoprolol-related heart block, 161
Mitral regurgitation, 145
Mobitz I block, 47, 48f
Mobitz II block, 49, 49f
Mobitz I second-degree heart block, 182b
Mobitz type II heart block, 151
Myocardial infarction (MI), 147, 212b
   atrial fibrillation, 143
   bundle branch block, 163
   cardiac biomarker, 138–139, 216
   chest pain, 213
   complications, 105, 149, 221
   ECG changes, 149, 222
   medication used, 219b
   papillary muscle rupture, 217
   recommended drugs after, 219
   reperfusion strategy after, 219
   risk factor(s), 212, 212b
Myocardial ischaemia, 79–82, 157, 215

N

Narrow- and broad-complex rhythms, 15f
Non-ST elevation myocardial infarction (NSTEMI)
   acute management, 208
   clinical features, 82
   ECG changes, 79–82, 82f, 208
   management, 82
   ST depression, 83f
   subendocardial infarcts, 76f, 209
   transmural infarction, 76f
Normal ECG variants, 179
   athletes, 96–99, 96b, 97f–98f
   paediatric cases, 99
   pregnancy, 99, 99b
Normal ECG waves, 13f
Normal PR interval, 192
Normal P wave, 41, 42f
Normal sinus rhythm, 11f, 35f

O

Oral contraceptive pills, pulmonary embolism, 204
Orthodromic circuit, atrioventricular nodal re-entrant tachycardia (AVNRT), 21, 25f
Osborn wave, 94, 95f

P

Pacemakers
   clinical features, 96
   definition, 94–96
   ECG findings, 96
   insertion complications, 105–106, 151b
   LBBB, 176
   management, 96

Pacemakers (Continued)
  modes, ventricular activity, 151
  NBG code for, 95t
  pocket haematoma, 151
  pocket infection, 151
  types, 95t
Paediatric cases, 99, 100f
Palpitations, atrioventricular nodal
    re-entrant tachycardia (AVNRT), 172
Papillary muscle rupture, myocardial
    infarction, 217
Pathological Q waves, 56, 57f
Peaked T wave, 87, 87f
Pericardial effusion, 61, 61f, 151
Pericardiocentesis, 211
Pericarditis, 210b
  causes, 83b
  causes of, 210–211
  clinical features, 84
  definition, 83
  ECG findings, 83, 84f, 84b, 210, 211b
  management, 84, 211
  ST elevation and PR depression, 84f
Permanent pacemaker insertion
  complete heart block, 187
  2:1 heart block, 201
Polycythaemia, pulmonary embolism,
    204
Polyuria, atrioventricular nodal
    re-entrant tachycardia (AVNRT),
    172
Poor R-wave progression, 56–57, 58f
Posterior infarct, 9f
Pracordial leads, 8f
PR and QT interval, 12
Precordial ECG lead placement, 6f
Precordial leads, 224f
Pre-excited atrial fibrillation, 174
  antiarrhythmic drugs, 116–117, 173
  long-term management options, 174
Pregnancy, 99, 99f, 99b
Previous ischaemia, significant Q
    waves, 198
PR interval, 225b
  atrioventricular block, 46–47
  definition, 46
  depression, 46
  electrophysiology, 46, 46f–47f
  interpretation, 46
  long, 46
  normal, 46
  normal conduction, 47f
  short, 46
Prolonged P wave, 43, 44f
Prominent Q waves, 179
Pulmonary embolism
  ECG changes, 204
  management, 205
  right bundle branch block (RBBB), 177
  risk factors, 204
Purkinje fibre, 2:1 heart block, 200
P wave, 225b
  absent, 41, 43f

P wave (Continued)
  definition, 41
  electrophysiology, 41
  interpretation, 41–43
  inverted, 41, 43f
  normal, 41, 42f
  normal ECG waves, 41f
  peaked, 44f
  tall, prolonged, 43, 44f

Q

QRS complex, 225b
  bifascicular block, 53f, 68f
  bundle branch blocks, 61–62
  components, 53
  definition, 53
  depolarisation, 53f
  electrophysiology, 53–54
  high-amplitude, 55, 56f
  individual waves, 53f
  interpretation, 54–57
  left-axis deviation, 38f
  left fascicular block
    anterior, 65, 66f
    posterior, 67f
  left ventricular hypertrophy (LVH),
    57–60
  low-amplitude, 56
  maximum normal duration, 179
  negative deflection, inferior leads, 157
  normal, 54
  normal cardiac axis, 35f
  pathological Q waves, 56
  pericardial effusion, 61, 61f
  poor R-wave progression, 56–57
  positive/negative, 36t–37t
  right-axis deviation, 39f
  right ventricular hypertrophy
    (RVH), 60–61
  transition zone rotation, 57, 58f
  trifascicular block, 68–69, 69f
  wide, 54
QT interval, 225b
  corrected QT interval (QTc), 71
    normal, 71, 71f–72f
  definition, 71
  electrophysiology, 71
  hypercalcaemia, 72
  hypocalcaemia, 72–74
  interpretation, 71–72
  long, 71–72
  prolonging factors, 153
  short, 71, 72b
Quadrigeminy, 32f
Quetiapine, 153
Q waves, 198
  myocardial infarction, 222
  significant, 198

R

Re-entrant arrhythmias, 14
Regular broad-complex tachycardia,
    22–25, 27f

Regular narrow-complex tachycardia,
    15–21, 18f
Repolarisation, 13
Retrograde conduction, 157
Rhythm, 13–15
Right-axis deviation, left posterior
    fascicular block, 38–39, 39f
Right bundle branch block (RBBB),
    62–64, 62f, 118–119, 176–178
  causes, 64b, 177
  clinical features, 64
  ECG changes, 177
  ECG findings, 63–64
  management, 64
Right ventricular hypertrophy (RVH)
  causes, 61b
  clinical features, 61
  definition, 60
  ECG findings, 60–61, 60f
  management, 61

S

Second-degree heart block, 47–50, 162
  2:1 atrioventricular block, 49, 50f–51f
  clinical features, 49
  ECG findings, 47–49
  management, 50
  Mobitz I block, 47, 48f
  Mobitz II block, 49f
Sepsis, atrial fibrillation, 142
Septal infarct, 9f
Septal myocardial infarction, 187
Shortness of breath, atrioventricular
    nodal re-entrant tachycardia
    (AVNRT), 172
Short PR interval, 46
Sick sinus syndrome, 29f, 113–114,
    167–168, 225b
  aetiology, 167–168
  clinical significance, 30
  definition, 29
  dual-chamber pacemaker, 196
  ECG findings, 29–30
  ECG patterns, 167
  management, 30
Sinus arrhythmia, 15
Sinus bradycardia, 225b
  ECG changes, 181
  possible causes, 180–181
  sick sinus syndrome, 167
Sinus tachycardia, 17, 18f
  clinical significance, 27–28
  definition, 27
  ECG findings, 27, 29f
  management, 28
  pericarditis, 210
Small Q waves, 179, 179b
Smartphone apps, 11, 11f
Smoking, myocardial infarction, 212
ST elevation myocardial infarction
    (STEMI), 75
  acute, 75
  anterior, 79f

ST elevation myocardial infarction (STEMI) (Continued)
  anterolateral, 79f
  clinical features, 77
  diagnostic ECG findings, 215
  ECG findings, 76–77, 77f
  immediate treatment, 217
  infarction sites, 77t
  inferior, 80f
  lateral, 80f
  and LBBB, 77b
  leads and arteries, 78f
  management, 77
  posterior infarctions, 77, 80f–81f
Stroke, 147, 155
ST segment, 225b
  acute coronary syndrome (ACS), 75
  Brugada syndrome, 84–85
  definition, 75
  depression, 75, 76b
  digoxin toxicity, 85
  electrophysiology, 75
  elevation, 75, 76b
  interpretation, 75
  isoelectric line, 76f
  normal, 75, 76f
  pericarditis, 83–84
Subendocardial infarcts, 76f, 209
Sudden cardiac death, 155
Supraventricular tachycardia, hypokalaemia, 194
Synchronised DC cardioversion, 156

T

Tachyarrhythmias, 225b
Tachycardia
  atrial tachycardia (AT), 17–19
  interpretation flowchart, 16f
  irregular broad-complex, 25–26
  irregular narrow-complex, 21–22
  regular broad-complex, 22–25
  regular narrow-complex, 15–21
  sinus tachycardia, 17, 18f
  ventricular, 23–25
Tachycardia–bradycardia syndrome, 30f

Tamponade, ventricular rupture, 221
Tented T waves, hyperkalaemia, 88
Third-degree heart block, 162
  clinical features, 50
  ECG findings, 50
  management, 50–52
Three-lead electrocardiogram (ECG), 5, 10f
Torsades de pointes, 185
  hypokalaemia, 194
  ventricular tachycardia, 26, 28f, 155
Transcutaneous pacing
  complete heart block, 187
  2:1 heart block, 201
Transmural infarction, 76f, 215
Trifascicular blocks, 68–69, 69f, 178
Trigeminy, 32f
Triggered activity, 14
Troponin I and T, 217
T wave, 226b
  definition, 87
  electrophysiology, 87
  hyperkalaemia, 88–89
  interpretation, 87–88
  inversion, 88, 88b
  normal, 87
  peaked, 87, 87f
  ventricular repolarisation, 87f

U

Unstable angina, 82
U waves, 90, 90f
  definition, 90
  ECG findings, 90
  hypokalaemia, 90–91, 91f

V

Vagal manoeuvres, 23f, 172
Valsalva manoeuvre, 157, 157b
Ventricular ectopic beat, 19, 31f
Ventricular ectopics, 122–123, 183–185, 185b
  complications, 184
  long QTc, 185
Ventricular escape rhythms, 30–31, 30f

Ventricular fibrillation (VF), 225b
  clinical significance, 25
  definition, 25
  digoxin toxicity, 202
  ECG findings, 25
  electrical defibrillation, 159
  hypokalaemia, 194
  long QTc, 185
  management, 25–26
Ventricular pacing, 96f
Ventricular tachycardia, 155, 225b
  blood pressure drop, 169
  clinical significance, 25
  definition, 23
  ECG findings, 27f
  electrical defibrillation, 159
  hypokalaemia, 194
  idiopathic, 169
  long-term management, 159
  management, 25
  non-sustained, 23
  prognosis, 170
  sustained, 23
  Torsades de pointes, 26
Ventricular trigeminy, 184
Verapamil-related heart block, 161

W

Wave morphology, 12
Wells score, pulmonary embolism, 205
Wenckebach rhythm
  complications, 183
  fatigue of AV node cells, 182
Wide-complex tachycardia, 153
Wide QRS complexes, 54, 55f, 175
Wolff-Parkinson-White (WPW) syndrome, 38, 151
  arrhythmia, 155
  AVRT, 165
  family history, 155
  risk factors, 154
  sudden cardiac death, 155
  ventricular ectopics, 184

X

Xanthopsia, digoxin toxicity, 202, 203